Preventing AIDS

Preventing
A I D S

The Design of Effective Programs

Ronald O. Valdiserri

RUTGERS UNIVERSITY PRESS
New Brunswick and London

Library of Congress Cataloging-in-Publication Data

Preventing AIDS : the design of effective programs / edited by Ronald O.
Valdiserri.
     p.   cm.
    Includes bibliographies and index.
    ISBN 0-8135-1433-9 (cloth)—ISBN 0-8135-1434-7 (pbk.)
    1. AIDS (Disease)—Prevention.   I. Valdiserri, Ronald O., 1951–
    [DNLM: 1. Acquired Immunodeficiency Syndrome—prevention &
control.   WD 308 P944]
RA644.A25P75   1989
616.97'9205—dc19
DNLM/DLC   88-36573
for Library of Congress   CIP

British Cataloging-in-Publication information available

FOR MY BROTHER, DR. EDWIN VALDISERRI

Contents

Introduction

Organized attempts to prevent the spread of human immunodeficiency virus (HIV) are essential components of our response to the AIDS (acquired immune deficiency syndrome) epidemic. This book will discuss the development of programs that seek to limit the transmission of HIV, especially those that target viral transmission through sexual intercourse and through needle sharing among intravenous drug users. Developing effective prevention programs for these targets requires that we (a) recognize and understand the behaviors that transmit the virus; (b) appreciate how solutions to previous epidemics of sexually transmitted diseases and past approaches to treating addictive drug use have influenced our current programmatic responses to AIDS; (c) become familiar with theories that both explain and predict human behavioral change; (d) develop an appreciation for the individual and group circumstances of the persons whom we wish to reach with our prevention programs; (e) analyze the strengths and limitations of the specific tools available to us for developing, implementing, providing, and evaluating AIDS prevention services; and (f) understand the barriers that can interfere with programmatic efforts to prevent the further spread of the human immunodeficiency virus.

This book contains a great deal of specific information about the individual and group circumstances of persons whose behaviors place them at increased risk for HIV infection. Its overall approach, however, emphasizes the commonality of theoretical and organizational issues relevant to AIDS-prevention activities for all of those at risk—rather than limiting its scope to a specific target group.

I have organized and presented this material so that it is accessible to a broad range of readers with different levels of experience and involvement in the AIDS epidemic. However, the book's decided focus is on program development and thus it is especially relevant to persons working within organizations and agencies that provide or are planning to provide AIDS-prevention services. This focus on programming is most apparent in Chapter Five, which reviews the American Public Health Association's criteria for the development of health-promotion and education programs, using a variety of American AIDS-prevention initiatives as examples.

Although AIDS-prevention programs is the focus of this book, the larger subject of HIV infection as a socially mediated phenomenon is recurrent throughout it. Regardless of the groups we consider as targets for prevention programs, whether gay men, intravenous drug users, minority women, or adolescent school dropouts, it soon becomes apparent that understanding their social circumstances is essential to providing effective and meaningful prevention services. In this context, social circumstances are defined in the broadest possible sense. They can refer to group norms that endorse riskful behaviors or social networks through which minorities communicate. They can describe economic circumstances that limit life-choice options or value judgments about behaviors that are controversial or poorly understood.

This approach is not meant to minimize the role of biomedical solutions to the problem of preventing HIV infection, but it does consider disease as more than a physical process. Disease can also be viewed as a social process; it can reflect how we live as a society, what values are important to us, how well we plan and allocate resources, and how thoroughly we understand the interrelations of our social and organizational "ecosystem."

As has been the case with many other health problems, even after we develop biomedical solutions to HIV infection, we will still require the support of society to implement them: societal resources will have to be allocated to cover the costs of providing these services and social systems will be called upon not only to distribute them but also, when necessary, to encourage their consumption. The screening of donated blood to prevent transfusion-associated HIV infection is an example of the interrelationship between technology and society in solving health problems. Although the ELISA test to detect HIV antibody has been available since 1985, in many countries of the developing world transfusion remains a common route of HIV infection. Health professionals in these countries are certainly aware of this mode of transmission and of the potential for eliminating it by screening donor blood, but societal resources are not always available to support and distribute screening technology. Therefore, although we assume that the future of AIDS prevention will include drugs to treat infected persons and render them noninfectious, we

continue to support the importance of understanding the larger social context of illness as essential for successful prevention programs.
In the same way that penicillin (a technologic solution to infection
with *Treponema pallidum*) has failed to eradicate syphilis, it is
equally unrealistic to assume that new drugs, by themselves, will
adequately address the prevention of HIV infection.

Finally, because this book aproaches the subject of HIV prevention
from the general perspective of health promotion, it is possible for
readers to apply the principles and standards outlined herein to a diverse variety of AIDS-prevention efforts. In a field where data accumulate daily, where questions exist about the efficacy of interventions, and where burgeoning biomedical research is likely to result
in improved methods to control and treat HIV infection, an approach
that stresses concepts, principles, and health outcomes is believed to
be more advantageous than one that highlights AIDS-prevention instructions in a "how to" format.

Note: The expressions "AIDS prevention" and "HIV prevention" are
used throughout this book to refer to preventing infection with human immunodeficiency virus.

Chapter 1

The Epidemiology of HIV Infection

Even before the discovery of the human immunodeficiency virus (HIV) and its general acceptance as the etiologic agent of the acquired immunodeficiency syndrome (AIDS), it was apparent that individuals with AIDS were demographically similar to persons with hepatitis B virus (HBV) infection, a blood-borne and sexually transmissible virus that causes liver disease. Gay and bisexual men reporting large numbers of sexual partners, intravenous drug users, recipients of blood transfusions, and hemophiliacs were identified as risk groups for AIDS, as they all had been previously characterized as groups at increased risk for HBV infection (Catterall 1978). This observation was one of the first clues to the transmission of HIV. From this observation flowed the hypothesis that the agent responsible for causing AIDS must be both sexually transmissible and also transmissible through exposure to infected blood or blood products. We now know that this original hypothesis was correct, and our understanding of the ways in which the virus can be transmitted has become more complete through several years of research and observation. AIDS is characterized as a *syndrome*, a medical term that means that infection with this human retrovirus can produce many different clinical outcomes (Redfield et al. 1986). We also know that this virus infects cells bearing the CD4 receptor, most notably the T helper lymphocyte (Seligmann et al. 1987). Because we can measure both the antibody response to HIV and the presence of viral antigens in the bloodstream, we are able to determine with a high degree of certainty whether an individual has been infected with HIV, even in the absence of demonstrable symptoms.

SEXUAL TRANSMISSION OF THE VIRUS

After its isolation in peripheral blood mononuclear cells (Barre-Sinoussi 1983; Gallo 1983), HIV was subsequently isolated in semen

1

(Ho 1984; Zagury 1984) and female genital secretions (Vogt 1986; Wofsy 1986), which explained its ability to be sexually transmitted. However, not all forms of sexual activity are considered to carry the same risk of infection. For instance, in gay and bisexual men, anal receptive intercourse with ejaculation has been shown to be the most common mode of transmission (Kingsley 1987; McCusker 1988; Winkelstein et al. 1987). In this respect, HIV infection resembles HBV infection, which was also found to be transmitted among gay men most frequently by this sexual behavior (Schreeder 1982). Originally, this finding was explained by the fact that the thin columnar epithelial cells lining the rectum sustained minute tears and disruptions during the act of intercourse, thus affording the virus easy access to the capillaries immediately beneath the mucosal surface. More recent evidence that HIV is capable of infecting the cells lining the lower intestine (Nelson 1988) provides a more direct explanation of this observed association.

Although most instances of homosexual HIV infection can be attributed to receptive anal intercourse with ejaculation, this does not preclude the possibility of alternate modes of homosexual transmission. Some studies have suggested that insertive anal intercourse also carries a small risk of infection (Kingsley 1987). While most studies have not identified a substantial HIV infection risk associated with homosexual oral intercourse (Kinglsey 1987; Lyman 1986; Winkelstein 1987), there is probably a finite, although extremely small, risk of transmission associated with this activity (Darrow 1987).

The early observation of a one-to-one male to female ratio among Africans with AIDS (Piot 1984) strongly suggested that the virus could be transmitted through heterosexual intercourse, a supposition that has subsequently been well established (Harris 1983; Piot 1987; Redfield 1985a). Vaginal intercourse with ejaculation is considered to be the primary mode of sexual transmission among heterosexuals, and has been replicated in a laboratory setting using chimpanzees (Fultz 1986). Although vaginal intercourse can result in bidirectional transmission (from an infected male to his susceptible female partner and vice versa), in the United States the virus appears to more frequently transmitted from an infected male to his female partner than it is in the opposite direction (Lefrere 1988; Padian 1987a). The presence of concomitant infection within the genitourinary tract (Anderson 1987) or the presence of ulcerations of the penile skin (Fast 1984; Greenblatt 1988) probably facilitates the heterosexual transmission of virus, and this explanation has been advanced to account for the more frequent observation of heterosexual infection in the developing world (Biggar 1986; Greenblatt 1988). Although some investigators have suggested a link between heterosexual anal intercourse and HIV infection (Bolling and Voeller 1987; Melbye 1985; Padian et al. 1987), this form of sexual activity is probably not as important in heterosexual transmission as it is in homosexual transmission (Fischl 1987b). One study reported that among female spouses of infected males, receptive oral intercourse was correlated with HIV seropositivity (Fischl 1987b), though it was not possible to prove conclusively that this was a mode of transmission, since none of the participants engaged in this behavior to the exclusion of vaginal intercourse. Furthermore, the previously mentioned laboratory study (Fultz 1986) was unable to infect a susceptible chimpanzee by oral exposure to HIV particles.

Although the occurrence of HIV infection among lesbians has been reported (Marmor 1986; Monzon 1987), it is considered to be a very unusual phenomenon. The rarity of HIV infection among lesbians is probably a manifestation of the low HIV seroprevalence within this group, as well as the relative inefficiency with which lesbian sexual activity can transmit the virus. Reports on the low frequency of other sexually transmitted diseases in this population support this interpretation (Robertson 1981). However, lesbians can become infected with HIV because of needle sharing in the context of intravenous drug use.

Unfortunately, it is often impossible to quantify the exact risk of infection associated with a specific sexual activity, especially if that activity is an unusual or rare means of transmission. Furthermore, the studies necessary to determine the risk attributable to a specific sexual activity would be extremely difficult to undertake from both an ethical and logistical perspective. The quintessential example of this quandary pertains to the risk of HIV infection as a result of prolonged intimate kissing with the exchange of saliva ("french kissing"). Because HIV can be recovered from the saliva of infected individuals (Groopman 1984), albeit infrequently and in low titers (Ho 1985), most researchers admit that it is theoretically possible for a person to become infected as a result of this activity, but that if it does happen at all, it is probably an extraordinarily rare phenomenon. Salivary enzymes and an intact squamous epithelium are significant local barriers to numerous microorganisms that might gain access to the blood stream through the mouth. In fact, laboratory tests have shown that the ability of HIV to infect blood cells can be completely inhibited by exposure of the virus to saliva (Fox 1988:

636), which suggests that saliva itself may play a role in preventing HIV infection through intimate kissing. In support of this hypothesis is the observation that HBV, a virus that is also found in the saliva of infected individuals, is not known to be transmitted by either intimate kissing or oral sexual intercourse (Schreeder 1982).

There is only a single case report in the medical literature of apparent salivary transmission of HIV. Salahuddin and his colleagues report the presence of HIV antibodies in a woman whose husband developed AIDS as a result of an unscreened blood transfusion (Salahuddin 1984). Evidently, the man became impotent after his surgical procedure, and kissing was the couple's sole reported sexual activity. Therefore, although french kissing is considered to be a highly unlikely route of viral transmission, clients should understand that any exposure to blood must be considered dangerous, and that bleeding gums and lesions of the oral mucosa that are not healed are potential sources of infection or portals for viral entry.

It is imperative that prevention programs educate clients about sexual activities that carry the greatest risk of HIV infection. Because it may not be possible to inform an individual of the exact risk of infection involved in each of the many sexual activities that humans may engage in, many sexual risk reduction guidelines present sexual behavior on a continuum from "no risk" through "some risk" to "high risk." Most high-risk activities are characterized by the exchange of blood, semen, or vaginal secretions between sexual partners. For homosexual men, these activities would include both insertive and receptive anal intercourse with ejaculation. For heterosexuals, vaginal and anal intercourse with ejaculation are considered to involve the most risk. Activities of intermediate risk *might* result in the exchange of body fluids, and would include oral sex for both homosexuals and heterosexuals. Activities classified as "no risk" or "safe" do not result in the exchange of body fluids, and include mutual masturbation, hugging, fondling, and massage.

TRANSMISSION OF THE VIRUS THROUGH NEEDLE SHARING

Among intravenous drug users the practice of sharing needles is an important mode of viral transmission (Chaisson 1987; Des Jarlais 1985; Friedland 1985), and the average monthly frequency of injections is an important independent risk factor for HIV infection in high-incidence areas (Marmor 1987). Although the practice of sharing needles varies regionally (Ginzburg 1984) and among ethnic groups (Brown et al. 1987), it is relatively common (Black 1986; Ginsburg 1984; Howard 1970), especially in "shooting galleries," where individuals can rent paraphernalia for injecting drugs ("works") (Chaisson 1987; Des Jarlais 1987; Friedland 1985). Needle sharing is partly explained by a limited supply of syringes and needles, which results from widespread statutes that make them available only through doctors' prescriptions (Lambert 1988a). However, it is probable that needle sharing also serves psychological and social functions for the participants, providing a means of socialization for newcomers, a way of achieving status and fraternity for group members, and a means of reinforcing group norms (Friedman 1986; Ghodse 1987; Howard 1970; Selwyn 1987).

Once HIV infection has been established in an intravenous drug user, it can be transmitted through sexual intercourse to both male and female partners. This route of transmission is considered to be critically important in the development of HIV infection within the heterosexual population. In a retrospective epidemiologic analysis of women with AIDS in the United States, the two most common risk factors were found to be a history of intravenous drug use or sexual relations with an intravenous drug user (Guinan and Hardy 1987).

PROSTITUTION AND HIV INFECTION

Prostitution has been identified as another consequential link between the intravenous drug user and the heterosexual population. Economically disadvantaged intravenous drug users, both male and female, may engage in prostitution to provide economic support for themselves and their addictions (Brunswick 1980; Drucker 1986). If infected with HIV, they are capable of transmitting the virus by engaging in high-risk sexual practices. Among a small sample of military personnel who were evaluated for HIV-related illness, more than half the subjects reported a history of sexual relations with female prostitutes (Redfield 1985b). In areas of the country where the prevalence of HIV infection among intravenous drug users is substantial, there is a high likelihood that economically disadvantaged female addicts are propogating the spread of HIV through prostitution. This does not mean that the only way female prostitutes can become infected with HIV is through intravenous drug use. Prostitutes have traditionally been identified as reservoirs of sexually transmissible infections, both in America (Brandt 1985) and in the developing world (D'Costa 1985; Meheus 1974), for the obvious reason that they have large numbers of sexual partners. Studies of HIV infection in Africa have identified female prostitutes as a high-risk group for infection (Kreiss 1986; Van de Perre 1985) and have documented a significant relationship between AIDS in heterosexual males and sex with female prostitutes (Clumeck 1985; Quinn 1986; Vittecoq 1987). In a study of Haitian males who have AIDS and who reside in the United States, heterosexual intercourse appeared to be the major mode of HIV transmission, and sexual contact with female prostitutes was found to be a significant risk factor (Fischl 1987a).

PERINATAL TRANSMISSION OF HIV

A major consequence of HIV infection in women is the potential for transmitting the virus to their offspring (Scott 1985). Perinatal transmission of HIV is thought to occur by three routes: in utero; during labor, as a result of exposure to infected maternal blood or uterine cervical cells (Pomerantz 1988); and after birth, as a result of breast-feeding (Friedland 1987). The relative frequencies of infection by each of these routes is unknown, though each is presumed to carry some risk. Transplacental transmission has been documented by the results of an autopsy study. A newborn, delivered of an infected mother by cesarean section, was found to have HIV-infected lymphoid cells (Lapointe 1985). Studies in America, Europe, and Africa indicate that not every infected mother will give birth to an infected child (Mann 1986a; Mok 1987; Scott 1985), and there is even a report in the medical literature of monozygotic twins, one of whom developed AIDS while the other was clinically, serologically, and virologically free of HIV infection three years after birth (Menez-Bautista 1986). Currently it is estimated that between 40 and 50 percent of infected mothers will have infected newborns (Friedland 1987:1131).

Human immunodeficiency virus has been isolated from breast milk (Thiry 1985), and a small number of cases of postnatal transmission have been reported (Bucens et al. 1988; Lepage 1987; Ziegler 1985). Although breast-feeding is a potential mode of HIV infection (Colebunders 1988), studies in Haiti demonstrate a relatively low risk of transmission (Stanback 1988), and it may be that the greatest risk of HIV infection through breast-feeding occurs if the mother or wet-nurse incurs a primary HIV infection during the postnatal period

(Ziegler 1988). In a European collaborative study of infants born to HIV-infected mothers, six of eleven infants were uninfected, despite breast-feeding for up to seven months, thus reinforcing the notion that this activity does not have a risk of infection comparable to intrauterine transmission (Senturia 1987). This issue of postnatal HIV transmission via breast-feeding is especially problematic in the developing world where alternatives to breast milk may be limited (Baumslag 1987). Because breast-fed infants have significantly lower rates of death from diarrhea and respiratory infections (Victoria 1987), there are serious concerns that proscriptions against breast-feeding will result in a dramatic increase in infant mortality.

HIV TRANSMISSION THROUGH
BLOOD TRANSFUSION

The development of a laboratory test to detect the presence of antibodies to the human immunodeficiency virus (Weiss 1985a) has virtually eliminated the possibility of HIV transmission as a result of whole-blood transfusion or the administration of blood-cell components, plasma, or clotting factors. Since the enzyme-linked immunosorbent assay (ELISA) test to detect HIV antibody became commercially available in 1985, all donated blood has been routinely screened, and this, together with the heat treatment of factor concentrate for hemophiliacs (Blomback 1987), has essentially interrupted this mode of transmission. Of course, among transfusion recipients and hemophiliacs who have already been infected, the virus can be transmitted to their sexual partners and offspring (Fischl 1987b; Kreiss 1985).

Reliance on the ELISA test alone, however, can occasionally result in falsely negative results, especially in the early stages of infection (Raevsky 1986; Ward 1988). With currently available methods for screening donated blood, estimates of the chances of receiving a falsely negative (that is, infectious) unit of blood range from approximately 1 in 40,000 (Ward 1988:477) to 1 in 250,000 (Bove 1987:244). The development of tests to detect the presence of HIV antigen, which appears earlier in infection than HIV antibody (Kessler 1987), may further reduce the already low risk of administering blood that falsely tests negative for HIV antibody. Optimism notwithstanding, transfusion-associated AIDS is still an important mode of HIV transmission in the developing world (Greenberg 1988; Mann 1986a;

Quinn 1986; Van de Perre 1987), where limited economical, technical, and personnel resources do not always permit the routine screening of blood (Quinn 1986).

VARIABLES IN THE RISK OF INFECTION

Another issue germane to the discussion of HIV transmission relates to the infectivity of the virus, or how often one must be exposed to the virus in order for infection to take place. The amount of virus to which one is exposed (that is, "the infectious dose") and the manner in which one is exposed to it both play a role in determining whether infection will result. As with other infectious diseases, the success of HIV infection depends on both an efficient means of transmission and an adequate infectious dose, and is influenced by a number of host and environmental factors (Haverkos 1987).

Among the female sexual partners of infected hemophiliacs, for example, transmission appears to be more frequent when the infected male has more severe, and perhaps more long-standing, HIV infection (Smiley 1988). The presence of genital ulcerations may also increase the probability that exposure to human immunodeficiency virus will result in infection (Greenblat 1988). Studies of the homosexual partners of men with AIDS suggest that the potential for sexual transmission of HIV may be greater "close to or after the onset of disease" (Osmond 1988:944). Clinical and serologic analyses of female sexual partners of infected men (Padian et al. 1987; Peterman 1988; Smiley 1988) and male sexual partners of other infected men (Grant 1987) have concluded that infection is not a certain outcome from a single sexual exposure. Although it is apparent that the number of sexual exposures to an infected partner increases the likelihood of infection, clients should be cautioned that infection with HIV may not require multiple exposures and can occur after a single sexual contact (May 1988; Peterman 1988; Staszewski 1987).

The preceeding discussion has focused on the major mechanisms by which HIV is transmitted, without specific consideration of the prevalence of infection within various target populations. In their work on the sexual transmission of enteric protozoa, Phillips and his colleagues (1981) hypothesized that the substantial prevalence of sexually transmitted enteric pathogens in homosexual men from New York City was due to a prevalent mode of sexual behavior that could efficiently transmit protozoa, in concert with a large reservoir of infection. Stated another way, and in the context of our discussion, in order for an individual to become infected with HIV, he must engage in a behavior known to be an effective means of transmission (for example, needle sharing or receptive anal intercourse without condoms) with an infectious partner. No activity between uninfected individuals carries risk for HIV infection.

Another major variable in risk of infection, therefore, relates to the endemic level of HIV infection within the target population. Based on fifty surveys conducted in twenty-three cities across the United States, the Centers for Disease Control estimated that between 20 and 50 percent of gay and bisexual men were infected with HIV as of January 1988 (Booth 1988:253). Consequently, sexually active gay men are very likely to encounter partners who are either knowingly or unknowingly infected with HIV. Because the level of infection within this population is so great, sex with large numbers of partners should not be considered a prerequisite for infection. Certainly, engaging in high-risk behavior with multiple partners increases a susceptible individual's chances of becoming infected, but homosexual men should not be led to believe that limiting sexual relations to a single partner confers protection against HIV infection. Risk reduction for homosexual men lies primarily in avoiding behaviors that are the most dangerous in terms of HIV infection (that is, receptive anal intercourse without condoms), rather than in emphasizing "promiscuity" as a risk factor.

In a review of twenty-two brochures on safe sex for homosexual men, Siegel and her colleagues found about half the brochures to be worded ambiguously and noted that they often suggested limiting or reducing the number of sexual partners as a way to reduce the risk of HIV infection (1986:242). While this recommendation is not technically incorrect, it probably misrepresents the benefit of limiting numbers of partners in many homosexual communities where the prevalence of infection is already extraordinarily high (De Gruttola 1986). A survey of condom use among gay and bisexual men revealed that men with a single nonanonymous partner within the past six months were less likely to use condoms for receptive anal intercourse than were men reporting multiple or anonymous partners (Valdiserri 1988). This finding might indicate that a man with a single partner minimizes the risk of acquiring HIV through receptive anal intercourse. Other researchers have also suggested that the persistence of high-risk behavior among gay and bisexual men may be due to an underestimation of risk (Jones 1987; Bauman 1987).

Among intravenous drug users, the prevalence of human immunodeficiency virus infection is not equally distributed across the

United States. Rates of infection in New York City and northern New Jersey range between 50 and 60 percent, while most other areas of the nation generally have rates of infection below 5 percent (Booth 1988:253). This implies that the probability of acquiring HIV infection, even among individuals engaging in high-risk behaviors (for example, needle sharing) varies geographically. Des Jarlais and Friedman believe that the "best single piece of information for predicting whether an individual IV drug user is likely to have been exposed to HIV is geographic location" (1987:67). Because the spread of HIV infection among heterosexuals is believed to be closely linked to infection among intravenous drug users, this information suggests that those areas of the nation with the highest prevalence of HIV infection among intravenous drug users will also have the most significant distribution of heterosexually and perinatally transmitted cases of AIDS. Results of ongoing serologic surveys and case surveillance seem to support this hypothesis (Curran 1988; Guinan 1987; Lambert 1988b; Schoenbaum 1987; Weinberg 1987).

The level of HIV infection among the estimated 15,500 Americans with hemophilia A or B is quite high. Approximately 70 percent of persons with hemophilia A (Factor VIII deficiency) who have been tested are infected with HIV, and 35 percent of tested persons with hemophilia B (Factor IX deficiency) are likewise infected (Centers for Disease Control 1987a:3). Unlike the situation for intravenous drug users, HIV infection among hemophiliacs is equally distributed throughout the United States, "reflecting the national distribution of the clotting factor concentrates they received before 1985" (Centers for Disease Control 1987a:3). Like the sexual partners of gay men, sexual partners of hemophiliacs need to realize that they are at increased risk of becoming infected with HIV, although heterosexual transmission in this group seems to be less frequent than it is among the sexual partners of male intravenous drug users (Ragni 1988).

IMPLICATIONS FOR PREVENTION PROGRAMS

The fact that the prevalence of HIV infection varies both geographically and across "risk groups" raises another consideration that must be addressed in AIDS prevention efforts. While, ultimately, it is the presence or absence of infection within a sexual or IV drug sharing partner, and not a specific behavior per se, that is the most significant variable in determining transmission to a susceptible individual, it remains the more prudent course for risk-reduction guidelines to focus on specific behaviors rather than on the geographic variance of infection. This is true for a number of reasons. Individuals who live in areas where the incidence of HIV infection is low may misconstrue their low probability of exposure to mean no likelihood of exposure and persist in behaviors that place them at risk of infection. Increasing rates of HIV seropositivity among both European and American intravenous drug users (Adler 1986; Brunet 1987; Macdonald 1987; Moss 1987) suggest that persons living in communities in which the level of infection has not yet "peaked," may experience an increasing risk of exposure as a function of time. Also, because of the mobility of our society, the boundaries between communities often become blurred, and we frequently come in contact with persons from areas of the country where AIDS is more common. An early study of riskful behaviors among gay and bisexual men from Pittsburgh, Pennsylvania, revealed that nearly half of the forty-eight men in the sample reported travel to and sexual relations with other homosexual men in New York City within the preceeding twenty-four months (Valdiserri 1984:259). Certainly, the long incubation period of HIV (that is, the interval of time between infection and onset of symptoms) increases the likelihood of an infected individual unknowingly transmitting the virus to sexual or intravenous-drug-using partners. Because the incidence of AIDS is suspected to increase with the duration of seropositivity (Goedert 1986), it is not currently possible to state with finality a mean incubation period. An estimate of four and one- half years has been suggested as the mean incubation period for transfusion-associated AIDS (Lui 1986), but other researchers have reported that incubation periods for transfusion-associated AIDS vary depending on the age of the subject, with children having shorter incubation periods than adults (Medley 1987). Lui and his colleagues (1988:1333) have calculated a mean incubation period of 7.8 years for AIDS in homosexual men.

This chapter has focused on the behaviors that are most dangerous in terms of HIV transmission, and has tried to give the reader an appreciation of the variables influencing the process of infection. Health care providers have not been included in the discussion because their occupational status, by itself, does not qualify them as a high-risk population. Numerous studies evaluating the potential for HIV infection of health care providers caring for patients with AIDS have found the risk to be quite low (Henderson 1986; Klein 1988; Lifson 1986; Mann 1986b). When occupational seroconversion does occur, it is usually associated with an accidental percutaneous exposure, for example, a "needle stick" accident (Weiss 1985b). Experimental laboratory workers exposed to highly concentrated solutions of virus are probably at greater risk of infection than workers in a hospital environment (Weiss 1988), but in all of these settings, the risk of occupational infection can essentially be nullified by adherence to universal precautions for all blood and body fluids (Centers for Disease Control 1987b).

While there are a number of issues pertaining to the long-term effects of HIV infection that can only be answered by the cummulative experience of years of observation, many of the important questions about the epidemiology of human immunodeficiency virus have already been answered. It is apparent and well documented that HIV is transmitted as a result of both heterosexual and homosexual intercourse, through the practice of sharing needles containing contaminated blood, and perinatally from mother to child. Evidence against casual transmission comes from studies of households where family members of persons with AIDS have been tested for evidence of infection (Fischl 1987b; Friedland 1986), and in a boarding school where classmates of infected French hemophiliacs were tested for the presence of antibody to HIV (Berthier 1986). Not one of these studies has uncovered a single case of infection from casual contact. An extensive field study of an American community with a high incidence of AIDS reconfirmed the importance of the previously described routes of transmission, and provided no evidence for insect transmission (Castro 1988). The fact that human immunodeficiency virus is inactivated by a number of commonly used disenfectants, including weak solutions of household bleach (Resnick 1986; Spire 1984), proves that it is not indestructible.

Yet, many people still believe that infection can result from casual contact or through insect vectors. A 1987 survey of some three thousand Americans over the age of eighteen found that. 36 percent of the sample thought that food from a restaurant where the cook had AIDS was a likely source of infection. Eighteen percent believed that working near a person with AIDS carried a risk of infection, and 35 percent thought that mosquitoes and other insects could spread the virus ("Survey Finds Wide AIDS Ignorance" 1988). Some of these misconceptions can be attributed to misinformation, misapplication of knowledge, or ignorance. For many, however, these responses may relate to irrational fears of AIDS or subconscious attitudes about the disease and its victims (Valdiserri 1987).

Discussions of AIDS prevention often include the caveat that individuals do not usually act solely on the basis of factual information,

1986. "Stability and Inactivation of HTLV-III/LAV Under Clinical and Laboratory Environments." *Journal of the American Medical Association.* 255(14):1887–1891.

Robertson, P., and Schachter, J. 1981. "Failure to Identify Venereal Disease in a Lesbian Population." *Sexually Transmitted Diseases* 8(2):75–76.

Salahuddin, S.Z., Groopman, J.E., Markham, P.D., Sarngadharan, M.G., Redfield, R.R., McLane, M.F., Essex, M., Sliski, A., and Gallo, R.C. 1984. "HTLV-III in Symptom-Free Seronegative Persons." *Lancet* ii:1418–1420.

Schoenbaum, E.E., and Alderman, M.H. 1987. "Antibody to the Human Immunodeficiency Virus in Women Seeking Abortion in New York City." *Annals of Internal Medicine* 107(4):599.

Schreeder, M.T., Thompson, S.E., Hadler, S.C., Berquist, K.R., Zaidi, A., Maynard, J.E., Ostrow, D., Jusdon, F.N., Braff, E.H., Nylund, T., Moore, J.N., Gardner, P., Doto, I.L., and Reynolds, G. 1982. "Hepatitis B in Homosexual Men: Prevalence of Infection and Factors Related to Transmission." *Journal of Infectious Diseases* 146(1):7–15.

Scott, G.B., Fischl, M.A., Klimas, N., Fletcher, M.A., Dickinson, G.M., Levine, R.S., and Parks, W.P. 1985. "Mothers of Infants with the Acquired Immune Deficiency Syndrome." *Journal of the American Medical Association* 253(3):363–366.

Seligmann, M., Pinching, A.J., Rosen, F.S., Fahey, J. L. Khaitov, R.M., Klatzmann, D., Koenig, S., Luom, N., Ngu, J., Riethmuller, G., and Spira, T.J. 1987. "Immunology of Human Immunodeficiency Virus Infection and the Acquired Immunodeficiency Syndrome." *Annals of Internal Medicine* 107:234–242.

Selwyn, P.A., Reiner, C., Cox, C.P., Lipshutz, C., and Cohen, R.L. 1987. "Knowledge About AIDS and High-Risk Behavior Among Intravenous Drug Users in New York City." *AIDS* 1:247–254.

Senturia, Y.D., Ades, A.E., Peckham, C.S., and Giaquinto, C. 1987. "Breast Feeding and HIV Infection." *Lancet* ii(8555):400–401.

Siegel, K., Grodsky, P.B., and Herman, A., 1986. "AIDS Risk Reduction Guidelines: A Review and Analysis." *Journal of Community Health* 11(4):233–243.

Smiley, M.L., White, G.C., Becherer, P., Macik, G., Matthews, T.J., Weinhold, K.J., McMillan, C., and Bolognesi, D. 1988. "Transmission of Human Immunodeficiency Virus to Sexual Partners of Hemophiliacs." *American Journal of Hematology* 28:27–32.

Spire, B., Barre-Sinoussi, F., Montagnier, L., and Chermann, J.C. 1984. "Inactivation of Lymphadenopathy-Associated Virus by Chemical Disinfectants." *Lancet* ii(8408):899–901.

Stanback, M., Pape, J.W., Verdier, R., Jean, S., and Johnson, W.D.1988. "Breast Feeding and HIV Transmission in Haitian Children." Abstract 501, proceedings from the *IV International Conference on AIDS*, Book 1, page 340.

Staszewski, S., Schieck, E., Rehmet, S., Helm, E.B., and Stille, W. 1987.

"HIV Transmission from Male After Only Two Sexual Contacts." *Lancet* ii(8559):628.

"Survey Finds Wide AIDS Ignorance." 1988. *New York Times*, January 30, 6.

Thiry, L., Sprecher-Goldberger, S., Jonckheer, T., Levy, J.A., Van de Perre, P., Henrivaux, P., Cogniauz-LeClerc, J., and Clumeck, N. 1985. "Isolation of AIDS Virus from Cell-Free Breast Milk of Three Healthy Virus Carriers." *Lancet* ii:891–892.

Valdiserri, R.O. 1987. "Epidemics in Perspective." *Journal of Medical Humanities and Bioethics* 8(2):95–100.

Valdiserri, R.O., Brandon, W.R., and Lyter, D.W. 1984. "AIDS Surveillance and Health Education: Use of Previously Described Risk Factors to Identify High-Risk Homosexuals." *American Journal of Public Health* 74(3):259–260.

Valdiserri, R.O., Lyter, D.W., Leviton, L.C., Callahan, C.M., Kinglsey, L.A., and Rinaldo, C.R. 1988. "Variables Influencing Condom Use in a Cohort of Gay and Bisexual Men." *American Journal of Public Health* 78(7):801–805.

Van de Perre, P., Carael, M., Nzaramba, D., Zissis, G., Kayihigi, J., and Butzler, J.P. 1987. "Risk Factors for HIV Seropositivity in Selected Urban Based Rwandese Adults." *AIDS* 1:207–211.

Van de Perre, P., Clumeck, N., Carael, M., Nzabihimana, E., Robert-Guroff, M., DeMol, P., Freyens, P., Butzler, J.P., Gallo, R.C., and Kanyamupira, J.B. 1985. "Female Prostitutes: A Risk Group for Infection with Human T-Cell Lymphotropic Virus Type III." *Lancet* ii(8454): 524–527.

Victoria, C.G., Vaughan, J.P., Lombardi, D., Fuchs, S.M., Gigante, L.P., Smith, P.G., Nobre, L.C., Teixiera, A.M., Moreira, L.B., and Barros, F.C. 1987. "Evidence for Protection by Breast Feeding Against Infant Deaths from Infectious Diseases in Brazil." *Lancet* ii(8554):319–322.

Vittecoq, D., Roue, R.T., Mayaud, C., Borsa, R., Armengaud, M., Autran, B., May, T., Stern, M., Chavanet, P., Jeantils, P., Modai, J., Rey, F., and Chermann, J.C. 1987. "Acquired Immune Deficiency Syndrome After Travelling in Africa: An Epidemiological Study in Seventeen Caucasian Patients." *Lancet* ii(8533):612–615.

Vogt, M.W., Witt, D.J., Craven, D.E., Byington, R., Crawford, D.F., Schooley, R.T., and Hirsch, M.S. 1986. "Isolation of HTLV-III/LAV from Cervical Secretions of Women at Risk for AIDS." *Lancet* i(8480): 525–526.

Ward, J.W., Holmberg, S.D., Allen, J.R., Cohn, D.L., Critchley, S.E., Kleinman, S.H., Lenes, B.A., Ravenholt, O., Davis, J.R., Quinn, M.G., and Jaffe, H.W. 1988. "Transmission of Human Immunodeficiency Virus (HIV) by Blood Transfusions Screened as Negative for HIV Antibody." *New England Journal of Medicine* 318(8):473–478.

Weinberg, D.S., and Murray, H.W. 1987. "Coping with AIDS: The Special Problems of New York City." *New England Journal of Medicine* 371(23):1469–1473.

In his outline of a "platform for action" against syphilis, he advocated the following: reporting all infected individuals to state or local health departments and tracing their sexual contacts to ascertain the source of infection; providing adequate funding to ensure the necessary resources for complete treatment of all cases and contacts; encouraging a cooperative effort between private physicians and public health agencies to ensure that all infected individuals received adequate treatment; educating the public about the means of transmission; and routine widespread serologic testing to identify all infected individuals in order to bring them to treatment (Parran 1937:247).

Parran's programmatic approach to syphilis control encouraged the wider dissemination of an existing technologic solution (neosalvarsan) by developing federally funded systems to identify cases and bring them to treatment. He advocated serologic testing during employment physicals, routine physical examinations, hospital admissions, life insurance examinations, marriage license applications, and prenatal examinations, as well as testing of "lawbreakers" (Parran 1937:248–251). He also recognized the importance of viewing syphilis as a disease rather than as a moral punishment (Parran 1937: 203); of maintaining patient confidentiality throughout the testing, contact tracing, and treatment process (p. 255); of engaging respected community leaders to promote his program (p. 165); of employing visible peer-group members in the provision of diagnostic services to blacks (p. 163); and of considering syphilis as a threat to the entire community rather than as a problem submerged within the less desirable strata of society (p. 267). Throughout his discussion runs the premise that a medical case finding and treatment model should be the primary response to syphilis prevention. Although he recognized that infection could be controlled by promoting condom use and postcoital prophylaxis, he did not advocate those measures.

Dr. Parran's contributions to syphilis control should not be minimized. He was instrumental in leading the attack against the "moralistic precepts" of the American Social Hygiene Association (Brandt 1985:136), an organization that promoted educational campaigns stressing "the menace of prostitution and promiscuity" rather than a public health approach to the control of sexually transmitted diseases (Brandt 1985:135). The course of action he outlined represented a major step forward in the control of syphilis, and his book helped to end the silence surrounding the subject of sexually transmitted diseases in the popular press. His approach was so

successful that his primary recommendations for controlling syphilis and gonorrhea are still in place today in most municipal health
departments. The other legacy of Dr. Parran's achievement is that
prevention of sexually transmitted diseases has come to be identified, for the most part, with early identification of cases and contacts, followed by subsequent referral and treatment, rather than the
promotion of behavioral change per se.

Thus, Dr. Parran's program of widespread testing to identify infected individuals and to bring them to treatment has had a major
historical influence on our current approach to AIDS prevention. The
essential difference, however, is that we do not yet have an effective
cure for HIV infection. Although zidovudine has been approved for
selective HIV-infected patients with advanced illness characterized
by *Pneumocystis carinii* pneumonia or symptomatic AIDS- related
complex (Brook 1987), and the drug does appear to decrease morbidity, improve clinical status, and decrease the rate of secondary infectious complications (Fischl et al. 1987b), it is not a cure for HIV
infection. Furthermore, treatment with this drug does not necessarily make the recipient noninfectious (Fischl et al. 1987b). Our current lack of an effective treatment for HIV infection that can render
the recipient noninfectious, together with the long time an individual can carry the virus and remain asymptomatic, suggests that
HIV prevention strategies will have to be appreciably different from
those suggested by Dr. Parran and must focus on a primary goal of
behavioral change rather than rely only on case identification. This
is perhaps the major reason why, in Brandt's words, "merely invok-
ing the public health approaches that have characterized antisyph-
ilis programs is unlikely to stem the tide of the AIDS epidemic"
(Brandt 1988:380).

It is not difficult to understand why public health programs have
traditionally deemphasized behavioral change as a strategy to prevent sexually acquired infections. When curative durgs and vaccines
are available, it is probably more efficient and cost-effective to identify cases of infection and bring them into treatment than it is to attempt to change sexual behaviors that would expose an individual
to infection. In Cutler's discussion of the history of venereal prophylaxis, he notes that the military did not promote the use of condoms
during the Korean conflict because they found that it was "cheaper
and easier" to treat incident infections than it was to "teach self-
protective behavior" (Cutler 1981:326).

Another reason for the emphasis on a medical model of prevention is the disparity in evolution between the behavioral and medi-

cal sciences. At this time, we have had more practical experience with eliminating microbial invaders from an infected host than we have with achieving lasting behavioral change as a result of planned interventions. Finally, there is the matter of consensus. While everyone would agree that infected individuals should receive treatment as a means of preventing further spread of disease, it is much more difficult to reach a consensus on what constitutes appropriate behavioral endpoints for the prevention of sexually transmitted diseases. Should programs encourage abstinence or promote prophylaxis? Dr. Parran reflected the mores of his time and underscored a debate that is still extant in American public health when he expressed his belief that monogamy within the confines of marriage is the only legitimate expression of sexual activity (Parran 1937:220). As such, prophylaxis was not actively encouraged by Dr. Parran, and the prevailing consensus was that fear of acquiring syphillis played an important role in discouraging sexual activity outside the confines of marriage (Brandt 1985:159).

Because HIV infection is first and foremost a sexually transmitted disease, programmatic efforts to prevent its transmission are often influenced by the traditional notion that promoting the prevention of venereal disease is tantamount to encouraging sexual activity by removing the fear of untoward consequences (Brandt 1985). Similar criticisms have been leveled at efforts to reduce the rate of unplanned teenage pregnancy by promoting contraceptive use (Lader 1987), and they echo Dr. Parran's sentiments: "the extensive use of contraceptives has removed the inhibitions of those who, restrained by fear rather than morality, might come under the category of casual or clandestine prostitutes" (Parran 1937:209). In part, resistance to the extensive promotion of condoms as a means of preventing HIV transmission reflects societal concerns that such efforts will result in increased sexual activity beyond the scope of socially accepted norms because it will minimize the fear of infection (Goldman 1987). A brief historical review of the role of condoms in preventing sexually transmitted diseases exemplifies this long-standing conflict between societal mores and public health objectives (Valdiserri 1988).

A HISTORICAL REVIEW OF CONDOM USE

The use of a penile covering made of linen to prevent the transmission of syphillis was first described by Fallopius in 1564 (Himes

1963:190). By the eighteenth century, condoms, which were then manufactured from the dried intestines of domestic livestock, were popularly recognized in Europe as a means of preventing venereal infections (Grose 1785, cited in Himes 1963:197). After Goodyear and Hancock achieved success with the vulcanization of rubber in 1843 (Sherris 1982:H123), the production of inexpensive condoms became a reality. A further modification of vulcanization, discovered in 1846 by Alexander Parks, improved condom production even further (Reed 1978:15). Continued improvements resulted from the introduction of liquid latex in the mid-1930s (Dalsimer et al. 1973: H-3) and by Food and Drug Administration quality control standards promulgated in 1938 (Shenefelt 1981).

Obviously, there is no reliable way to determine how effective the earlier versions of condoms were in preventing transmission of venereal pathogens. It is almost certain, however, that the eighteenth-century varieties fashioned from the dried entrails of sheep and other livestock were far inferior to modern varieties manufactured from latex. Concerns about the efficacy of these early prophylactics explain, in part, the resistance of the medical community to promoting them as a reliable means of preventing infection. Astruc's treatise on venereal disease, translated into English in 1737, presents the notion of relying on a condom for protection against syphilis as absurd:

> I hear from the lowest debauchees who chase without restraint after the love of prostitutes, that there are recently employed in England skins made from the soft and seamless hides in the shape of a sheath, and called condoms in English, with which those about to have intercourse wrap their penis as in a coat of mail in order to render themselves safe in the dangers of an ever doubtful battle. They claim, I suppose, that thus mailed and with spears sheathed in this way, they can undergo with impunity the chances of promiscuous intercourse. But in truth they are greatly mistaken. (Astruc 1737, cited in Himes 1963:196).

In addition to concerns about efficacy, there were objections to promoting the use of condoms on moral grounds. In 1788, Cristoph Girtanner referred to the condom as a "shameful invention which suppresses and annihilates completely the only natural end of cohabitation, namely procreation" (Girtanner 1788, cited in Himes 1963:196). Throughout its recorded history, the recognition that the condom could prevent conception often resulted in resistance to its promotion as a means of preventing sexually acquired infections. In

1940, Dr. Woodbridge Morris, then general director of the Birth Control Federation of America, criticized the American Social Hygiene Association for excluding any specific mention of condoms as a means of preventing sexually acquired infections. He accused the organization of minimizing the importance of the condom in controlling venereal disease because it "happens to be a method of contraception" (Brandt 1985:159). During the Second World War, the United States Army recognized the condom as "the only practical mechanical protection against venereal infection" (Coates et al. 1960:197) and required post exchanges to stock condoms of approved quality, a move which was criticized by a numer of civilian and church groups. Their criticisms were based on two factors: that the condom was a method of contraception and that extensive promotion would "incite to promiscuity" (Coates et al. 1960:196).

Surgeon General C.E. Koop, in tacit recognition that sexual abstinence will not be an acceptable option for everyone who might be at risk for HIV infection, has identified condoms as an essential means of protecting oneself or a partner from the virus (Koop 1986). Yet, there are critics who believe that promoting condoms as a means of preventing HIV infection is unethical and misleading because there remains a risk of infection even when condoms are used, and because programs that promote them as a means of achieving safer sex may disuade individuals from reducing their number of sexual partners or abstaining from sex (Emanuel and Emanuel 1987). Some have suggested that individuals should forgo insertive intercourse completely rather than rely on a method that is not entirely effective (Kelly and St. Lawrence 1987). Objections to advocating condoms as a means of preventing HIV infection, while generally less vehement, are nonetheless reminiscent of past diatribes that denounced the use of condoms as prophylactics because of the fear that their promotion would result in increased sexual activity (Valdiserri 1988).

Technologic advances have resulted in a vastly improved condom, capable of preventing the laboratory transmission of a number of viral pathogens, including human immunodeficiency virus (Conant et al. 1986; Van de Perre et al. 1987), herpes virus (Conant et al. 1984), hepatitis B virus (Minuk et al. 1987), and cytomegalovirus (Katznelson et al. 1984). Nonetheless, it is important to emphasize that condom use as a method of preventing HIV infection does have an associated failure rate. Condom failure can result from inconsistent or improper use (Trussell and Kost 1987); occasional product failure, as when a condom ruptures (Free et al. 1980); or condom slippage, so that its seminal contents are spilled in the body. In Fischl's study of the heterosexual transmission of human immuno-deficiency virus, she documented, in a follow-up period of twelve to thirty-six months, that 10 percent of seronegative spouses (one person in her sample) continuing vaginal intercourse with seropositive partners became infected with HIV—even though they reported using condoms. This rate of seroconversion was, however, substantially lower than the 86 percent of originally seronegative spouses who became infected while continuing to have unprotected vaginal intercourse with infected partners (Fischl et al. 1987a:641). In another study, nearly three thousand HIV seronegative gay men were followed at six-month intervals for two years, to determine whether the use of condoms reduced the risk of HIV seroconversion. The investigators noted that among men with more than eight different partners in the previous twelve months, "the seroconversion rate was 9.5 times higher for those men using condoms with none of their partners" compared to those men who used condoms with all of their partners (Detels et al. 1988:214). The investigators concluded that condoms provided "significant but not complete" protection against HIV infection (Detels et al. 1988:214). Analysis of the efficacy of condoms in preventing pregnancy, although not completely analogous to their efficacy in preventing HIV infection, reveals a failure rate ranging from 2 to 14 percent (Trussell and Kost 1987:257).

There are ways to minimize the occurence of HIV infection as a result of condom failure, most notably by teaching everyone who relies on them as prophylactics to use them consistently and correctly. Latex condoms are generally superior to natural membrane condoms as barriers to viral transmission because the natural membrane condom may permit the leakage of small virus particles (Lytle et al. 1988). Condoms should never be used more than once, and they should always be lubricated with water-based lubricants rather than oil-based lubricants or saliva (Sherris 1982). Oil- based lubricants,.especially those containing mineral oil, can cause deterioration of the condom within two to five minutes of use (Voeller et al. 1988). Men who wear condoms should be instructed to grip the condom firmly to the base of the penis upon withdrawal to avoid condom slippage. Because of the possibility of condoms rupturing during use (Cohn et al. 1988), especially if they are improperly or inadequately lubricated, it is recommended that they be used in conjunction with virucidal lubricants containing nonoxynol-9, an agent that has been demonstrated to destroy HIV in vitro (Hicks et al.

1985; Rietmeijer et al. 1988). Men who continue to engage in sexual practices that are particularly efficient in the transmission of HIV (vaginal and anal intercourse), even with the use of condoms, should be advised to withdraw the penis from their partners prior to ejaculation (Valdiserri et al. 1988).

From a public health perspective, the issue is not whether condom-protected intercourse is "safer" than forgoing insertive anal and vaginal intercourse; it is not, and should never be presented as such. However, it is important to recognize that there are situations in which individuals may be unwilling to abstain from vaginal or anal intercourse, and for those individuals information about the appropriate way to use condoms is absolutely essential.

Barriers to the widespread promotion of condoms as a primary means of avoiding HIV infection harken back to historical fears that such efforts will have a contrary effect on disease control by presenting the condom as a way to have sex without associated risk. Value judgements about the behaviors in question may also impede the acceptance of condom promotion as a legitimate public health response to AIDS. Continued debate about the appropriateness of advertising contraceptives on network television (Holden 1987; Lader 1987) and religious controversy about the morality of educating youth about condoms as a means of preventing AIDS (Ostling 1987) are reminiscent of earlier cited objections against condom use. Both criticisms have had a significant negative impact on the widespread adoption of a medically recognized method of prophylaxis, effective against a broad host of venereal infections (Stone et al. 1986).

A BRIEF HISTORY OF INTRAVENOUS DRUG USE

In the same way that reviewing programmatic responses to past epidemics of venereal disease provides a historical perspective on the current public health response to AIDS, a brief review of the history of intravenous drug use in this country is helpful in understanding long-held attitudes about the other major behavioral mode of HIV transmission—needle sharing among intravenous drug users. Few examples of the evolution of public thought, policy, and legislation relating to a health problem are as fascinating as the story of narcotic drugs in America.

Since ancient times, opium has been recognized as a reliable analgesic. By the early 1800s, most medical texts and home remedy compendiums listed recipes for laudanum, a solution of opium in water or alcohol (Morgan 1981:3), and many of the best-selling elixirs and tonics of the early nineteenth century contained opium (Morgan 1981:2). The principal analgesic alkaloid of opium, morphine, had been isolated in 1806 by the German chemist W.A. Serturner (Rublowsky 1974:127). Not until 1853, however, did technology produce the implement that now plays such an important role in the transmission of HIV among intravenous drug users—the hypodermic syringe (Rublowsky 1974:129). By the 1870s, the hypodermic syringe was standard equipment for most physicians, and, "like other products of the therapeutic revolution, its sale was unrestricted" (Morgan 1981:22). As a result of the extensive use of parenteral morphine by army doctors during the Civil War (Rublowsky 1974:129), the widespread therapeutic application of morphine for conditions as diverse as "sciatica, cholera, asthma, sunstroke, and hernia" (Morgan 1981:24), and the ease with which both morphine and syringes were available to the general public (often through mail-order catalogues) (Morgan 1981:26), addiction soon came to be recognized as a significant medical problem.

Toward the end of the nineteenth century, concerns about the increasing nonmedical use of opiates converged with popular sentiment that opiate use represented a "moral failing" (Morgan 1974:19). Opium was seen as a serious threat to the vitality of American society (Morgan 1981:51), and the prominent association of opium use with immigrant Chinese laborers reinforced the notion that it was a decadent foreign vice (Morgan 1981:49).

In what was to be one of many futile attempts to develop a medical treatment for opiate addiction, heroin, first synthesized in England in 1874 (Austin 1978:199) was used to treat the symptoms of morphine withdrawal and was initially hailed as a cure for addiction (Rublowsky 1974:130). Although the medical profession, cautious as a result of the disaster caused by the widespread prescription of morphine, did not overuse heroin, it was easily obtained in most drug stores and soon became popular among drug users. In the years preceeding the First World War, heroin use was a significant problem in several major urban centers in America (Morgan 1981:95).

Although medical science came to recognize the addictive properties of narcotic drugs, popular sentiment tended to view narcotic addiction as a willful act, and the print media described it in terms of "dissipation," identifying it with "wayward youth, irresponsibility, and crime" (Morgan 1981:96). It was in this spirit that the first major piece of federal domestic legislation dealing with narcotic control, the Harrison Act, was passed in 1914. The law had

ventions to apply. One wonders, for example, whether the analogies that compare high-risk behaviors in AIDS with habits such as smoking are overblown. If so, theories and findings from such comparisons may not all be useful. Even in the case of IV drug users, the behavior that puts people at risk for AIDS is not drug use per se, but a drug culture that promotes needle sharing. For most people, unprotected intercourse seems a form of "gambling" behavior, although more work in this area is needed. Both seat belt use and unprotected intercourse may be habitual to some degree—yet on each entry into a car, and with each sexual encounter, a person has a realistic opportunity to choose or reject protection.

Accurate characterization of behaviors that carry a high risk of transmitting HIV as "gambles," "habits," or "central to a person's life," carries major implications for the selection of applicable theories and for designation of interventions that are most cost-effective. Here are two illustrations of this point. Gay men know a great deal about the dangers of sexually-acquired HIV infection, and in the face of the AIDS epidemic, numerous studies report drastic declines in numbers of partners and in practices that carry a high risk of sexual transmission (Fox et al. 1987; Joseph et al. 1987; Martin 1987; Valdiserri et al. 1989). In the face of risk, many gay men will reduce the number of "gambles" they take; they will decide to reduce their number of partners and to increase their use of condoms. One might claim that cognitive and decision-making theories explain these observations, although fear arousal could also play a role. However, a residual group of men may still be engaging in high-risk behavior on a regular basis. Their high-risk behavior may be an important part of their life-style and thus be resistant to change. A different theoretical framework, based either on a "habit" analogy or on the assumption that high-risk behavior is of central importance to these people, is necessary in order to explain their risk-taking behavior and to develop an appropriate intervention for them.

The second illustration involves the female sexual partners of male IV drug users. It is estimated that 80 percent of these women are not drug users themselves (Mondanaro 1987). Even if these women want to protect themselves from HIV infection, the choice may not be theirs alone to make. Their partners must also be persuaded to clean their drug paraphernalia and to use condoms. If neither effort works, someone may need to persuade these women to leave their relationships (Staver 1987). These women are very much at risk, yet their situation may be of central importance in their lives. Even a superficial analysis leads to the conclusion that no one theory is adequate to address their prevention needs. Closer study of the needs of these women is vital if we are to understand how to begin to intervene with them (Nelkin 1987).

As these examples show, the sequencing of theories in "blueprinting" needs to begin simply, with cognition, and become more complex as a broader range of forces are considered.

COGNITIVE AND DECISION-MAKING THEORIES

In general, the assumption underlying cognitive and decision-making theories is that people are processors of information. These theories focus on biases in thinking that might prevent people from acting rationally, and work on the assumption that many behaviors, attitudes, and beliefs can be explained without considering emotion or motivation. Although they may be limited in this respect, cognitive and decision-making theories can be extremely useful for understanding AIDS interventions, especially in the area of risk communication.

Decision Theories

Decision theories rest on the assumption that people are "rational actors," that is, that they will make choices they believe will increase their likelihood of obtaining valued goods or experiences and avoiding negative experiences (Abelson and Levi 1985). This framework has been applied to health under the names risk communication (Slovic et al. 1987), protection motivation theory (Rogers 1975), and the theory of subjective expected utility (Sutton 1982). In the context of AIDS prevention, these theories assume that a decision maker who knows which behaviors are risky in terms of viral transmission would choose to reduce or eliminate those behaviors because he or she perceives that they increase the likelihood of HIV infection (Fischhoff 1988a).

However, theories of decision-making are complicated, and their application to AIDS prevention is not as simple as this description implies. The person engaging in high-risk behavior may perceive that good experiences will result from it and must weigh the positive and negative consequences of the behavior. Intravenous drug users want their drug and may be compelled to share a needle in order to inject it. Prostitutes want to make money from sex and may not be willing to lose a client who refuses to wear a condom.

A second qualifier to the rational decision maker model is that we often operate under conditions of uncertainty. The choices we make are seldom certain to result in the consequences we seek or to prevent those we wish to avoid. For example, a woman may want to have sex with a man she believes is an intravenous drug user. That individual may or may not be infected with HIV. The truth is unknown to the woman, and the probability of his being infected depends, in part, on the prevalence of HIV infection among IV drug users in that community. A strict rational-actor theorist will predict that the woman will operate to maximize her utilities: that is, she will have sex if she values it and if her perception of the probability of her partner being infected is sufficiently low. She will avoid sex if she perceives the probability of HIV infection to be high, or if she does not value sex with this individual very much.

In decision-making theories, high-risk behavior is seen as a series of gambles, as it is in the case of seat belt use. Any single episode of unprotected car travel has a probability of resulting in a serious accident. Over many episodes, this probability is cumulative—one in three over a lifetime (Warner 1983). A similar cumulative probability is at work in high-risk behavior related to HIV infection.

This analogy leads us to the third problem with a utility maximizing approach: people often fail to act on the basis of probabilities. Even if one assumes that people are able to change easily, they may have difficulty thinking in terms of probabilities, and their perception of risk depends in part on the way in which the issue is framed (Nisbett and Ross 1980; Kahneman and Tversky 1973). For example, college students view condoms' safety differently depending on whether the information focuses on success (for example 95% percent safe) or failure (5 percent failure rate) Fischhoff and Svenson 1988). People also simplify risks; they regard behavior as "safe" or "unsafe," and they do not view safety as being a continuum (Fischhoff, in press). In addition, people often underestimate the cumulative probability of illness or injury (Fischhoff, in press). Some theorists would say that more complete information on probabilities would produce more rational action (Edwards 1977). Others argue that consistent biases in risk perception might best be addressed on their own terms (Fischhoff and Svenson 1988).

A fourth problem is that organisms, whether people or laboratory rats, often find it difficult to maximize utility when they must delay gratification (Logan 1965; Rachlin and Green 1972). Delaying gratification means rejecting a short-term reward, at the time it is offered, in order to obtain greater rewards later. People find it especially difficult to delay gratification when their attention is on the short-term reward (Mischel and Ebbesen 1970). This is a problem in many areas of behavioral change, including smoking cessation and weight control. We will return to this issue in discussing the theory of operant conditioning, but an example germane to AIDS prevention makes the point here. IV drug users may value their lives and not want to get AIDS (Ginzburg et al. 1986). Nevertheless, their wish to avoid AIDS is unlikely to help them choose safer behavior at the very moment when they are frantic for a "fix" and do not have clean "works".

Theory of Risk Communication

In spite of these difficulties, the study of people's interpretation of risk communication has proven very useful for prevention. For example, we are discovering important and consistent cognitive biases in people's interpretation of probabilities. These biases permit us to be more effective in risk communication (Fischhoff, in press). Some authors are now concluding that people's interpretation of risk can sometimes be more sensible and rational than the original wording of a probability statement describing that risk (Slovic et al. 1987).

According to available studies, people perceive greater danger when a risk is both unknown and dreaded. Unknown risks are characterized by the following: they are not observable, they are unknown to those exposed, their effects are delayed, the risk is new and unknown to science. Dreaded risks are not controllable, globally catastrophic, have fatal consequences, do not effect all people equally, pose a danger to future generations, have increasing effects over time, are not easily reduced, and may be involuntarily incurred by the population (Slovic et al. 1981).

The public's perception of AIDS is that it is a very great risk, in part because it is both unknown and dreaded, as defined here (Nelkin 1987). Incidentally, this fearful characterization may help explain "AIDS hysteria," although hysteria is hardly a decision-making concept. A search for control over a dreaded risk may help explain many of the mistaken beliefs that abound about HIV transmission and the inappropriate precautions sometimes taken by people encountering persons with AIDS.

Theories of decision making are especially helpful in understanding personal feelings of invulnerability. People may understand the probability of danger for others who behave in dangerous ways, but minimize the risk for themselves when they behave in the same way. For example, a person may overestimate his own driving skill if he has driven for years without experiencing an accident (Slovic 1987). He may also be less likely to wear seat belts for this reason. In the same way, people engaging in high-risk behaviors who, to date, have not experienced any negative effects, may develop a low expectation that such behavior could place them at risk for HIV infection. This mind set would help to explain why some people who test negative for HIV continue to engage in riskful behavior or are less likely to modify sexual practices when compared to known seropositives (Fox et al. 1987).

The Health Belief Model

A prevalent application of decision theories to health behavior is the Health Belief Model (Becker 1974; Rosenstock and Kirscht 1979). The Health Belief Model includes several families of variables that predict behavior:

a. Perceived susceptibility or vulnerability to a health threat

b. Perceived severity of the consequences of a disease or health threat

c. Perceived effectiveness of protective actions

d. Perceived costs of or barriers to protective actions

e. Cues to action, such as physician advice or symptoms

f. Demographic, structural, and social/psychological factors that "enable" behavior.

These variables are hypothesized to have a multiplicative relationship to each other. For example, the likelihood of condom use as a means of preventing HIV infection will be greater when people perceive themselves as susceptible to HIV infection, perceive the consequences of infection as very severe, perceive protective action as very effective, see few costs or barriers to self-protection (such as embarrassment over condom purchases), have a cue to action (for example, a reminder of protective behaviors when dating), and are enabled to protect themselves (for example, have the opportunity to get condoms).

Numerous studies indicate that these dimensions are important for explaining and predicting health-related behavior. However, the Health Belief Model has several specific weaknesses. Howard Leventhal, one of the original developers of this model, cites seven (Leventhal et al. 1980). First, he notes that perceived severity does not predict behavior very well. In several studies, preventive action was not more likely against a severe condition than against a less severe condition. Second, although the model predicts behavior, only a modest amount of the statistical variance in responses is accounted for by the model. In practitioner terms, a large amount of health behavior is not explained by the model. Third, people often fail to behave in line with their beliefs, even if there is a cue to action and the behavior is enabled by outside forces. Fourth, as mentioned above, people do not behave strictly in terms of probabilities. This suggests the need for an improved definition of the susceptibility dimension. Fifth, only health beliefs and motives are considered in this model. However, other beliefs and issues are important to the person who is engaging in high-risk behavior. For example, prostitutes make their living through sex with multiple partners, many of whom are anonymous. They may themselves be iv drug users. In spite of a desire to avoid becoming infected with HIV, they may not be vigilant about safer sex practices when using alcohol and drugs (Mondanaro 1987). A sixth problem is that we know very little about how health beliefs develop and about what maintains them. In fact, this model offers few explicit suggestions for intervention, except to provide information to people. A final problem is that beliefs may or may not precede behavior. It can sometimes be demonstrated that behavior precedes beliefs (Leventhal et al. 1980).

The Health Belief Model is the dominant model of health-related behavior among public health professionals at the present time. However, it is limited for the reasons given. While it has value, the practitioner should explore other models, since a recurrent finding in health promotion studies is that information alone is often inadequate to get people to change health-related behavior (Bartlett 1981; Green et al. 1980; Winett 1986). There is evidence that this is equally true for gay men and AIDS prevention. Knowledge of HIV and its transmission is extremely good in several cohorts studied—yet riskful behavior persists (Valdiserri et al. 1989; Research and Decisions Corporation 1984).

Theory of Reasoned Action

Another cognitive model of behavior change is the theory of reasoned action, which is useful to the AIDS prevention effort since it provides information about the linkages between knowledge, beliefs, attitudes, and behavior (Fishbein and Ajzen 1975; Ajzen and Fishbein 1980). In general, we assume that providing information will change beliefs, attitudes, and, ultimately, behavior. However, the causal linkages between these three concepts are tenuous (Kiesler et al. 1969). In particular, researchers find no associations, or very weak ones, between attitudes and behavior, a situation that has been "the scandal of the [social psychology] field for half a century" (McGuire 1985: 251). These weak associations are especially sobering in health education, where researchers frequently find that health information campaigns produce large changes in knowledge, modest changes in attitudes, and few changes in behavior (Bartlett 1981).

The theory of reasoned action holds that a person's intention to act is the immediate determinant of behavior. Four factors affect this intention: the person's attitude toward the behavior, or evaluation of it; the person's beliefs about the behavior; the person's perception of subjective norms (beliefs about what significant others will think of the behavior); and the value the person places on approval by others. This theory bears some resemblance to the other theories described in this section, in that expected utility of the behavior is represented by one's belief about outcomes (Fishbein and Ajzen 1975; Ajzen and Fishbein 1980). However, it adds an additional dimension to behavior in that it recognizes the influence of subjective norms—albeit in a totally cognitive, information-processing way. This theory would predict that a gay man who values the approval of his peers, believes that they endorse safer sex, and also believes that safer sex can be enjoyable, would be more likely to engage in safer sex compared to men who do not have these beliefs. In fact, one study shows the single attitudinal predictor of gay men's change toward safer sex to be the perception that peers approved safer sex (Joseph et al. 1987). This perception was also important in a marketing study conducted in San Francisco (Research and Decisions Corporation 1984). These findings indicate that activities to promote safer sex should concentrate on strengthening beliefs that peers will accept safer behaviors.

LEARNING THEORIES

Learning theories emphasize the identification of environmental conditions leading to the acquisition and maintenance of behavior. Identifying these conditions provides the health educator with unique tools for behavior change. Two general types of learning theory are current: the theory of operant conditioning, which does not make any assumptions about cognitive processes, and social learning theory, which does make such assumptions.

Theory of Operant Conditioning

The advantage of operant theory is that it does not rely on events inside the person in order to explain behavior. Rather, the task is to discover the environmental reinforcement factors that are maintaining behavior (Ferster and Skinner 1957; Skinner 1969). In the context of AIDS prevention, an operant conditioning approach is probably most helpful in giving persons who engage in high-risk practices control over their behavior by helping them to recognize and manage reinforcement factors. Operant conditioning principles may seem manipulative or menacing to some, but utilized properly, they can empower people to protect themselves. For years practitioners of behavioral medicine have been helping people with such life-style-related health problems as smoking, adherence to medication, or obesity by applying a modified operant conditioning approach (Brownell 1982; Chesney 1984; Pechacek 1979).

The operant approach rests on the analysis of three components that together constitute *contingencies of reinforcement:* behavior, reinforcer, and discriminative stimulus. Behaviors are defined by the individual or the behavior analyst, and in the context of AIDS prevention might include use or nonuse of condoms, visiting bathhouses for sex, sharing needles, or engaging in or abstaining from sex. A reinforcer is any consequence of a selected behavior that increases the frequency of that behavior. Positive reinforcers (for example, sexual pleasure) increase behavior when they are present, while negative reinforcers (for example, fear of unwanted pregnancy) increase behavior when they are withdrawn. Secondary reinforcers exert their effect through long association with primary reinforcers (for example, money is associated with many primary reinforcers) (Skinner 1969). Punishment, on the other hand, decreases or eliminates a selected behavior through either the removal of positive reinforcement or the presentation of aversive events. Behavior can be modified by making reinforcers or punishment *contingent* on the behavior.

A discriminative stimulus or cue is anything that sets the occasion for a response and reinforcement. One behavioral technique is to control the stimuli in the person's environment so that these cues are no longer available. For example, a hypertensive individual who needs to avoid salt might remove saltshakers from the table (Chesney 1984). Self-monitoring is also an important part of the operant approach, since contingencies of reinforcement vary from person to person and are identified only through observation. So, for example, smokers are urged to spend time identifying the situations that prompt them to smoke (for example, drinking their morning coffee or visiting a bar) so that these situations can be avoided or changed. In the context of AIDS prevention, self-monitoring would reveal the individual circumstances that increase or maintain the frequency of high-risk behaviors. For example, visiting "shooting galleries" may set the occasion for riskful behavior for some IV drug users, since they know they are more likely to share needles or fail to clean needles before using them there. Gaining control over the stimulus might consist of avoiding shooting galleries, and that is one action a health educator or outreach worker would recommend.

In terms of explaining behavior, the strength of the operant approach—attention to the environmental contingencies—may also be its major weakness. Leventhal, Meyer, and Gutmann (1980) point out that because contingencies of reinforcement are based on observation, we do not know what makes them effective, how long they will stay in force, and under what conditions a general class of reinforcement will be effective. Because of this uncertainty, behavior therapies tend to "throw in the kitchen sink", that is, to include any and all techniques that have been shown to be reinforcing or to provide stimulus control in other settings. For example, a behavior therapy might include all of the following: self-monitoring of an unwanted behavior, controlling stimuli that prompt the behavior, sensitizing the person to associate the behavior with unpleasant events, enlisting social support to reinforce a lower rate of the behavior, and making behavioral contracts in which the person receives reinforcement (for example, money) for refraining from the behavior. However, it may be that some of these activities are unnecessary, and careful study might show that only a few key elements are required to modify behavior. The reason to look for key components is that we would not have to dilute treatments with nonessential and cost-ineffective components.

"Kitchen sink" therapies are not the exclusive domain of operant conditioning, by any means. Many psychotherapies incur this criticism. There is, moreover, another side to the controversy. Therapy and counseling are by nature multifaceted, and therapists may have a legitimate interest in including anything that might be effective in helping clients change. Also, identifying key components of interventions is possible only when effective interventions are available. Especially in AIDS prevention, it may be premature to test individual components of interventions until we can gain a better idea of overall interventions that work. Nevertheless, practitioners will ultimately be better served by such theories when they can pinpoint the effective elements of prevention interventions.

Social Learning Theory

We do not need to experience reinforcement directly in order to learn about contingencies of reinforcement. We can also observe others and hear about their experiences. This cognitive process distinguishes cognitive learning theory from operant theory (Bandura 1977b). Social learning theory returns to the cognitive theorist's assumption that individual perceptions about the environment determine what is reinforcing and whether reinforcements can be obtained. Social learning theory has an advantage over some of the theories outlined so far in that it can explain the source of these perceptions. Social learning theory takes into account thoughts about oneself in addition to one's direct learning and posits that such thoughts mediate the relationship between information and action. Emerging from social learning theory are several concepts that are highly relevant to preventive behavior: self-efficacy, stages of behavior change, explanation of relapse, and self-regulation.

SELF-EFFICACY

Self-efficacy refers to individuals' perceptions that they are or are not capable of performing a behavior (Bandura 1977a; 1986). People begin with an appraisal of their efficacy for successfully performing a behavior and revise that appraisal in light of their success or failure. Behavior therapies and health education can affect these appraisals (Chesney 1984). People attribute success and failure to four possible factors: their own ability, their effort, the difficulty of the task or situation, or luck. This causal attribution affects self-efficacy. For example, someone who attributes failure on a task to lack of ability is likely to perceive lower self-efficacy to perform that task. Someone who attributes failure to a lack of effort is more likely to try again in spite of the negative experience (Weiner et al. 1972). The perception of self-efficacy may be specific to a task or generalized to many aspects of a person's life, but it is based on experience and it is modifiable.

The self-efficacy concept has contributed greatly to our understanding of changes in some health behaviors, such as smoking (Pechacek and Danaher 1979). Changes in perceptions of self-efficacy predict progression through stages of change in life-style (DiClemente 1986). Changes in self-efficacy occur in four general ways: through personal experience, through the experiences of people similar to oneself; through verbal persuasion, and, to some degree, from physiological states (Bandura 1977a; 1986). Self-efficacy perceptions can be changed by others, as is seen in the treatment of phobias (Bandura et al. 1982).

Persons engaging in high-risk behaviors may have reason to doubt their self-efficacy to protect themselves from HIV infection. Perceptions of self-efficacy may be relatively low because the self-protective behaviors and the situations involved are not familiar (Bandura 1986). Also, individuals who have tried to change their behavior in the past and failed are likely to perceive low self-efficacy. Finally, information about the dangers of HIV infection may create fear or alarm. Such emotional arousal can contribute to doubts about self-efficacy under some conditions (Maddux and Stanley 1986).

The self-efficacy theory gives some clues to designing interventions that might overcome peoples' self-doubt. First, role models can provide target groups with evidence that self-protection can be successful. The use of role models may be extremely important in cohesive groups, such as members of gay networks. Among Hispanic intravenous drug users, both network building and role models are important elements of prevention campaigns (Jimenez 1987). Even for apparently isolated people, information from similar but positive role models may provide empowerment. For example, women who are partners of IV drug users are generally isolated from each other (Mondanaro 1987). Intervention in this group might consist of providing contact with women in similar situations who have succeeded in initiating condom use with their partners, have persuaded partners to clean needles, or have left their partners because they were unwilling to modify their behavior. Although a single exposure to a positive role model may not produce immediate behavior change, in conjunction with other supportive interventions it may eventually help the at-risk person to modify his or her behavior.

A second implication of self-efficacy and of social learning theory is that providing people with skills for behavior change will improve their self-efficacy and, therefore, their persistence in maintaining behavior change. For example, smoking prevention interventions utilize peer support, positive role models, and social skills building, so that children can effectively resist pressure from their peers to smoke (McCaul and Glasgow 1985). By imparting social skills, counselors are increasing the likelihood that refusals will be successful, and after success, children will perceive increased self-efficacy to refuse cigarettes. In the same way, condom use by gay men has been increased in situations that emphasize peer support for safer sex, and skills training has helped facilitate discussion of safer sex among partners (Valdiserri et al. 1989).

STAGES OF BEHAVIOR CHANGE

Many of the theories we have described are presented as though behavior change was an all-or-nothing affair. However, behavior change is often a gradual process, with identifiable stages. This has been studied best in the additive behaviors, in which five stages are identified: precontemplation, in which people do not seriously consider protecting themselves; contemplation, in which they begin to consider self-protection and may seek out information about the hazard and self-protection; short-term self-protection, in which the person tries self-protection but may relapse into riskful behavior; recidivism, in which people have returned to riskful behavior but may try self-protection again; and long-term self-protection (DiClemente 1986; DiClemente and Prochaska 1985; DiClemente et al. 1985). This sequence of stages is applicable to AIDS prevention. For instance, at the stage of precontemplation, individuals engaging in high-risk behaviors may not even contemplate behavior change. However, at the contemplation stage, they begin to think about it, appraise their ability to avoid high-risk behaviors, and seek information about self-protection. Short-term behavior change is likely to be fairly simple for most individuals at risk, provided our assumption is correct—that riskful behavior is more akin to a gamble than a habit for most people. Recidivism may occur if behavior change is more difficult than an individual imagined, if perceived peer support is lacking, or if social skills for avoiding high-risk behaviors are not adequate. Longer-term behavior change occurs as people gain skill and increased self-efficacy for less dangerous behaviors.

The advantage of viewing self-protection as a process of behavior change is that we may be able to identify forces that move people forward in the process. For example, advice from health providers may move individuals from the precontemplation to the contemplation stage, provided that health professionals are a credible source of information. As people seek information and appraise their ability to change, positive role models may assist them in moving toward short-term changes. Observation and verbal change are predominant in the contemplation stage, while personal action and the results of action are important at later stages. Role models probably help at the contemplation stage, but skills building and success experiences matter at later stages.

The AIDS-prevention specialist has to decide whether to intervene at one stage or at several stages. If, for example, people deny that AIDS could be a problem for them, then prevention strategies might focus on moving people from the precontemplation to the contemplation stage. If, in contrast, individuals acknowledge their personal risk of HIV infection, then the intervention might be aimed at inducing action. As a third possibility, it may be that most at-risk people are trying to change, but some are having difficulty or experiencing negative consequences. In this case, skills building would be appropriate.

EXPLANATION OF RELAPSE

Relapse into dangerous behaviors fits closely with a self-efficacy model. As Schunk and Carbonari (1984) note, any change to new behavior is likely to meet with initial failures, or "slips." If these "slips" are attributed to a lack of ability or to the difficulty of maintaining behavior change, the person is likely to perceive lower self-efficacy and to relapse to the dangerous behavior (Brownell et al. 1986; Marlatt and Gordon 1980). If the person sees improvement over time, however, any "slips" are likely to be interpreted as temporary setbacks, and self-efficacy to change behavior will increase. Consider the example of two gay men who have resolved to use condoms during all future episodes of anal intercourse. One forgets to use a condom after receiving health education and interprets this "slip" as a temporary setback, with no implications for his future ability to act protectively. The other man, however, is a diffident person who has trouble asserting himself with new sexual partners. He fails to bring up the subject of condoms prior to sex, does not use a condom during sex, and attributes this "slip" to his own lack of ability to assert himself and to the difficulty of insisting on condom-protected intercourse. If enough "slips" occur, he may relapse permanently into unsafe sex.

SELF-REGULATION

A second theoretical construct emerging from social learning theory is that of self-regulation (Leventhal et al. 1980). To the processes listed earlier, self-regulation theory adds the hypothesis that people generate implicit theories about their bodies and about health and illness. Self-regulation consists of four steps: extracting information about the environment, generating a representation of illness dangers, planning and acting, and monitoring or appraising the effects of coping reactions. Self-regulation theory would explain nonadherence to hypertension medication, for example, by saying that the nonadherent individual has a mistaken theory about the relation-ship between symptoms, medication, and hypertension.

When the external danger to health is vague and not well under-stood, the illness representation that is generated is likely to be erro-neous (Leventhal et al. 1980; Fischhoff, in press). Representations of illness are also influenced by social learning. Thus, we think of mo-tor vehicle injuries in terms of "flaming crashes," and in the last century death from tuberculosis was considered "romantic." Al-though they probably have seen individuals with AIDS in the media, many people do not personally know someone with AIDS. Therefore, images of AIDS and AIDS prevention may be colored by unrealistic as-sumptions about the cause and transmission of HIV infection. When people do become personally familiar with AIDS, fear sometimes increases, perhaps because of vivid images of a brutal and uncontrol-lable disease.

A major implication of this theory, therefore, is that AIDS-preven-tion efforts need to tap into these cognitive representations of ill-ness danger in more effective ways, and to help people develop accurate representations of the danger, which will, in turn, assist them in coping. To study the representations of illness, we must re-fer back to the individual's perception of risk, and to the expression of fear as seen in theories of fear arousal.

THEORIES OF FEAR AROUSAL, MOTIVATION, AND EMOTION

Classic theories of motivation differ greatly from cognitive and de-cision-making theories in that they assume that a variety of pro-cesses inside the person cause behavior. More recently, theories of emotion, especially fear, have been integrated with the cognitive theories to provide explanations of behavior that address observed effects in a more satisfactory way. Most work that is directly related to health has focused on the emotion of fear, although anger and emotional coping are also important explanatory factors in these theories.

Managing fear and other emotions is a central problem in risk communication, especially about AIDS. Some fear is inevitable because health professionals, the media, and other information sources are describing the dangers posed by high-risk behavior. Vul-nerable people (for example, those who have engaged in riskful behavior) are likely to experience relatively more fear in the face of this communication, especially if they continue to engage in these behaviors (Leventhal and Watts 1966). Although fear can motivate behavior change, it can also produce dysfunctional effects which may interfere with behavior change. Therefore, risk communication must strike a balance between the positive and negative effects of fear.

Theories of Fear

FEAR AS A DRIVE

Two conceptions of fear are currently prevalent. The first conception, derived from the classical drive theories of experimental psychology, views fear as an aversive internal state that will cause the individual to act in ways that reduce fear (Hovland et al. 1953). In this model, a threatening stimulus, such as risk information, arouses fear. Because fear produces discomfort, people are motivated to eliminate it. Self-protective behavior is a means of coping with this emotion. If this behavior reduces fear or other negative emotions, the response becomes more probable because fear reduction is reinforcing (Hovland et al. 1953; Leventhal et al. 1980; Sutton 1982). A variety of other models of fear arousal have expanded on this idea (Janis 1967; McGuire 1968). However, research findings conflict with the theory of fear as a drive and suggest that the underlying processes are not so simple (Leventhal et al. 1980; Sutton 1982).

FEAR AS A SET OF RESPONSES

The second conception of fear views it as a repertoire of potential responses that an individual manifests when in a fearful state (Averill 1987). This repertoire is quite large. In some circumstances, we may "freeze" in the face of danger, while in others, we act rationally to avoid danger, and only after the danger is over do we tremble uncontrollably, faint, collapse, or weep. In different circumstances, we may deny the danger, or become angry, or engage in problem solving to avoid the danger. This view of fear as a repertoire of responses is an important development, for many reasons. For example, it can explain why fear can occur in the absence of an immediate danger or stimulus, since cognitive processes can generate fears. Also, it can incorporate the cutural and experiential determinants of how fear will be expressed. Furthermore, by studying which fear responses appear under which conditions, we may come closer to ensuring that AIDS information will produce "constructive" fear responses.

Viewing fear as a set of responses also improves our understanding of long-held fears. Individuals who are at increased risk of HIV infection may live with the fear of infection for long periods of time, especially if they have been unsuccessful at modifying their behavior. They are not in a state of acute fear that is the focus of the drive models, so that a drive cannot explain their actions very well. Unlike immediate short-term fears, long-term fears are more likely to be fairly important aspects of an individual's thinking and action, and to influence core psychological processes such as personality, values, and memory. One implication of this model is that when people have long-term fears, a one-time prevention campaign will not affect behavior very much unless it addresses these core processes effectively. For example, individuals with long-term fears of cancer from occupational exposures have been anecdotally observed to attribute many ailments to their exposures and may experience reactions ranging from survival guilt to stress disorders.

OTHER THEORIES OF FEAR AROUSAL

Researchers have developed other theories to account for the effects of fear-arousing communications. Two are cognitive in nature: Rogers' (1975) protection motivation theory and Sutton's (1982) theory based on subjective expected utilities are consistent with the decision-making theories described earlier; both state that people will act rationally to protect themselves from danger. Leventhal (1970; Leventhal and Everhart 1980) proposes a model of fear-arousing communications in which two processes occur at the same time: danger control and fear control. Danger control is largely cognitive and involves making a plan for self-protection. Fear control involves coping with an unpleasant feeling. Relaxation training, avoiding thoughts about the feared event, or drinking alcohol to reduce anxiety are examples of fear-control responses (Sutton 1982). Some of these fear-control methods turn out to be very important in explaining dysfunctional reactions.

EFFECTS OF FEAR-AROUSING COMMUNICATIONS

Studies of fear-arousing communications ordinarily vary the amount of fear imagery in a persuasive communication and then examine subsequent behavior. For example, if the investigators are attempting to persuade people of the value of dental hygiene, they might compare the behavioral effects of a graphic depiction of severe dental disease to those resulting after exposure to a depiction which is less anxiety provoking. This type of research is relevant to AIDS prevention in two ways: first, it can tell us what will happen if we frighten the targets of prevention programs, and second, it may tell us something about how people react to fear of AIDS, in general.

Many studies find that the greater the fear generated in a person or group, the more self-protective behavior results (Leventhal 1970; Sutton 1982). This finding is consistent with the model of fear as a drive, which predicts that self-protective behavior is a means of reducing fear. However, other findings cannot be explained by the drive model. For instance, regardless of the level of fear generated by communications, people show greater acceptance of the recommended behavior if they perceive it as effective (Sutton 1982). This finding does not fit the drive model of fear, but does fit the decision-making theories. Also, protective behavior and persuasion are greater when people get specific, concrete instructions on how to protect themselves (Leventhal et al. 1980; Sutton 1982). However, people may continue to report fear in spite of these specific instructions—even though the drive model states that fear should dissipate (Sutton 1982). Perceived or actual susceptibility to a feared event should increase self-protective behavior according to several theories. However, increased susceptibility does not consistently interact with high fear to increase such behavior.

NEGATIVE SIDE EFFECTS OF FEAR

Leventhal, Meyer, and Gutmann (1980) list several reasons why fear arousal should be used with caution in dealing with any risk communication. First, they note that high-fear messages are not always superior to low-fear messages in motivating behavior change. This suggests that we need to have a better understanding of the ways in which health problems are represented in people's imagery. For example, in some studies the proposed solutions to health related problems (X rays, surgery, innoculation) may themselves generate substantial fear. In the same way, it is clear that HIV antibody testing is feared by many individuals at increased risk for HIV infection, since the consequences of testing positive for HIV antibody involve not only the high likelihood of developing AIDS but also may include discrimination and stigmatization. These latter problems would be eased by antidiscrimination legislation, but would not disappear altogether.

A second problem noted by Leventhal and his colleagues (1980) is that fear can cause anger in people and lead them to disregard health messages if they think the messages are manipulative. Shilts (1987) describes such reactions to early AIDS warnings in that gays often ascribed political motivations to risk communication. Also, the authority figures providing AIDS-prevention messages may be linked with authority figures who in the past have stigmatized or otherwise penalized behaviors associated with increased risk. For example, will the IV drug user differentiate between the public health worker and the police? That, of course, is one reason why outreach workers are most effective if they are from the same neighborhoods and same backgrounds as the intravenous drug users.

A third dysfunctional reaction described by Leventhal and his colleagues (1980) is that people may become fatalistic or resigned to health dangers because they feel helpless to protect themselves. A fourth dysfunctional reaction, which Leventhal and his colleagues believe to be rare, involves denial of the danger posed in the fear communication. Since these four reactions are especially dysfunctional for prevention, they deserve more attention here.

Viewing fear as a repertoire of responses casts some light on the potentially negative consequences of fear-arousing communications. If people are predisposed to respond in a particular way when in a fearful state, and if no concrete guidance is given, a fear-arousing message should only reconfirm and strengthen existing attitudes and behaviors. Fear-arousing messages would therefore have the potential to result in no behavioral change or, worse, negative side effects. Conceptualizing fear as a set of responses posits that social learning and norms of behavior determine the ways in which people express fear. Averill (1987) notes that if we understood clearly the social rules for expressing fear, we could design better prevention strategies. The explanation of long-term fears as core processes also helps us to understand helplessness and denial reactions.

EXPLAINING HELPLESSNESS

People who perceive that they have little control over their lives are more likely to react in a helpless manner. This may be due to low self-esteem (Leventhal et al. 1966); a perception that health matters are beyond one's control (Wallston and Wallston 1978); or "learned helplessness," an expectation that self-protective efforts will not be successful (Abramson et al. 1978). These last two explanations have been elaborated as theories that relate to health in their own right.

of one's freedoms are threatened, and when there are implications for future threats to freedom, as well. Effects of reactance include the direct reassertion of freedom through behavior; a greater liking for the threatened behaviors; aggression toward the source of the threat; and indirect reassertions of freedom if actual reassertion has become impossible.

The application of this theory to AIDS prevention is straightforward. For example, gays have been struggling for several important freedoms, including the freedom to express their affectional preferences, for decades. Not all gay men define sexual freedom as sex with many people. However, expression of sexual freedom in this sense became an integral part of gay identity and socialization, and was central to discussions of civil rights in the 1970s (Shilts 1987). Now, health professionals are telling gays to limit their sexual behavior, not exchange bodily fluids, and use condoms. The threat to freedom is very great, since a fatal disease could result. The implications for the future are also very great, since no cure is in sight. Therefore, some gay men are bound to experience reactance. Reactance can take the form either of rejecting health messages or of accepting them but continuing to engage in unsafe sex. An important component of AIDS prevention in the gay community has therefore been a redefinition of gay identity that includes safer sex. This constitutes a reassertion of the centrally important freedoms involved, although unsafe sex per se is eliminated.

Reactance can even result from one's own decisions among alternatives. Thus, individual gay men can experience reactance even after thay have generally committed themselves to safer sex. The individual makes such a choice at each encounter, so that reactance is a possible response at any time.

Group Process

Theories of social influence and of reactance set the stage for a discussion of group process. Group decision making is frequently used to facilitate behavior change, whether for ideological reasons, financial considerations, or beliefs about the efficacy of group presentations as opposed to individual ones. The AIDS-prevention specialist is likely to employ group process in some fashion in the course of his or her attempts to encourage less riskful behavior. Therefore, a detailed discussion of group decision making and attitude change is in order.

AIDS-prevention programs may utilize group process in several ways. Group process is essential to planning, both for decision making and marketing. The prevention specialist may be an outsider to the target group and may lack important insights into the barriers and facilitators influencing self-protective behavior. For gaining support and advice from influential community members, there may be no superior technique to the nominal group method (Rossi and Freeman 1985). Focus groups are a marketing tool that can provide these insights (National Cancer Institute 1979). Group process can enhance community involvement efforts and empower people to carry out their own preventive activities. Finally, there are many reasons to believe that groups at increased risk of HIV infection will not generally respond to an outside prevention expert or to any authority figure who has not established credentials as someone who is useful to them. Democratic group process may help such experts establish their credibility.

Much attention has been devoted to group decision making by leaders who employ a democratic style. Called democratic social engineering by some (Graebner 1986), this form of social influence was introduced during the early years of the century as an alternative both to laissez-faire and authoritarian styles of leadership. Key to the concept is its focus on the group as "coparticipants in a problem-solving process, in which . . . the member will be open to influence from the leader to the degree he perceives the leader is open to influence from him" (Lippit 1985).

A notable study of the democratic style of group decision making was conducted during World War II by Kurt Lewin, whose interest led to the foundation of the National Training Laboratory and to the study and technology of group dynamics. Lewin set up an experiment to compare the effectiveness of authoritarian and democratic styles of leadership. The goal of his study was to persuade housewives to serve organ meats (heart, kidney, liver) to their families in support of rationing in the war effort. Some groups heard a lecture by an expert on the subject. Others took part in group discussions in which women expressed their own opinions about the need to change food habits, took over responsibility for doing something about the problem, and expressed the reasons they and their families had rejected organ meats. The expert was not introduced until late in the group discussion. The group discussions proved superior to the expert lecture in influencing housewives' decisions to use these meats (Marrow 1969).

Subsequent studies of leadership style yielded mixed results—

where she encounters publicity for an outreach program targeted to persons at increased risk of HIV infection (exposure to a channel of communication). She decides that this information may apply to her, so she attends to it. She is attracted by the outreach worker's presentation, which does not make judgements about her choice of partner. She understands that she is in danger of becoming infected with HIV because the presentation is simple and to the point. She starts thinking about related matters, such as her partner's use of drugs, how she would like him to take care of his health, and how bad it would be to have an infected child. She decides to learn more about how to avoid infection by persuading her partner to use condoms and not to share needles, trying to get her partner into treatment and, if necessary, leaving her partner. She is not sure whether she agrees with all of the outreach worker's information, but she does remember it. That night, as her partner is about to visit a "shooting gallery," she tries to remember what the outreach worker told her about the danger of sharing needles. She decides to mention this to her partner and does so. He rejects this information. She assesses her situation and wonders what to do next. Is her relationship with him worth the risk of infection?

In the example above, notice that the chain of outputs could fail at any stage and that later outputs would not be affected by the prevention communication. This is of central importance because for any given populations we expect that effects will be attenuated at each stage of the process—that is, a smaller and smaller percentage of people will move successfully to the next stage. Understanding this problem will help to overcome the "great expectations" that people hold for communications. For example, at family planning clinics, AIDS information is competing with information on birth control, and the woman might not attend to the outreach worker's AIDS presentation. If she did not attend, then she would not remember it and would not act on the basis of it. Alternatively, she might attend to the information, remember it, and decide to pass the information along to her partner, but postpone the discussion for fear of an argument, or fail to provide him with a clear communication herself.

On the positive side, however, one seldom hears a general health message only once. Repeated exposure to AIDS-prevention messages may have a cumulative effect on behavior change, as they appear to do for other health behaviors (Schachter 1982). Although people may not attend to an AIDS-prevention communication on one occasion, they may attend to it in the future. In our previous illustration, for example, a sustained outreach effort at a family planning clinic could, in fact, contact a person more than once. Our hypothetical client may not act immediately, but the accumulation of AIDS-prevention information may eventually lead her to self-protective action.

A final implication of this sequence of outputs is that one must consider cost-effectiveness in terms of the final output, that is, self-protective action. From the sequence just described, we can identify those points in the process where an increase in the power of communication or other aspects of intervention would translate into a cost-effective increase in self-protective action. For example, the outreach worker may prove more effective in terms of net risk reduction if he or she concentrates attention on communicating *how* to protect oneself—as several theories would predict (Leventhal et al. 1980). This might result in each worker reaching fewer targets, but would prove to be more cost-effective for the ultimate objective of net risk reduction (Leviton, forthcoming; Weinstein and Stason 1976).

McGuire (1985) lists additional findings on communication and persuasion that may be relevant to AIDS prevention. *Sources* will increase in efficacy the more credible, attractive, and powerful they are (1985:264). However, output responses will differ along with these three characteristics: increasing source credibility results in informative influence; increasing source attractiveness results in normative influence; and increasing the power of the source results in compliance (Kelman 1958).

Messages will be differentially effective depending on the positive or negative nature of the arguments or appeals. Threats will produce more compliance, but positive appeals are recalled better and behavior change is more likely in the longer term (McGuire 1985: 269). If health threats are involved, a negative approach tends to prompt coping with fear or stress, as described earlier, while a positive approach tends to prompt coping with the danger (Leventhal and Nerenz 1983). Message clarity, use of metaphors, drawing explicit conclusions, sticking to one's strongest arguments, dealing with the opposing arguments, and doing so early in a persuasive attempt, all enhance persuasiveness (McGuire 1985:269–273). Results of studies on some presentation and content issues are mixed, since some psychological processes are competing against others. Persuasion increases with the first few repetitions of an argument, but attention and interest decline with further repetition (1985:274), and overloading the audience with information impedes persuasion. Presenting information at or below the reading level of the target

FIGURE 2. Hypothetical Process of Risk Reduction for At-Risk Individuals

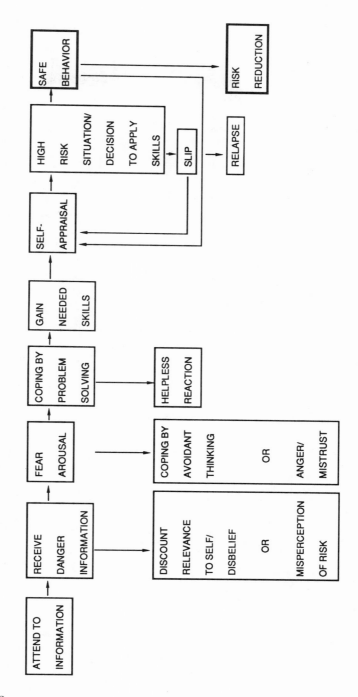

79

TABLE 1. Facilitators, Barriers, and Risk-Reduction Strategies

Theory	Facilitators	Barriers	Strategies
Cognitive theories	High expectation of outcome Protection Motivation	Low expectation of outcome	Change expected outcomes: (a) riskful behavior causes infection (b) reducing riskful behavior lowers chances of infection
	Perceived vulnerability	Poor understanding of probabilities Low perception of personal danger	Clear risk communications Personalized risk information
	Realistic mental representation	Unrealistic mental representation	Create effective, realistic image of disease
Fear arousal	Motivates protective action	Fear of recommended actions (for example, testing) Helplessness Denial or avoidant	Information on how to avoid feared consequences Effective means of self-protection Focus attention on solutions Avoid perceived manipulation

		thinking Anger External loss of control Fatalism about health	Intensive counseling and personal contact Counteract myths
Social influence and communication	Minimal loss of freedoms Influence by attractive group members Influence by informed leaders Rationale to change Cue to action	Larger loss of freedoms	Reinterpret freedoms Utilize indigenous outreach workers Utilize democratic group processes Health providers' advice Repeated media messages
Learning theories	Stimulus control	Proximity to desired riskful behavior	Behavior modification (where needed)
	High perceived self-efficacy Success experiences	Low perceived self-efficacy Failure experiences Relapse	Increase self-efficacy: Skills training Positive role models and their success Persuasive communications Attribute success to ability and failure to poor effort and situation

AIDS risk-reduction programs will be more effective if planning includes involvement by relevant members of the at-risk population (Figure 1). Focus groups provide information on culturally appropriate materials; community involvement gains credibility, ensures availability of positive role models for self-protection, and lowers mistrust and potential anger over the risk communication. The availability of the program is announced through several channels: mass media, word of mouth, and outreach worker activity. At this point, some individuals who have engaged in high-risk behaviors in the past may decide that the danger of infection warrants a change —especially if media and word of mouth sources have provided these individuals with specific recommendations on what behaviors to avoid or modify. The risk-taking behavior of these individuals is probably characterized best as a series of "gambles," and new information helps them maximize utilities. The prevention program can now focus attention on more intensive efforts for those at-risk individuals whose behavior is more resistant to change.

The outreach worker who is an indigenous community member provides a positive role model and credible information source. Such a person may be more effective than other health workers in persuading at-risk individuals to participate in intensive counseling interventions. (Only a portion of the target group will participate, however; the reasons relate to psychological barriers described below.) Individual or group counseling allows health workers to gain social influence and impart information in a persuasive, clear manner. Habitual behaviors can be addressed in counseling, as well as ways to modify them successfully. Counseling may also prepare people who have engaged in riskful behavior for HIV antibody testing, if this is to be a part of the intervention. Feedback on test results would be accompanied by counseling to explain the significance of results and to outline steps that infected people can take to avoid infecting others and to preserve their own health insofar as is possible. Counseling and testing may lead to some reduction of riskful behavior by the participants. The impact of the prevention program itself may decline over time to an unknown extent, although for gay men, trends toward decreased riskful behavior have been dramatic, overall. To guard against decay of program effects, participants may receive further program support in their decision to reduce risk, and program intervention may accumulate over time. Notice that at each stage there is attenuation of effects, as was described earlier with regard to communications theory.

Figure 2 outlines the process of HIV risk reduction for an at-risk individual. Table 1 presents a set of hypothesized barriers and facilitators for AIDS risk reduction in this process. From this listing, strategies for intervention can be derived. The early stages are an abbreviated communications model, in which attention to a risk communication may result in perception of danger, or in misperception of risk information, discounted relevance to self, or failure to believe the source of the information. If the individual does perceive danger, fear arousal may result, especially in people who feel especially vulnerable. Coping with fear arousal will occur first, and may result in avoidant thinking. Anger may also result if the source is perceived as manipulative or untrustworthy. If the individual moves on to problem solving as a coping strategy, his or her initial appraisal of self-protection ability may be low—or a belief in universal helplessness may be preexisting. Helpless reactions may result, with possible impaired learning of new skills. Individuals who can apply problem solving to the learning of new skills will appraise their ability to apply those skills. Facing a high-risk situation, the individual will weigh the costs and benefits of safer behavior, or of riskful behavior (which has it own attractions). The individual will make a decision on how to act. If a "slip" results, the individual may reappraise his or her ability as lowered and eventually relapse into habitual unsafe behavior. If safer behavior results, the individual will be strengthened in a high appraisal of capability and eventually may reduce or eliminate unsafe behavior on a permanent basis.

This chapter has synthesized theories of health behavior and behavior change with current information about behaviors that put people at risk for HIV infection. Its goal has been to develop a framework for analysis and intervention that practitioners can use in developing AIDS-prevention programs. The synthesis has focused on the character of behaviors riskful for infection, the causes of those behaviors, and effective interventions. We have yet to gain a complete understanding of these behaviors. However, the framework presented here can be applied in conjunction with social marketing strategies to design theoretically sound interventions that incorporate existing knowledge about human behavioral change.

REFERENCES

Abelson, R.P., and Levi, A. 1985. "Decision Making and Decision Theory." In G. Lindzey and E. Aronson (Eds.), *Handbook of Social Psychology.* 3rd Edition. New York: Random House.

84   Theoretical Foundations of AIDS Prevention

Abramson, L., Seligman, M., and Teasdale, J. 1978. "Learned Helplessness in Humans: Critique and Reformulation." *Journal of Abnormal Psychology* 87:49–74.

Ajzen, I., and Fishbein, M. 1980. *Understanding Attitudes and Predicting Social Behavior.* Englewood Cliffs, N.J.: Prentice-Hall.

Averill, J.R. 1987. "The Role of Emotion and Psychological Defense in Self-Protective Behavior." In N.D. Weinstein (Ed.), *Taking Care: Understanding and Encouraging Self-Protective Behavior.* Cambridge: Cambridge University Press.

Bandura, A. 1977a. "Self-Efficacy: Toward a Unifying Theory of Behavioral Change." *Psychological Review* 84:191–215.

Bandura, A. 1977b. *Social Learning Theory.* Englewood Cliffs, N.J.: Prentice-Hall.

Bandura, A. 1986. "Self-Efficacy Mechanism in Human Agency." *American Psychologist* 40:359–373.

Bandura, A., Reese, L., and Adams, N.E. 1982. "Microanalysis of Action and Fear Arousal as a Function of Differential Levels of Perceived Self-Efficacy." *Journal of Personality and Social Psychology* 43:5–21.

Bartlett, E.E. 1981. "The Contribution of School Health Education to Community Health Promotion: What Can We Realistically Expect?" *American Journal of Public Health* 71:1384–1391.

Baumeister, R.F., and Scher, S.J. 1988. "Self-Defeating Behavior Patterns Among Normal Individuals: Review and Analysis of Common Self-Destructive Tendencies." *Psychological Bulletin* 104:3–22.

Becker, M.H. (Ed.). 1974. "The Health Belief Model and Personal Health Behavior." *Health Education Monographs,* 2(4).

Brehm, J.W. 1966. *A Theory of Psychological Reactance.* New York: Academic Press.

Brownell, K.D. 1982. "Obesity: Understanding and Treating a Serious, Prevalent, and Refractory Disorder." *Journal of Consulting and Clinical Psychology,* 50:820–840.

Brownell, K.D., Marlatt, G.A., Lichtenstein, E., and Wilson, G.T. 1986. "Understanding and Preventing Relapse." *American Psychologist* 41:765–782.

Calnan, M.W., and Moss, S. 1984. "The Health Belief Model and Compliance with Education Given at a Class in Breast Self-Examination." *Journal of Health and Social Behavior* 25:198–210.

Chesney, M. 1984. "Behavior Modification and Health Enhancement." In J.D. Matarazzo, S.M. Weiss, J.A. Herd, N.E. Miller, and S.M. Weiss (Eds.), *Behavioral Health: A Handbook of Health Enhancement and Disease Prevention.* New York: Wiley.

Cook. T.D., Gruder, C.L., Hennigan, K.M., and Flay, B.R. 1979. "History of the Sleeper Effect: Some Logical Pitfalls in Accepting the Null Hypothesis." *Psychological Bulletin* 86:662–679.

Denniston, R.W. 1986. "Cancer Knowledge, Attitudes and Practices Among

Black Americans." In C. Mettlin and G.P. Murphy (Eds.), *Cancer Among Black Populations.* New York: Alan R. Liss.

Deutsch, M., and Gerard, H.B. 1955. "A Study of Normative and Informational Social Influence Upon Individual Judgment." *Journal of Abnormal and Social Psychology* 51:629–636.

DiClemente, C.C. 1986. "Self-Efficacy and the Addictive Behaviors." *Journal of Social and Clinical Psychology* 4:302–315.

DiClemente, C.C., and Prochaska, J.O. 1985. "Processes and Stages of Self-Change: Coping and Competence in Smoking Behavior Change." In S. Shiffman and T.A. Wills (Eds.), *Coping and Substance Abuse.* San Diego, Calif.: Academic Press.

DiClemente, C.C., Prochaska, J.O., and Gibertini, M. 1985. "Self-Efficacy and the Stages of Self-Change of Smoking." *Cognitive Therapy and Research* 9:181–200.

Eagly, A.H., and Carli, L.L. 1981. "Sex of Researchers and Sex-Typed Communications as Determinants of Sex Differences in Influenceability: A Meta-Analysis of Social Influence Studies." *Psychological Bulletin* 90:1–20.

Edwards, W. 1977. "Use of Multi-attribute Utility Measurement for Social Decision Making." In D.E. Bell, R.L. Keeney, and H. Raiffa (Eds.), *Conflicting Objectives in Decisions.* New York: Wiley.

Ferster, C.B., and Skinner, B.F. 1957. *Schedules of Reinforcement.* New York: Appleton-Century-Crofts.

Festinger, L. 1950. "Informal Social Communication." *Psychological Review* 57:217–282.

Fiedler, F.E. 1964. "A Contingency Model of Leadership Effectiveness." In L. Berkowtiz (Ed.), *Advances in Experimental Social Psychology.* New York: Academic Press.

Fischhoff, B. 1988a. "Decision Making on AIDS." Invited paper presented at the Vermont Conference on Primary Prevention, Burlington, Vt., Sept.

Fischhoff, B. In press. "Psychology and Public Policy: Tool or Tool Maker?" *American Psychologist.*

Fischhoff, B., and Svenson, O. 1988. "Perceived Risks of Radionuclides: Understanding Public Understanding." In M.W. Carter (Ed.), *Radionuclides in the Food Chain.* New York: Springer Verlag.

Fishbein, M., and Ajzen, I. 1975. *Belief, Attitude, Intention, and Behavior.* Reading, Mass.: Addison-Wesley.

Flay, B.R. 1985. "Psychosocial Approaches to Smoking Prevention: A Review of Findings." *Health Psychology* 4:449–488.

Folkman, S., and Lazarus, R.S. 1980. "An Analysis of Coping in a Middle-Aged Community Sample." *Journal of Health and Social Behavior* 21:219–239.

Fox, R., Odaka, N.J., Brookmeyer, R., and Polk, B.F. 1987. "Effect of HIV Antibody Disclosure on Subsequent Sexual Activity in Homosexual Men." *AIDS* 1:241–246.

Ginzburg, H., French, J., Jackson, J., Hartsock, P.I., MacDonald, M., and Weiss, S. 1986. "Health Education and Knowledge Assessment of HTLV-III Diseases Among Intravenous Drug Users." *Health Education Quarterly* 13:373–382.

Gostin, L., and Curran, W.J. 1987. "AIDS Screening, Confidentiality, and the Duty to Warn." *American Journal of Public Health* 77:361–365.

Graebner, W. 1986. "The Small Group and Democratic Social Engineering, 1900–1950." *Journal of Social Issues* 42:137–154.

Green, L.W., Kreuter, M.W., Deeds, S.G., and Partridge, K.B. 1980. *Health Education Planning: A Diagnostic Approach.* Palo Alto, Calif.: Mayfield.

Heider, F. 1958. *The Psychology of Interpersonal Relations.* New York: Wiley.

Hovland, C.I., Janis, I.L., and Kelley, H.H. 1953. *Communication and Persuasion.* New Haven, Conn.: Yale University Press.

Janis, I.L. 1967. "Effects of Fear Arousal on Attitude Change: Recent Developments in Theory and Experimental Research." In L. Berkowitz (Ed.), *Advances in Experimental Social Psychology.* Volume 3. New York: Academic Press.

Jimenez, R. 1987. "AIDS: Primary and Secondary Prevention Strategies Targetting Hispanics." Houston: AIDS Foundation Houston.

Jones, E.E., Kanouse, D.E., Kelley, H.H., Nisbett, R.E., Valins, S., and Weiner, B. 1972. *Attribution: Perceiving the Causes of Behavior.* Morristown, N.J.: General Learning Press.

Joseph, J.G., Montgomery, S.B., Emmons, C.A., Kessler, R.C., and Ostrow, D.G. 1987. "Magnitude and Determinants of Behavioral Risk Reduction: Longitudinal Analysis of a Cohort at Risk for AIDS." *Psychology and Health* 1:73–96.

Kahneman, D., and Tversky, A. 1973. "On the Psychology of Prediction." *Psychological Review* 80:237–251.

Kahneman, D., Slovic, P., and Tversky, A. (Eds.) 1982. *Judgment Under Uncertainty: Heuristics and Biases.* Cambridge: Cambridge University Press.

Kelman, H.C. 1958. "Compliance, Identification, and Internalization." *Journal of Conflict Resolution* 2:51–60.

Kiesler, C.A., Collins, B.E., and Miller, N. 1969. *Attitude Change: A Critical Analysis of Theoretical Approaches.* New York: Wiley.

Kiesler, C.A., and Kiesler, S.B. 1969. *Conformity.* Reading, Mass.: Addison-Wesley.

Kotler, P. 1979. *Marketing for Non-Profit Organizations.* Englewood Cliffs, N.J.: Prentice-Hall.

Lefcourt, H.M. 1976. *Locus of Control: Current Trends in Theory and Research.* Hillsdale, N.J.: Lawrence Erlbaum Associates.

Leventhal, H., Jones, S., and Trembly, G. 1966. "Sex Differences in Attitude and Behavior Change Under Conditions of Fear and Specific Instructions." *Journal of Experimental Social Psychology* 2:387–399.

Leventhal, H., and Watts, J. 1966. "Sources of Resistance to Fear-Arousing Communications on Smoking and Lung Cancer." *Journal of Personality* 34:155–175.

Leventhal, H. 1970. "Findings and Theory in the Study of Fear Communications." In L. Berkowitz (Ed.), *Advances in Experimental Social Psychology*. Volume 5. New York: Academic Press.

Leventhal, H., and Everhart, D. 1980. "Emotion, Pain, and Physical Illness." In C.E. Izard (Ed.), *Emotions and Psychopathology*. New York: Plenum.

Leventhal, H., Meyer, D., and Gutmann, M. 1980. "The Role of Theory in the Study of Compliance to High Blood Pressure Regimens." In R.B. Haynes, M.E. Mattson, and O.E. Tillmer (Eds.), *Patient Compliance to Prescribed Antihypertensive Medication Regimens: A Report to the National Heart, Lung, and Blood Institute*. Washington, D.C.: U.S. Department of Health and Human Services.

Leventhal, H., and Nerenz, D. 1983. "Representations of Threat and the Control of Stress." In D. Meichenbaum and M. Jaremko (Eds.), *Stress Reduction and Prevention: A Cognitive Behavioral Approach*. New York: Plenum.

Leviton, L.C. Forthcoming. "Can Organizations Benefit from Worksite Health Promotion?" *Health Services Research*.

Leviton, L.C., Valdiserri, R.O., Lyter, D.W., Callahan, C.M., Kingsley, L.A., and Rinaldo, C.R. Forthcoming. "AIDS Prevention in Gay and Bisexual Men: Evaluation of Attitude Change from Two Risk Reduction Interventions."

Lippit, R. 1985. "The Small Group and Participatory Democracy: Comment on Graebner." *Journal of Social Issues* 42:155–156.

Logan, F.A. 1965. "Decision Making by Rats: Delay Versus Amount of Reward." *Journal of Comparative and Physiological Psychology* 59:1–12.

Lyter, D.W., Valdiserri, R.O., Kingsley, L.A., Amoroso, W.P., and Rinaldo, C.R. 1987. "The HIV Antibody Test: Why Gay and Bisexual Men Want or Do Not Want to Know Their Results." *Public Health Reports* 102(5):468–474.

McCaul, K.D., and Glasgow, R.E. 1985. "Preventing Adolescent Smoking: What Have We Learned About Treatment Construct Validity?" *Health Psychology* 4:361–387.

McGuire, W.J. 1968. "Personality and Attitude Change: An Information-Processing Theory." In A.G. Greenwald, T.C. Brock, and T.M. Ostrom (Eds.), *Psychological Foundations of Attitudes*. New York: Academic Press.

McGuire, W.J. 1985. "Attitudes and Attitude Change." In G. Lindzey and E.

Aronson (Eds.), *Handbook of Social Psychology*. 3rd Edition. New York: Random House.

Maddux, J.E., and Stanley, M.A. 1986. "Self-Efficacy Theory in Contemporary Psychology: An Overview." *Journal of Social and Clinical Psychology* 4:249–255.

Marlatt, G.A., and Gordon, J.R. 1980. "Determinants of Relapse: Implications for the Maintenance of Behavior Change." In P.O. Davidson and S.M. Davidson (Eds.), *Behavioral Medicine: Changing Health Lifestyles.* New York: Brunner/Mazel.

Marrow, A.J. 1969. *The Practical Theorist: The Life and Work of Kurt Lewin.* New York: Basic Books.

Martin, J.L. 1987. "The Impact of AIDS on Gay Male Sexual Behavior Patterns in New York City." *American Journal of Public Health* 77:578–581.

Massey, V. 1986. "Perceived Susceptibility to Breast Cancer and Practice of Breast Self-Examination." *Nursing Research* 35:183–185.

Matarazzo, J.D., Weiss, S.M., Herd, J.A., Miller, N.E., and Weiss, S.M. (Eds.). 1984. *Behavioral Health: A Handbook of Health Enhancement and Disease Prevention.* New York: Wiley.

Mischel, W., and Ebbesen, E.B. 1970. "Attention in Delay of Gratification." *Journal of Personality and Social Psychology* 16:329–337.

Mondanaro, J. 1987. "Strategies for AIDS Prevention: Motivating Health Behavior in Drug Dependent Women." *Journal of Psychoactive Drugs* 19:143–149.

Moscovici, S. 1985. "Social Influence and Conformity." In G. Lindsey and E. Aronson (Eds.), *The Handbook of Social Psychology.* 3rd Edition. New York: Random House.

National Cancer Institute. 1979. *Pretesting in Health Communications.* Washington, D.C.: U.S. Department of Health and Human Services.

Nelkin, D. 1987. "AIDS and the Social Sciences: Review of Useful Knowledge and Research Needs." *Reviews of Infectious Diseases* 9(5):980–986.

Nisbett, R., and Ross, L. 1980. *Human Inference: Strategies and Shortcomings of Social Judgement.* Englewood Cliffs, N.J.: Prentice-Hall.

Norman, M.G., and Tudiver, F. 1986. "Predictors of Breast Self-Examination Among Family Practice Patients." *Journal of Family Practice* 22:149–153.

Pechacek, T.F. 1979. "Modification of Smoking Behavior." In N. Krasnegor (Ed.), *The Behavioral Aspects of Smoking.* National Institute on Drug Abuse Research Monograph 26. Rockville, M.D.: U.S. Department of Health, Education and Welfare.

Pechacek, T.F., and Danaher, B.G. 1979. "How and Why People Quit Smoking." In P.C. Kendall and S.D. Hollon (Eds.), *Cognitive-Behavioral Interventions: Theory, Research and Procedures.* New York: Academic Press.

Prochansky, H.M. 1981. "Uses and Abuses of Theory in Applied Research." In L. Bickman (Ed.), *Applied Social Psychology Annual.* Volume 2. Beverly Hills, Calif.: Sage.

Rachlin, H., and Green, L. 1972. "Commitment, Choice, and Self-Control." *Journal of the Experimental Analysis of Behavior* 17:15–22.

Research and Decisions Corporation. 1984. *Designing an Effective AIDS Prevention Campaign Strategy for San Francisco: Results from the First Probability Sample of an Urban Gay Male Community.* San Francisco, Calif.: Research and Decisions Corporation.

Rogers, E.M., and Shoemaker, F.F. 1971. *Communication of Innovations: A Cross-Cultural Approach.* 2nd Edition. New York: Free Press.

Rogers, R.W. 1975. "A Protection Motivation Theory of Fear Appeals and Attitude Change." *The Journal of Psychology* 91:93–114.

Rogers, R.W., and Mewborn, C.R. 1976. "Fear Appeals and Attitude Change: Effects of a Threat's Noxiousness, Probability of Occurrence, and the Efficacy of Coping Responses." *Journal of Personality and Social Psychology* 34:562–566.

Rosenstock, I.M. 1974. "The Health Belief Model and Preventive Health Behavior." *Health Education Monographs* 2:354–386.

Rosenstock, I.M., and Kirscht, J.P. 1979. "Why People Seek Health Care." In G.C. Stone, F. Cohen, and N.E. Adler (Eds.), *Health Psychology.* San Francisco: Jossey-Bass.

Ross, M., and Fletcher, G.J.O. 1985. "Attribution and Social Perception." In G. Lindzey and E. Aronson (Eds.), *Handbook of Social Psychology.* 3rd Edition. New York: Random House.

Rossi, P.H., and Freeman, H.E. 1985. *Evaluation: A Systematic Approach.* Beverly Hills, Calif.: Sage.

Rothman, J. 1979. "Three Models of Community Organization Practice, Their Mixing and Phasing." In F.M. Cox, J.L. Erlich, J. Rothman, and J.E. Tropman (Eds.), *Strategies of Community Organization.* Itasca, Ill.: Peacock.

Rotter, J.B. 1966. "Generalized Expectancies for Internal Versus External Control of Reinforcement. Psychological Monographs, 80(609).

Schachter, S. 1951. "Deviation, Rejection and Communication." *Journal of Abnormal and Social Psychology* 46:190–207.

Schachter, S. 1982. "Recidivism and Self-Cure of Smoking and Obesity." *American Psychologist* 37:436–444.

Schunk, D.H., and Carbonari, J.P. 1984. "Self-Efficacy Models." In J.D. Matarazzo, S.M. Weiss, J.A. Herd, N.E. Miller, and S.M. Weiss (Eds.), *Behavioral Health: A Handbook of Health Enhancement and Disease Prevention.* New York: Wiley.

Shilts, R. 1987. *And the Band Played On: Politics, People and the AIDS Epidemic.* New York: St. Martin's Press.

Silver, R., and Wortman, C. 1980. "Coping with Undesirable Life Events." In J. Garber and M.E.P. Seligman (Eds.), *Human Helplessness.* New York: Academic Press.

Skinner, B.F. 1969. *Contingencies of Reinforcement: A Theoretical Analysis.* New York: Appleton-Century-Crofts.

Slovic, P., Fischhoff, B., and Lichtenstein, S. 1987. "Behavioral Decision Theory Perspectives on Protective Behavior." In N.D. Weinstein (Ed.), *Taking Care: Understanding and Encouraging Self-Protective Behavior.* Cambridge: Cambridge University Press.

Slovic, P., Fischhoff, B., and Lichtenstein, S. 1981. "Informing the Public About the Risks of Ionizing Radiation." *Health Physics* 41:589–598.

Solomon, D.S., and Maccoby, N. 1984. "Communication as a Model for Health Enhancement." In J.D. Matarazzo, S.M. Weiss, J.A. Herd, et al. (Eds.), *Behavioral Health: A Handbook of Health Enhancement and Disease Prevention.* New York: Wiley.

Staver, S. 1987. "Minority Women Grappling with Growing AIDS Problem." *American Medical News* November 6, 59–63.

Suls, J., and Fletcher, B. 1985. "The Relative Efficacy of Avoidant and Non-avoidant Coping Strategies: A Meta-Analysis." *Health Psychology* 4:249–288.

Surgeon General of the United States. 1987. *Surgeon General's Report on Acquired Immune Deficiency Syndrome.* Washington, D.C.: U.S. Department of Health and Human Services.

Sutton, S.R. 1982. "Fear-Arousing Communications: A Critical Examination of Theory and Research." In J.R. Eiser (Ed.), *Social Psychology and Behavioral Medicine.* New York: Wiley.

Valdiserri, R.O., Lyter, D.W., Leviton, L.C., Callahan, C.M., Kingsley, L.A., and Rinaldo, C.R. 1989. "AIDS Prevention in Homosexual and Bisexual Men: Results of a Randomized Trial Evaluating Two Risk Reduction Interventions." *AIDS* 3 (1):21–26.

Wallston, B.S., and Wallston, K.A. 1978. "Locus of Control and Health: A Review of the Literature." *Health Education Monographs* 6:107–117.

Wallston, K.A., and Wallston, B.S. 1982. "Who Is Responsible for Your Health? The Construct of Health Locus of Control." In G.S. Sanders and J. Suls (Eds.), *Social Psychology of Health and Illness.* Hillsdale, N.J.: Lawrence Erlbaum Associates.

Warner, K. 1983. "Bags, Buckles and Belts: The Debate over Mandatory Passive Restraints in Automobiles." *Journal of Health Politics, Policy and Law* 8:44–75.

Weiner, B., Heckhausen, H., Meyer, U., and Cook, R.C. 1972. "Causal Ascriptions of Achievement Behavior: A Conceptual Analysis of Effort." *Journal of Personality and Social Psychology* 21:239–248.

Weinstein, M.C., and Stason, W.B. 1976. *Hypertension: A Policy Perspective.* Cambridge, Mass.: Harvard University Press.

Wicklund, R.A. 1974. *Freedom and Reactance.* Potomac, Md.: Lawrence Erlbaum Associates.

Winett, R.A. 1986. *Information and Behavior: Systems of Influence.* Hillsdale, N.J.: Lawrence Erlbaum Associates.

Zaltman, G. 1983. "Theory in Use Among Change Agents." In E. Seidman (Ed.), *Handbook of Social Intervention.* Beverly Hills, Calif.: Sage.

Chapter 4

Identifying the Targets of AIDS Prevention

Understanding the theoretical bases of health behavior is prerequisite for creating effective AIDS-prevention programs. Especially important is the realization that people's behavior does not depend simply on the presence or absence of accurate information. A common misconception about health-related behaviors is that positive, or healthy, behaviors can be induced merely by informing individuals of the dangers of unhealthy behaviors. Examples of this fallacy are plentiful. Many have been discussed in the previous chapters, and readers can probably think of examples in their own lives. It is essential to recognize the multivariate nature of human behavior and to reiterate that programs for HIV prevention must not limit themselves to modalities that are purely informational. Public education campaigns are an integral component of our response to preventing HIV infection, but they should not represent the totality of our response. At a minimum, they provide our citizenry with basic information about the cause of AIDS, the ways in which HIV is transmitted, and the means by which an individual can prevent infection with the virus. Whether or not they are capable of modifying behavior among persons whose actions place them at risk for HIV infection is somewhat more problematic.

Reviews of our past experience with the success of media campaigns in altering health-related behaviors have concluded that aside from "some notable exceptions," the mass media have a "limited potential for changing behavior" (Manoff 1985b:68). This does not mean that the modality is defective or the concept worthless; Manoff suggests that difficulties in measuring behavioral impact, poor message design, misidentification of target audience, and failure to recognize and neutralize "resistance points" may be common reasons why media campaigns often have less than spectacular results (p. 69).

Consider, for example, media campaigns against cigarette smoking. Analysis of their effects on behavior suggest what kinds of programs are likely to succeed. Ben-Sira studied the ability of a mass media health campaign to promote smoking cessation among Israeli adults and concluded that it had minimal success in motivating smokers to change their behavior but did serve an important primary reinforcing function for heavy smokers who decided to quit but anticipated difficulties in doing so (1982:833). As a secondary consequence, he noted, the campaign was also successful in motivating nonsmokers to persuade smokers to attempt to give up their unhealthy habit (p. 833).

Flay reviewed forty mass media campaigns designed to influence cigarette smoking behavior and found that "mass media health-promotion programs can be more effective than many academics may have thought" (1987:153). He concluded that "intensive television and radio programming of high frequency, extended reach, and long duration can produce behavioral effects" (p. 155). He also observed that media campaigns aligned with community programs to promote smoking cessation were likely to improve the effectiveness of the media programming (p. 156). In his analysis, public service campaigns that failed to produce the desired behavioral effects may have been ineffective because they relied upon announcements of questionable quality that were shown infrequently and at times of the day when the audience size was small.

Public education campaigns might appear simple to carry out. In reality, they are not. Although the potential contribution of the mass media as an effective tool in AIDS education has been widely recognized (Dan 1987; Hastings and Scott 1987; Hogan 1988; Sherr 1987; Watney 1987), it has also been documented that AIDS-education media campaigns can cause considerable anxiety (Hastings and Scott 1987), even among those who are at minimal risk for HIV infection (Anderson et al. 1987; Holman et al. 1987). After the British media campaign "AIDS: Don't Die of Ignorance," conducted in the latter part of 1986 and early 1987, "large numbers of patients with no known risk were so worried that they requested a test" (Anderson et al. 1987:1429). A similar demand was noted by the Health Department of Western Australia after their "Grim Reaper" media campaign in 1987 (Holman et al. 1987; Morlet et al. 1988). If public education campaigns result in increased demand for AIDS prevention, counseling, and testing services by individuals who are at minimal or no risk for infection, the overall cost of these programs will escalate, which means that the cost of identifying those who are truly at risk will increase.

Therefore, we must distinguish between (1) campaigns intended for a general audience, aiming to provide basic information about AIDS and HIV transmission, and (2) campaigns targeted to individuals who are at increased risk of infection, aiming to clarify the behaviors that place people at risk and to help people modify their behaviors so that the risk is minimized. Obviously, the goal of public education campaigns will change dramatically when an effective agent to treat HIV is developed. Then, a primary objective will be to identify all infected individuals and bring them to treatment.

Because the risk of becoming infected with HIV varies on the basis of behavior, geography, and circumstance, and given the emotionally charged nature of the illness, it may not be possible to employ media campaigns to provide information about AIDS without inadvertently causing a certain degree of anxiety. Although it is not possible to prevent the "worried well" from seeking out AIDS-prevention services, targeting the message for a specific audience can minimize untoward or unintended consequences, and will ensure that the intervention or service will reach the individuals for whom it is intended. Financial realities mandate that we distribute prevention resources where they have the greatest likelihood of producing desired results.

If AIDS media campaigns can result in anxiety among individuals who have less than one chance in a hundred of becoming infected, imagine the anxiety they engender in populations where the prevalance of infection might be one in five or greater (Booth 1988). Among groups that have a substantial rate of HIV infection, media-delivered risk-reduction messages about AIDS can serve to reinforce individuals' perceptions of their risk of AIDS and may thus result in excessive levels of fear. More is at stake than the discomfort experienced by a person who is frightened by the message—though that is not an inconsequential variable. Fear can induce "resistance" to acceptance of the AIDS-prevention message. In order to neutralize fear-generated resistance to health-promotion messages, the message needs to offer specific instructions as to how the undesired outcome may be avoided (Leventhal et al. 1983; Job 1988).

There are other potential "resistance points" to media-delivered AIDS-prevention messages, and their identification has been cited as "a major purpose of qualitative research in advance of strategy and message development" (Manoff 1985a:189). Unlike interpersonal communication, mass media communication is not interactive; thus campaigns carried out over the media must anticipate, in advance, potential resistance to their message. The informational content of a message can easily be preempted by strong "conative and emotive factors" (p. 196). To ensure adequate dissemination of the message, presentations should be made using multiple media and should be delivered at different times over a relatively long period (Flay et al. 1980). Furthermore, campaigns must be "sufficiently tailored to take into account the different educational needs and attitudes" of their target audiences as well as regional differences in disease prevalence (Temoshok et al. 1987:59)—especially since age and educational levels can influence beliefs about the transmission of HIV (Heaven 1987).

Conducting preliminary research to identify the target audience is now widely recognized as necessary preparation for developing a media campaign (Flay et al. 1980; Manoff 1985a; Mendelsohn 1973). In reality, any program that has as its goal the prevention of HIV infection, whether it be media delivered or institutionally based, must identify its target population prior to program design and implementation. Identification, in this context, does not merely mean description of persons who are at risk for HIV infection; that is common knowledge at this point in the epidemic. Instead, it is best considered to entail a comprehensive and in-depth understanding of the group members for whom prevention services are intended.

What we learn by studying the special characteristics of a group or subculture at increased risk for HIV infection not only helps us identify its members but also helps us design prevention programs that the group will find relevant, realistic, and acceptable. Just as knowledge by itself may not cause a person to change behavior, merely providing prevention services, especially if they tend to emphasize behavioral proscriptions in the absence of options, does not guarantee that they will be accepted by the target audience. A conscious effort must be made to provide services that members of the target group will perceive as beneficial from their vantage point. Some segments of society find this orientation distasteful because it seems to condone or affirm circumstances or life-styles they disapprove of. Nonetheless, it is essential that prevention programs be based on this standard. This approach is not unique to the AIDS epidemic, and the significance of applying market research principles to health programs has been formally recognized since the 1960s (Kotler and Levy 1969).

Social marketing refers to the "design, implementation, and control of programs seeking to increase the acceptability of a social idea or cause in a target group," and "utilizes concepts from market segmentation, consumer research, concept development, communication facilitation, incentives, and exchange theory to maximize target group response" (Kotler 1984:25). The process of social marketing can be categorized as market research, product development, the use of specific incentives to increase the level of the desired behavior, and facilitation (that is, how to make it easier for people to change their behavior) (Kotler 1984). It has been employed in the recruitment of gay men into AIDS education and research projects (Silvestre et al. 1986), in the promotion of condoms as contraceptives in the developing world (Fox and Kotler 1980:28), and in heart disease prevention programs, among others (p. 29).

Social marketers use their knowledge of a population to promote a particular behavior or service ("the product") that will further their own agenda (for example, improve the health status of a target group, or, in our instance, prevent the transmission of HIV). Central to this activity, however, is the philosophical orientation that the "product" must be acceptable to the target group. Quite simply, this philosophy is based on the importance of addressing "consumer wants, needs, expectations, and satisfactions" in the marketing process (Murphy 1984:89). Stated another way by the American Public Health Association, "a health promotion program should reflect a consideration of the special characteristics, needs, and preferences of its target group members" (Ad Hoc Work Group . . . 1987:90).

In the specific area of AIDS prevention, whether we subscribe to the constructs of social marketing or to the American Public Health Association's criteria for the development of health promotion and education programs, it is apparent that understanding the groups we wish our programs to reach is absolutely essential for successful planning, implementation, and outreach. The remainder of this chapter will therefore be devoted to a discussion of the groups whose members are at increased risk for HIV infection. We will focus on group rather than individual characteristics, with the realization that even within groups, the degree of HIV risk is modulated by individual circumstances.

In this country, and in most areas of Europe, homosexual men account for the majority of diagnosed cases of symptomatic HIV infection. Many of the special considerations in promoting AIDS prevention in this population relate to the fact that homosexuals are a socially stigmatized group. Throughout the history of Western civilization, homosexuals have been the subject of legal discrimination and social disapproval that is strongly based in religious traditions about the unacceptability of their behavior (Karlen 1980; Marmor 1980). Although the media response to AIDS has had the secondary effect of attenuating commonly held taboos about the discussion of gay male sexual behavior, it would be naive to assume that the discrimination, myths, and fears that have long characterized society's reaction to this group have evaporated.

Among the most tenacious and widely held misconceptions is that homosexuality is a life-style of choice and, as such, represents a moral failing (Warren 1980:125). Unlike minority status that is based on physical characteristics or racial identity and that is predetermined at birth, gays are judged "guilty" of consciously selecting a minority sexual orientation that is anathema to society. This myth relates to ongoing confusion about the genesis of homosexuality. As noted by Marmor, "many people still tend to think of homosexuality either as a pattern that is freely chosen by a conscious act of will or as something that is 'caught' from others, either as a result of seduction or by an 'infectious' imitation or 'modeling'" (1980:19). In reality, the basic factors leading to a homosexual orientation are probably established "before the age of six, well before the school years even begin" (Marmor 1980:20). The belief that an individual can choose to be either heterosexual or homosexual is an overly simplistic model for analyzing this complex area of human behavior. It does not coincide with clinical observations of human sexual preference as a continuum from exclusive same-sex preference through bisexuality to exclusive opposite-sex preference. Granted, most sexual behavior, unless it can be categorized as compulsive, does have a prominent voluntary component. However, for the adult homosexual, the primary choice appears to be in the decision to suppress, repress, or integrate into one's adult life a homosexual orientation—not to "become" heterosexual or remain homosexual.

Viewing homosexuality as willful sexual misconduct rather than as a legitimate, albeit minority, sexual orientation, has profound implications for program planners who are attempting to prevent the transmission of HIV within this population. AIDS educators who consider homosexual behavior as an expression of choice may fail to appreciate the psychological significance and self-affirming function that sexual expression holds for their clients. They may find it difficult to understand or accept that for some gay men, the freedom to express their sexual preference transforms sexual behavior into much more than an emotional experience or libidinous release. Failure to recognize and incorporate this perspective into the philosophy of the program can result in prevention programs whose sole message is that sexual behaviors that can lead to infection should be avoided, rather than that clients have options in modifying their behaviors to minimize the possibility of viral transmission. Programs that dictate or flatly proscribe behaviors for their clients, rather than assist them in modifying their behaviors, are likely to have only limited success because they will not be accepted by many of the individuals they need to reach.

Controversy over the advocacy of condoms for anal intercourse exemplifies this debate. One school of thought holds that the prevention message should be that anal intercourse be completely avoided. The opposing view is that the message should stress the danger of this behavior with regard to infection risk, advocate its elimination from "casual" sexual encounters, and promote the use of condoms for every episode of anal intercourse. We suggest that a message limited to advocating avoidance will be less effective than one that recognizes the potential importance of this behavior for certain clients. To make this point in a different way, consider the feasibility of preventing HIV infection among heterosexuals by advocating the complete avoidance of vaginal intercourse. While some clients would follow this advice, others, especially those who perceive their chances of becoming infected to be minimal, would consider it too great a restriction. Therefore, prevention messages for gay men should not place the value system of the educator above the value system of the client; such messages should recognize and affirm the importance of the client's sexual orientation (McKusick et al. 1985). Programs that do not subscribe to these principles will have only limited success in attracting clients because they will be labelled by the target population as "insensitive" to its needs.

During adolescence, most homosexuals are acutely aware of the pervasive societal disapproval of homosexual behavior. While some adolescents may describe themselves as gay or bisexual (Remafedi 1987c:328), many others will suppress or repress their homosexual impulses (Malyon 1981:326). This makes it extremely difficult, if not impossible, to integrate same-sex affectional orientation into the burgeoning adult personality. The internalization of societal homophobia "often causes protracted dysphoria and feelings of self-contempt"; to adjust, the adolescent homosexual commonly compartmentalizes his sexual desires (p. 324), and conceals his sexual identity from family, friends, and classmates. This highly developed skill takes on the sigificance of a survival strategy. As Warren points out in her analysis of homosexuaity and stigma, the positive consequence of this adaptation is a "close-knit and highly significant gay community"; the negative side is a "paranoid style of living in the straight world" and anxiety about disclosure (Warren 1980:128).

The homosexual's fear of societal censure in response to his sexual orientation is likely to intensify as a consequence of epidemic HIV infection. This will make it difficult for prevention programs to reach individuals who are homosexually active but highly "clos-eted" (that is, extremely secretive about their sexuality). The hesi-tancy of some gay men to share information about their sexuality, even when it is necessary for medical evaluation purposes, was dem-onstrated by Ross (1987), in his study of heterosexual and homosex-ual Australian men attending a veneral disease clinic. He concluded that homosexual men "appear to be much more reticent about dis-cussing personal issues with others, including attending medical personnel" (p. 178). Unfortunately, the homosexual patient's re-luctance to share personal information with health care providers is not just the result of "paranoia" but may often reflect his accurate awareness of underlying negative attitudes held by physicians, nurses, and medical students toward homosexuality (Kalman et al. 1987; Kelly et al. 1987).

Understanding the temporal process by which a gay identity is ac-quired is germane to our discussion at this point, for the adolescent homosexual represents an important target for AIDS education. Most retrospective studies of gay men identify the awareness of same-sex attraction occurring at approximately thirteen years of age, while self-designation as gay generally occurs between the ages of nine-teen and twenty-one; disclosure to significant others follows be-tween the ages of twenty-three and twenty-eight (Remafedi 1987b: 223). Dank documented an average of six years between the "time of first sexual feelings toward persons of the same sex and the decision that one was a homosexual" (1971:182).

As was indicated earlier, during adolescence many homosexuals cope with their sexual feelings by compartmentalizing them, leav-ing them unresolved until a future date. This "developmental mor-atorium" implies that adolescent homosexuals will not have the same opportunities for "extensive social involvements and interper-sonal attachments with peers" as do their heterosexual counterparts (Malyon 1981:326). Being unable to interact with other homosexual youth precludes the "extensive experimental behavior" that other adolescents undertake to learn the roles expected of them as adults (p. 326). According to Malyon, "the result of these missing develop-mental experiences is that a complete resolution of the adolescent identity crisis is precluded" (p. 326). In fact, the high level of sexual activity that accompanies the "coming-out" process for many male homosexuals may be a manifestation of the delayed experimenta-tion that categorizes the usual adolescent period for heterosexual males (Hanley-Hackenbruck 1988; Malyon 1981).

Even during the years prior to self-acceptance, however, the adolescent male homosexual is likely to have some sexual experience with same-sex partners (Troiden 1979). Saghir and his colleagues, in a survey of eighty-nine self-identified gay men, reported that 86 percent had "homosexual contacts" before the age of fifteen, including anal intercourse in 19 percent of their respondents (1969:222). Many of these encounters were with adult males. Other researchers have found that it is not unusual for homosexually active adolescents to have partners who are older than themselves (Remafedi 1987a). Adolescents who are exploring their homosexuality, especially with a partner who is older (and therefore more likely to have been previously infected with HIV) are at increased risk for HIV infection. Inexperience and confusion about their sexual feelings will make it difficult for them to translate their knowledge of AIDS prevention, if they have such information, into appropriate self-protective behavior (for example, condom use).

Homosexuals, unlike heterosexuals, do not undergo an "anticipatory period" of socialization (Dank 1971:182). Parents and teachers do not prepare them for their role in gay society, and they enter it with many of the same negative stereotypes, apprehensions, and fears that are held by heterosexuals. When gay men do "come-out" (identify themselves as homosexual), gay bars are the first contact with organized homosexual society that many are likely to encounter (Dank 1971:187). In the language of sociology, gay bars are the places where newly self-recognized homosexual men first learn about the prevalent group norms of their subculture.

Because the phenomenon of coming out is associated with both the commencement of regular sexual activity (Troiden 1979:367) and regular attendance at gay bars (Dank 1971), it represents a critical period during which uninfected gays can be easily reached—in an environment that is familiar and nonthreatening to them—and educated about the prevention of HIV infection. Not only can these establishments serve as focal points for the dissemination of AIDS prevention information, they can also provide ingress for the introduction of new group norms relating to safer sexual behavior. In order to reach the population of men attending gay bars, it will be necessary for health educators to collaborate with leaders from the gay community and with community-based organizations providing services for gay men.

The use of gay social organizations to promote the prevention of sexually transmissible diseases is not a new concept. A related approach was described over a decade ago, when officials of a municipal public health department conducted routine screening for

syphilis and gonorrhea in gay bathhouses (Judson et al. 1977). Developing linkages with pre-existing networks within a target population, whether these are formal (community-based organizations)
or informal (opinion/community leaders), is a necessary component
of outreach, regardless of the target, and underscores the importance
of involving the target population in the development of health-promotion services.

In addition to using gay social organizations as a site for outreach
and prevention services, it is advisable to incorporate an institutional component into outreach activities, especially in nonurban
areas of the country where the male homosexual population is not
highly concentrated or well organized and gay social organizations
are limited. Publicly funded clinics for the diagnosis and treatment
of sexually transmitted diseases (STD) can play a pivotal role in
reaching sexually active gay men with information about the prevention of HIV infection.

Health care providers in these settings may require training that
desensitizes them to the subject of male homosexual behavior, addresses stereotyped perceptions about gays, affirms the importance
of confidentiality, and trains them to interview and educate clients
in a nonjudgmental manner. This type of staff training is just as important as training that provides information about the basics of
viral transmission, pathogenesis, and disease prevention. Although
there will be instances when a client's sexual orientation is suggested by a medical diagnosis (for example, herpetic or gonococcal
proctitis), practitioners who have a stereotyped image of gay men
are likely to make incorrect assumptions about their clients' sexual
preference and may consequentially fail to provide information to
those who need it.

The preceding discussion has emphasized the group characteristics of gay men, without much attention to individual differences. But sexual preference, like other human characteristics, is
best viewed as a continuum that is influenced by a number of variables, including age, personality, culture, and environmental milieu. Therefore, a primary responsibility of program planners
developing AIDS-prevention initiatives is to appreciate and understand the degree of diversity within the homosexual population and
to modify their outreach and intervention approaches to coincide
with the different circumstances and developmental stages along
the continuum of human sexual preference. Especially important is
the realization that men may engage in same-sex behavior but not
define themselves as homosexual (Dank 1971; Isay 1988; McKusick

et al. 1985: 230). In a study of 604 men attending public and private clinics for sexually transmitted diseases in Sweden, Finland, Ireland, and Australia, Ross found that those men who are less likely to report their homosexual activity expected "the most negative reaction to their homosexuality" and believed in "more conservative sex roles for males and females" (1985:83). Some men may be sexually active with both men and women (Smith 1987). In a study of participants engaging in sex in public restrooms, Humphreys (1970) found that 54 percent of the participants were married middle-class men with children (cited in Marmor 1980:270).

Cultures strongly influence self-definition of homosexuality. In societies where "cross-gender behavior produces strong emotional negative reaction in large segments of the population," gender roles are strongly dichotomized (Carrier 1980:108). In such cultures, men who engage in insertive sexual practices with other men (for example, insertive oral and/or anal intercourse) do not generally consider themselves, nor are they considered, to be homosexual—as long as they are not *exclusively* involved in homosexual behavior (Carrier, 1980). This phenomenon has been observed in Mexico, Greece, and Brazil, and is strongly associated with the cultural value of machismo, that is, hypermasculinity as an ideal of male social behavior (Carrier 1980:108). Its relevance to AIDS prevention is that we should anticipate encountering similar perceptions among members of American ethnic groups where the cultural ideal of machismo is still widely held (Gayle 1987). African-American and Hispanic men who have sex with other men may not identify themselves as "gay," and prevention programs targeted to a "gay" audience will not succeed in attracting them. Even men from these two groups who are exclusively homosexual in orientation may not self-identify as being "gay" because they feel that this designation negates their racial and ethnic heritage. These issues will be discussed in more detail later in this chapter. For now, we will consider the group characteristics of intravenous drug users, and how they affect outreach for AIDS-prevention programs.

Intravenous (IV) or subcutaneous administration is associated with a number of drugs, although heroin, cocaine, and amphetamines are among those most commonly administered in this manner (Ginzburg et al. 1988:187). Persons who use illicit intravenous drugs can also be considered as a discrete subculture, with their own "structured sets of values, roles, and status allocations" (Friedman et al. 1988:202). The norms of this subculture are shaped by two powerful variables: the illegality of drug use and the physiologic realities of dependency and withdrawal among individuals who are addicted to the drugs they use. Intravenous drug users, like homosexuals, are a highly stigmatized group and are "feared, mistrusted, and disliked" (Friedman et al. 1986:385). Unlike the gay community, they often lack the group-specific resources to generate a community-based response to AIDS, either in terms of prevention programs or in caring for those already infected (Ginzburg et al. 1988:186). There are exceptions to this generalization, most apparent in the efforts of ex-users who have become active in combatting the spread of HIV infection among current users (Friedman et al. 1988:210). However, this lack of a sense of community is a rather pervasive consequence of the active user's overwhelming need to procure an expensive, illegal, and scarce product. Competition for and procurement of this commodity results in expertise at manipulative skills (Carpi 1987:22) and in widespread mistrust, not only of non-drug-using society but also of other drug users (Des Jarlais and Friedman 1987b:253).

While manipulative skills serve an important survival function for the active user and are acceptable subcultural norms within that context, they are impediments to the development of a community-based response to AIDS in this group. The amalgam of marked economic disadvantage, manipulative survival skills, and the physiologic need to procure an illegal substance poses a substantial barrier to drug users as a group promoting AIDS prevention to the degree that has been achieved in the gay community (Des Jarlais and Friedman 1987a). This barrier can also interfere with exogenous attempts to promote prevention within this group, especially given the drug user's mistrust of authority—another adaptation to a lifestyle that is, by definition, at odds with the law.

Des Jarlais and Friedman identify the extensive reliance on oral communication as a characteristic of this subculture, both as a prudent adaptation to an illegal activity and also because of widespread deficits in reading and writing abilities observed among economically disadvantaged drug users (1987b:254). This implies that dissemination of information about AIDS-prevention services, as well as specific behavioral recommendations to prevent the transmission of the virus, may have to be presented orally rather than in writing. While this increases the probability that the message will be received, it will also increase program costs. These same authors also note that members of this subculture may express varying commitments to its values, depending on the current status of their addiction, that is, whether they are actively using drugs, in treatment, or contemplating treatment (Des Jarlais and Friedman 1987b:254). Strategies for targeting and promoting AIDS prevention among intravenous drug users must be tailored to encompass all of these categories.

Prevention programs for individuals who are in treatment or awaiting treatment are likely to be easier to implement than those directed at active users, since the target population is identifiable with minimal effort, readily accessible, and existing organizational structures can be used as the framework for delivering this additional service. These programs may also have a greater probability of success, since drug users in treatment have already expressed a tangible desire to modify their behavior. Obviously, removing or minimizing the variable of dependency as an overriding behavioral influence and controlling the need to inject intravenous drugs (as in the case of treating heroin addiction with methadone maintenance) greatly reduce the risk of acquiring or transmitting HIV by this means. But, these interventions do not eliminate the possibility of transmission occurring, especially if the individual relapses or continues to inject nonopiate drugs, such as cocaine. Also, intravenous drug users in treatment may already be infected and can transmit HIV to their sexual partners if they do not take appropriate precautions.

For the reasons outlined above, a great deal of emphasis has been placed on the expansion of existing treatment facilities for intravenous drug users who wish to terminate their addiction (Boffey 1988; Booth 1988; Drucker 1986; Weinberg and Murray 1987). Although it is likely that such expansion will take place as a consequence of the AIDS epidemic, it is unlikely that the ongoing debate about how to "treat" intravenous drug use will be resolved in the near future (Newman 1987). However vehement this debate becomes, it does not in any way minimize the importance of utilizing all existing drug treatment programs to gain ready access to individuals who are at risk of becoming infected with or transmitting HIV.

Although most intravenous drug users will have some contact with a drug treatment program during the course of their addiction, in New York City it is estimated that "only between 15 and 20 percent of current addicts are enrolled in care" (Drucker 1986:176). In order for AIDS-prevention services to reach drug users who are not currently in treatment, it will be necessary to access a variety of organizations that are used by these individuals and their sexual partners. Primary health care facilities, emergency rooms, publicly funded clinics for the treatment of sexually transmissible diseases, contraceptive care clinics, shelters for runaway youths, unemployment agencies, corrections institutions, municipal courts, and programs within state departments of health and welfare are examples of the kinds of agencies providing services to the intravenous drug user. Staff from these organizations can be trained to evaluate individuals for a history of IV drug use and to provide prevention information to persons they determine to be at risk.

Identifying the organizations providing services to intravenous drug users is not synonymous with a comprehensive outreach effort. To be successful, such an effort would require centralized administrative direction that intersects all of the various departments and organizations involved. This objective is not impossible to achieve, but would be quite difficult, especially when one is dealing with bureaucratic structures that may not be favorably disposed to the superimposition of external authority. Widespread staff training in the area of intravenous drug use and skills training for conducting interviews on highly personal and potentially taboo topics such as illegal drug use and sexual behavior are other prerequisites that would require substantial administrative effort and additional, often nonbudgeted, resources.

Based on our knowledge of the drug-using subculture's pervasive mistrust of authority and the value it places on maintaining secrecy in its dealings with the non-drug-using world, it is likely that many at-risk individuals will pass through service organizations without being recognized, even if a widespread, comprehensive program to identify intravenous drug users is successfully implemented. Even after individuals are identified as IV drug users on the basis of clinical or historical information, we can not assume that they will attend to the AIDS-prevention information being provided. As outlined in Chapter Three, communication is a complex process, influenced by various input and output factors. For instance, the service provider may fail to establish a suitable rapport with the client, or the client may not be comfortable enough with the surroundings to be able to attend to the prevention message. As an example of the importance of "context" in health promotion, Worden and his colleagues found that the supportive "context" of a women's club environment was more significant in influencing knowledge about and frequency of breast self-examination than were variations in program content (1983:331). It is likely, therefore, that outreach to intravenous drug users will include a prominent, noninstitutionally based component.

Using a direct word-of-mouth outreach strategy by entering into the subculture of the active IV drug user is an approach that has been pioneered by ADAPT, the Association for Drug Abuse Prevention and Treatment. This community-based organization employs volunteers who are familiar with the drug subculture, often because they are ex-users themselves. They travel into neighborhoods where intravenous drug use is prevalent, establish networks of communication with users and their significant others, and provide practical information about preventing the transmission of HIV. Because of their familiarity with the subculture and their acceptance by the target population, they can interact with dealers, pushers, and current users in a meaningful way, and are able to provide their services in locales where they are most needed, often in "shooting galleries." Although such outreach is more expensive, time consuming, and possibly more controversial than outreach through established organizations or media channels, it has the potential of resulting in greater efficacy, since the outreach worker is perceived as both an advocate and a peer.

In attempting to reach intravenous drug users with an AIDS-prevention message, one must recognize the diversity of the target group, not just in terms of demographic characteristics but also in terms of their "investment" in their addiction. It is not enough to offer treatment for the addiction, since this "product" will not be equally desirable to all drug users. Although many of these individuals can probably be induced to enter treatment programs, we must expect that there will be significant numbers who are not yet willing to give up their drug use. In this circumstance, planners must develop a service or "product," as the social marketing lexicon has it, that is perceived as beneficial by the client who is still injecting drugs (Kotler 1984). In conventional marketing, product characteristics, packaging, concept, and position are adjusted to increase the likelihood of sale; in social marketing, program benefits are designed to attract the targeted client.

Many public health officials consider the test for the HIV antibody, which will be discussed in detail in a later chapter, as such a product. There is some evidence to suggest that among some intravenous drug users, offering a free, confidential antibody test to determine the presence or absence of HIV infection would be perceived of as a desirable "product" (Carlson and McClellan 1987; Lewis and Galea 1988). Unfortunately, there is not a great deal of information on the behavioral outcomes of HIV testing of intravenous drug users, although there is some suggestion that its results can be beneficial (Des Jarlais 1987a:73). Testing may not, however, be the ideal "product" for every user. Some who test negative may interpret it to mean that they will never become infected or that their prior behaviors have been acceptably safe. Those who think they are already in-fected may not believe that the test will add any additional useful information, or they may fear that they will be unable to cope with the diagnosis of HIV infection at a time when there is no curative treatment. To the planner who is trying to develop an acceptable "product," relying solely on the HIV antibody test is neither prudent nor warranted. As part of the strategy to promote AIDS risk reduction among intravenous drug users, much consideration has been given to the specific behavior of needle sharing and how prevention efforts might focus on modification of this activity as a "product" of the service.

Needle sharing has been widely described as both a practical con-sequence of the economic and legal milieu of the intravenous drug user and also as a manifestation of the values held by this group (Black et al. 1986; Howard and Borges 1970; Brown et al 1987; Ghodse et al. 1987; Selwyn et al. 1987). Because of the obvious and important role that this behavior plays in the transmission of HIV, strategies to minimize this route of infection in active users by ei-ther advocating the cleansing of needles and syringes with a solu-tion of common household bleach (Chaisson et al. 1987; Froner 1987) or by making sterile needles and syringes readily available to active users (Des Jarlais and Hopkins 1985; Lohr 1988; Schmalz 1988) have been proposed as "products" of prevention campaigns. These approaches will be explored in greater detail in later chapters, but for our purposes it is important to realize that there are often highly charged objections to such proposals because of the percep-tion that they will encourage illegal drug use and because of fears that they may not be effective at interrupting transmission (Cook 1987; Kerr 1988). These objections must be resolved in the context of well-planned and controlled clinical trials, for until there is some definite evidence of benefit, or lack thereof, the controversy is likely to continue unabated. However, from a social marketing perspec-tive, these proposals are likely to be considered highly beneficial by targeted users who are not prepared to enter treatment to end their addiction—especially given the apparent increased demand for "clean" needles that has been spurred by the fear of AIDS (Des Jarlais and Hopkins 1985:1476). The debate about the role of free sterile needles in combatting the spread of HIV infection underscores some of the problems faced by social marketers who develop "products" to promote changes in health status or to attract individuals into health promotion programs. Because of related social issues, social marketers have "less flexibility in shaping the product" than do their commercial counterparts (Bloom and Novelli 1981:83).

Female sexual partners of male intravenous drug users are an especially important target for AIDS-prevention activities because of their risk of sexually acquired infection and their ability to transmit infection to their offspring. As Des Jarlais and Friedman report, almost 80 percent of male intravenous drug users in New York City report female sexual partners who did not inject drugs themselves (1987b:261). Avenues to access these women will be different from those that are designed for active drug users. Publicly funded contraceptive and prenatal care clinics, and other state and local social service agencies for women and children, are examples of organizations that provide services for the female sexual partners of IV drug users and that can be incorporated into a social service net to identify women who are in need of information about preventing the transmission of HIV.

Women who regularly use intravenous drugs themselves are thought to represent between 30 and 40 percent of the total population of intravenous drug users (Drucker 1986:171). Outreach to this population will incorporate many of the strategies outlined above, with special emphasis on correctional facilities and courts of law. This is because a substantial proportion of female intravenous drug users support themselves by prostitution (Drucker 1986:171). This does not mean that all female prostitutes are IV drug users or that all women who use IV drugs engage in prostitution. Nonetheless, the strength of this association is such that female prostitutes are a fertile target group for outreach to identify IV drug users, to encourage treatment for drug problems, and to intervene to prevent infection by and transmission of HIV.

It is essential that we not limit our discussion of targeting prevention efforts to individuals who are already using drugs. Des Jarlais and Friedman identify persons who have not yet begun using drugs as a primary focus for AIDS prevention (1987a:71). Intervening to prevent the onset of intravenous drug use, thereby eliminating the possibility of transmission through needle sharing, is in many ways preferable to undertaking AIDS-prevention efforts with active users, or even with persons already in treatment, since it precludes the problems of recidivism, likely to accompany withdrawal in the former group, and treatment failure in the latter. Prevention of the onset of drug use as a strategy to prevent the transmission of HIV is likely to result in consensual approval because of its wide-based appeal to many divergent segments of the population and because of its other health-related and social benefits. Therefore, it is relevant to our discussion to understand the variables associated with drug use in order to develop a profile of individuals who are at risk for this behavior. Many of the data that follow are generic in that they deal with all manner of drugs, both legal and illicit. Although few studies are limited only to drugs that are administered intravenously, the information is still helpful in arriving at generalizations that can be used to guide program planners in the identification of groups at risk for this behavior.

A multitude of surveys and prospective and retrospective studies on drug use target adolescence as a critical time to affect future drug-using behaviors (Kandel and Logan 1984; Newcombe et al. 1986; Murray and Perry 1985; Raveis and Kandel 1987; Yamaguchi and Kandel 1984). As a transition from childhood to adulthood, adolescence is a critical window during which many health-related behaviors are shaped. It is also a time of increased threat to physical and emotional health and well-being. The popular cultural icon of the awkward adolescent moving from childhood to adulthood under the knowing scrutiny and patronage of the loving adults who surround him in many ways belies the turbulence and danger inherent in this transitional state. Not only are adolescents at increased risk for the initiation of licit and illicit drug use, they are also at risk for unplanned pregnancy (Hofferth et al. 1987; Jones et al. 1985; Robbins et al. 1985; Scott 1983; Zelnik and Kantner 1979) and even more disturbing, they are the only age group in which mortality has risen since 1960 (Goleman 1987:13), primarily as a result of suicide, homicide, and accidental death (Brody 1988). Because of their propensity for risk taking (Baumrind 1985; Goleman 1987; Lewis and Lewis 1984) many adolescents engage in "socially disruptive and health-endangering behavior" (Baumrind 1985:14) before they are "capable of understanding the causal relationship between an act and the nonreversibility of its consequences" (Lewis and Lewis 1984:584). According to Lewis and Lewis, risk taking among adolescents tests the strength of the individual's affiliation with his social group, influences the child's adult identity formation, and functions as a mechanism by which adolescents learn more about the norms of different subcultures (1984:580). These risky behaviors are often mediated by the influence of peers (Baumrind 1985; Goleman 1987; Lewis and Lewis 1984).

As described above, adolescent risk-taking behaviors have the potential for resulting in a variety of health problems, not just drug use. Adolescent hemophiliacs, for example, have the same propensity to engage in risk-taking behaviors as do unaffected adolescent males (Senft et al. 1981:90). In the case of adolescent hemophiliacs who are infected with HIV, risk-taking behavior may manifest as unprotected sexual intercourse. Although the implementation of donor screening, donor HIV antibody testing, and heat treatment of clotting factor concentrate has essentially nullified this route of HIV infection among hemophiliacs, the hemophiliac who is already infected is capable of transmitting HIV to his sexual partners. With this particular population, unlike many of the others we have discussed, we do not face difficulties in identifying our targets; their illness has forced many of them to be actively enrolled in treatment programs. However, there may be significant difficulties in attempting to induce adolescent hemophiliacs to modify their sexual behaviors to prevent viral transmission (Kolata 1988). Denial used as an adaptive mechanism (Zeltzer et al. 1980:136), decreased feelings of masculinity and sociability (Handford and Strickler 1982:232), and the existence of a heritable chronic illness that is capable, in itself, of creating a stigma (Simon 1982:246), even without the additional burden of HIV seropositivity, may all act as barriers to promoting sexual risk reduction among HIV-infected adolescents with hemophilia.

Because adolescence is characterized by a propensity to engage in risk-taking behaviors, and is described developmentally as a transitional state during which previously accepted parental and authoritative values are questioned and tested (Baumrind 1985:14), many researchers consider adolescent experimentation with drugs, both licit and illicit, to be "statistically normative"—although most adolescents who experiment with drugs do not become chronic users (Baumrind 1985:31; Murray and Perry 1985:236). Of the demographic factors associated with adolescent drug use, age and sex differences are the most important. The likelihood and degree of drug use increases with age during adolescence, and adolescent males are more likely to use drugs, both legal and illegal, than females (Murray and Perry 1985:237). Early age of drug use onset is especially important in predicting subsequent abuse (p. 237). Compared to white youths, northern black inner-city youths begin using drugs at an earlier age, and are more likely to use "hard" drugs (Brunswick 1980:457).

Social and environmental factors also play a role in adolescent drug use, especially if the adolescent coexists with highly visible models in his environment who are using drugs (Murray and Perry 1985:238). These models can be peers (Clayton and Ritter 1985; Kandel 1985; Murray and Perry 1985) or family (Murray and Perry 1985). Not surprisingly, ease of obtaining drugs in the child's environment is also associated with increased drug use (Murray and

Perry 1985:237). In terms of intrapersonal factors, adolescents who have a greater chance of using drugs, compared to controls, tend to be more unconventional, more spontaneous, and less likely to place value on traditionally accepted avenues for achievement (Murray and Perry 1985:238). Researchers have also found that illicit drug use can serve a self-medicating function for some adolescents (Yamaguchi and Kandel 1984:679). Behavioral factors associated with drug use include sexual activity, delinquency of various forms, and declining academic performance (Murray 1985:238). Drug use is also associated with a high rate of abseenteeism and with dropping out of school (Brunswick 1980:468; Leary 1988), two categories in which minority youth are overrepresented (Brunswick 1980:468). Programs for homeless youth report a substantial rate of substance abuse (National Network of Runaway and Youth Services 1985:14).

From the preceding, it is apparent that many factors are associated with adolescent drug use. The association of a specific variable with drug use does not necessarily imply a causal relationship; in some instances the association may be temporal, and in others, both the variable in question and the drug-using behavior may be associated with another common factor. For example, while the high rate of absenteeism from school may be a direct result of drug use, it may also mean that adolescents who miss more school than average are more likely to spend time in activities that put them in contact with drug users. Likewise, declining academic performance may be a result of drug use, or may precede it; adolescents who do not perform well in school may use drugs to bolster their self-esteem or to cope with the stresses of their failure. What is clear, however, is that no one single factor can be used as a marker for drug use—nor is there a formula to predict which adolescents who admit to using drugs will develop substance abuse problems. In the words of Newcombe and his colleagues, "there is not one particular and specific reason that accounts for all types of drug use and is applicable to all types of drug abusers" (1986:529). Drug use is best considered a multifactorial problem that is influenced by psychosocial and environmental elements. Adolescents' increased risk for drug use relates to their propensity for taking risks. Also, drug use among adolescents may play a functional role (Murray and Perry 1985:250; Newcombe et al. 1986:529). Among the proposed functions ascribed to drug use in adolescence are social acceptance for younger adolescents and stress reduction for older adolescents (Murray and Perry 1985:250). We also know that the risk for initiation to most illicit drugs, other than cocaine, is minimal after the age of twenty-one (Kandel and Logan 1984:660).

The importance of these variables as they pertain to the prevention of HIV infection is in their ability to suggest which adolescents are at increased risk for the onset of illicit drug use and which may progress to the intravenous self-administration of drugs. Although drug use is not limited to any particular class or race, these variables suggest that economically disadvantaged inner-city youth are at increased risk. This presumption is confirmed by the fact that African-Americans and Hispanics, who account for a significant portion of the poor inner-city population, are overrepresented in samples of intravenous drug users when compared to their prevalence in the general population.

Data from the Treatment Outcome Prospective Study (TOPS), which were derived from three national annual cohorts of intravenous drug users between 1979 and 1981, documented that Caucasians, who make up 74 percent of the general population, accounted for 45 percent of the IV users in the study group, while African-Americans, who account for 13 percent of the general population, accounted for nearly 40 percent of the cohort, and Hispanics, who make up 13 percent of the general population, accounted for approximately 14 percent of the cohort (Ginzburg 1984:208). In 1982, the National Institute on Drug Abuse conducted a survey of drug abuse treatment facilities, which revealed that of clients in the New York City standard metropolitan statistical area, 32 percent were white, 40 percent were black, and 28 percent were Hispanic (National Institute on Drug Abuse 1982, cited in Centers for Disease Control 1986:665). The increased frequency of black intravenous drug users, compared to their frequency in the general population, has been observed since shortly after World War II (Chambers and Moffett 1970:188). Next to African-Americans, Mexican-Americans are the largest ethnic minority group among the population of addicted opiate users in the United States (Desmond and Maddux 1984:317). When compared to Caucasian and African-American addicts, Mexican-American addicts have more severe educational and occupational deficits (Desmond and Maddux 1984:340). As one might expect from these statistics, a majority of persons who have developed AIDS as a result of HIV infection through needle sharing or heterosexual contact (often through an infected IV drug using partner) are African-American or Hispanic (Bakeman et al. 1986:191; Centers for Disease Control 1986:655).

These observations should not be interpreted to imply that every African-American and Hispanic adolescent is at increased risk for intravenous drug use or that only minority youth will develop substance abuse problems. The observations and figures presented here are not meant as generalizations or to perpetuate stereotypes, but rather to help planners target individuals who are at increased risk for developing HIV infection, in this instance, because of their increased risk of intravenous drug use.

The frequent association of IV drug use with economic disadvantage serves as a persistent reminder that intravenous drug use is as much a socioeconomic problem as it is a medical one. The incidence of drug use among minority inner-city youth mirrors the rise in joblessness and poverty in America's inner cities (Wilkerson 1988: A12). Sociologists use the term "underclass" to refer to the segment of American society that is perpetually poor, confined to the inner city, and predominantly nonwhite. America's underclass is growing; between 1970 and 1980, the number of impoverished African-Americans rose by 24 percent, and the number of impoverished Hispanics rose by 73 percent (Wilkerson 1988:A12). Brunswick suggests that the black inner-city adolescent who is faced with the same needs for "expanded competence and mobility" as his middle-class peers, but who has "less opportunity for achievement in socially desirable channels," may initiate drug use in order to fulfill a "business or occupational function" (Brunswick 1980:450).

For the program planner assigned the task of preventing HIV infection by preventing the onset of intravenous drug use, these findings suggest that two important targets are (1) economically disadvantaged minority youth and (2) children living in "dysfunctional" families who are at increased risk for running away from home (National Network of Runaway and Youth Services 1985:2). Developing successful interventions for these groups will not be easy, especially given our inability to modify disadvantageous social environments quickly. However, it is possible to utilize the school system to reach these youths before they begin to use drugs.

Drug use prevention programs should begin in grade school. This recommendation is based, in part, on research showing that inner-city African-American youths tend to initiate drug use at an earlier age than Caucasians. In Brunswick's study of black youths from Harlem, the average age of initiation to illicit drugs was thirteen (1980:457). Desmond and Maddux report that the onset of daily opiate use for Mexican-Americans usually begins prior to the age of twenty (1984:321). The other rationale for early and aggressive programs for grade school children is that by the time school absenteeism becomes a problem, the adolescent may already be using drugs (Brunswick 1980:468; Leary 1988:A24; Murray and Perry 1985:238). In the case of runaways, it is crucial to educate youth about the risk of both drug use and HIV infection before they become "lost" to the system. By the time the child has left home, he or she may already be involved in both iv drug use and prostitution (National Network of Runaway and Youth Services 1985:25), behaviors that can lead to HIV infection and continued transmission of the virus. School-based programs relating to the prevention of HIV infection should not limit themselves to drug-use prevention alone, but should also discuss the prevention of the sexual transmission of HIV.

A consideration of the special circumstances of race and ethnicity as they pertain to AIDS prevention is an important component of outreach, and is not limited to discussions of minority adolescents who are at increased risk for the initiation of illicit drug use. If prevention campaigns present AIDS as a "gay white disease," outreach into minority communities will suffer, especially in areas where the incidence of AIDS is currently low and the target group has limited exposure to community members who have contracted the disease (Mays and Cochran 1987:224). Although this perception will change as the number of people of color who are diagnosed with AIDS increases, it is imperative that prevention initiatives emphasize the relevance of AIDS as it pertains to minorities and that media that are used to promote AIDS prevention employ language and visual images that reinforce this message (Gayle 1987). We cannot expect African-Americans and Hispanics to identify with the threat of AIDS if the public service announcements and other media messages warning them of the dangers of this disease are carried only by white men and women.

Within minority communities, outreach techniques need to vary depending on the risk behavior that one is targeting. For example, homosexual men of color, especially men of a lower socioeconomic status, may identify with their racial/ethnic group more strongly and more fundamentally than with persons who share the same sexual orientation. This means that efforts to appeal to African-American and Hispanic men whose same-sex behavior puts them at risk for HIV infection may have to focus on their self-identification as racial/ethnic minority group members rather than as gay men. Because of strong cultural ties with fundamentalist religions (Mays and Cochran 1987:229) and the prevailing cultural ethos of machismo (Gayle 1987:77), African-Americans are often quite negative about the subject of homosexuality, and many African-American homosexuals remain "closeted," passing as heterosexuals (Williams 1986:417). Hispanic men are also raised in a culture that places great importance on the ideals of machismo and procreation, so that Hispanic men who engage exclusively in same-sex relationships are subject to extreme disapproval.

While homosexuality is generally regarded in an unfavorable light across most groups within our society, among racial and ethnic minorities same-sex preference represents an additional "liability," in terms of their relationship with the majority population and also in their dealings with heterosexual minority peers. It is not coincidental that homosexual men who are members of racial and ethnic minorities are often highly secretive about their sexual preferences and do not generally choose to share that aspect of their identity with other minority group members who are heterosexual. This heightened degree of stigmatization in concert with the lower socioeconomic resources of many minority group members has resulted in a paucity of "visible and formal organizational networks" among homosexuals of color (Williams 1986:412).

Because of the lack of extant formal networks among minority homosexual groups, dissemination of information about HIV infection and prevention may require more time and more specific targeting techniques than has been the case with white, middle-class gay men who live in urban areas and who have many social and informational networks available to them. In 1985, Williams surveyed sixty-two African-American homosexual men from Detroit about AIDS and found that they were "generally uninformed about who is at risk for AIDS" (1986:417). Only eight of her sixty-two respondents correctly specified that HIV is transmitted through blood and semen (Williams 1986:417). A report comparing cases of early syphilis in DeKalb County, Georgia, from 1981 to 1985, on the basis of race, demonstrated that early syphilis among African-American men with same-sex partners had risen, while the rate in Caucasian men had decreased (Landrum et al. 1988). Although there are many ways to explain these findings, they do suggest that prevention messages aimed at white gay men are not having an impact on black men with same-sex partners.

These findings suggest that informal communication networks should be used to disseminate AIDS prevention information to homosexual men of color and that outreach to these target groups should rely extensively on a noninstitutionally based strategy, with peer-mediated delivery, often in settings where these men socialize, whether bars, bathhouses, or social clubs. While it is advisable to incorporate the institutional participation of social service and health organizations into a comprehensive effort to provide AIDS-prevention information to homosexual men of color, it is imperative that the staff members of these agencies receive training that sensitizes them to the culturally relevant issues, and that they be provided with skills training enabling them to interview and educate clients

effectively. Because of the added cultural liabilities incurred by minority men who identify themselves as gay, it is also advisable that
organizationally based prevention programs be designed so that a
client does not have to admit to homosexuality in order to receive
prevention services.

As indicated earlier, in societies where machismo is a prevalent cultural ideal, the insertive partner in a same-sex encounter
does not necessarily identify himself as homosexual. Given the
documented risk of HIV infection associated with insertive anal intercourse (Kingsley et al. 1987), and recognizing that bisexual African-American and Hispanic men will not be reached by messages
designed for an exclusively homosexual target, it will be necessary
to modify outreach strategy to these men to emphasize the relative
risk associated with specific sexual practices rather than emphasizing the gender of the sexual partner. Because bisexual men of color
may be unwilling to share their proclivities with other minority
men who are bisexual, this outreach should not rely extensively on
informal communication networks, but should instead utilize institutional settings where these men work and receive health care and
other social services, or where they congregate with other minority
men for the purpose of socialization. AIDS-prevention information
and services should be presented in a gender neutral manner so that
these men will not have to fear disclosure in order to have access to
these services.

Presently, African-American and Hispanic women account for
nearly three-fourths of all diagnosed AIDS cases in women in the
United States (Guinan and Hardy 1987:2040). Intravenous drug use
or sexual contact with a male intravenous drug user are the most
frequent modes of HIV infection in these women (Guinan and Hardy
1987:2040). Although we have discussed outreach strategies for female drug users and for female partners of IV drug users, it is important to recognize that consideration of race and ethnicity must also
modulate outreach initiatives to women.

Horowitz, in her study of inner-city Hispanic women from Chicago, discovered that the use of birth control by a single woman is
associated with negative cultural values because it is seen as an "explicit indication to engage in sexual intercourse," and because it
negates the cultural importance of motherhood (1981:249). According to her analysis, premarital sexual activity is at odds with prevailing cultural mores that endorse virginity at marriage, submission to
men, and motherhood. However, premarital sexual activity is accepted if it is perceived to be the unplanned consequence of "uncon-
trolled passion" between two people who are in love (p. 249). Hence,

it may be very difficult to suggest that unmarried Hispanic women use condoms with their male sexual partners as a means of protecting against HIV infection. Because of the value placed on procreation, it may be even more difficult to suggest that married Hispanic women consider the use of condoms with husbands who are at risk for HIV infection. The importance and esteem associated with the role of motherhood in the African-American community (Randolph and Gersche 1986:12) might also interfere with attempts to promote the use of condoms for AIDS prevention.

Inner-city, low-income black women face many of these same barriers. Despite their expanded role in the day-to-day managerial aspects of their households, these women may still manifest very traditional values in their dealings with male sexual partners, including husbands. In Randolph and Gersche's discussion of black adolescent pregnancy, they emphasize the distinction between the "strength" of an African-American woman in the matrix of her extended family and the attribute of dominance, explaining that strength is not always associated with dominance, especially in terms of relationships with men (1986:12).

Because of traditional values that militate against women questioning the motives of men in regard to sensitive topics such as sexuality, a major barrier to AIDS-prevention efforts targeted to women, especially minority women, may be the women's inability to determine whether or not their male partners have a history of behaviors that would place them at increased risk for HIV infection. Women who are raised with strong cultural taboos against discussing topics pertaining to sexuality or questioning the motives of their men, may find it impossible to broach the topic of AIDS prevention. Even if they understand how HIV is transmitted, women who are married to bisexual men may have no knowledge of their husbands' extramarital same-sex relationships and may assume that they are "safe." Women who are involved in sexual relationships with intravenous drug users may also be unaware of their partners' habits—and even if they are aware, they may be uncomfortable asking questions about needle-sharing activities. Because of these circumstances, it may be more appropriate to emphasize the dangers of perinatal transmission of HIV as a motivation for both men and women to participate in AIDS-prevention programs. This approach capitalizes on the esteemed position that children hold in our society. By presenting AIDS-prevention outreach efforts as an attempt to prevent disease in children, both men and women may be motivated to overcome the cultural barriers outlined above.

As a general impediment to minority outreach for AIDS prevention, we must appreciate that minorities, because of their longstanding history of having suffered discrimination and oppression, do not
always perceive institutions and governmental agencies as supportive, but may instead consider them intrusive and view them with
mistrust and suspicion (Hays and Mindel 1973:52). Local health departments initiating community-based AIDS-prevention programs
for African-Americans and Hispanics may encounter difficulties because of this perception. This mistrust, which is often mistakenly
viewed as a lack of concern, may be intensified if minority members
are not employed in visible decision-making positions within the
initiating health organizations. A 1987 survey of community-based
AIDS service providers conducted by the National AIDS Network
reported that a majority of the agencies surveyed revealed only "limited success and many difficulties in providing AIDS education services to people of color" (National AIDS Network 1987:9). Among
the reasons given were "limited success in involving minorities in
agencies and programs, lack of contacts in minority communities,
and unsuitability of educational materials for use in minority communities" (National AIDS Network 1987:9).

Target group members should be involved in planning AIDS-prevention programs. By relying on direct input from leaders in the
targeted community and by incorporating social science research
that addresses behavior, mores, and related health and social problems that are of consequence to members of that community, AIDS-
prevention programs can improve their chances of reaching their
intended audiences. The importance of involving the target population in the design and implementation of AIDS-prevention programs
is relevant to all of the specific target groups we have discussed in
this chapter. To put it most simply, these are the very persons who
know the most about their own behaviors and who can, consequently, add essential insight to the overall program process.

Experts in the field of health promotion have defined health
education as "learning experiences designed to assist individuals,
groups, or communities in the voluntary control of their own health
as they define it" (Ad Hoc Work Group . . . 1987:89). However, such
an orientation is, frankly, at odds with the longstanding tradition
of paternalism in health care. As care givers we are often more prone
to tell our clients what is "best" for them rather than ask for such
information from them. For example, care givers working with intravenous drug users, may subconsciously feel that their clients
have abdicated any right to participate in health-related decisions

because their addiction is irresponsible behavior. Adolescents may be perceived of as too naive to be able to contribute in a meaningful way to important decisions about how to improve their health. Gay organizations promoting condom use as an alternative to unprotected anal intercourse may be seen as misguided because they are endorsing continued sexual activity, albeit modified, rather than abstinence. These generalizations suggest some of the potential reactions organizations may encounter when they empower their targets to participate actively in program development.

From a social science perspective, involving target members in the design and implementation of prevention programs is a strategy that capitalizes on social networks. A social network is the constellation of individuals in a person's social environment and can be described on the basis of size (number of people), density (the extent to which individuals in the network communicate with one another independent of the focal person), durability (stability of the network), dispersion (how easily the focal person can make contact with members of the network), homogeneity (extent to which members share social characteristics); frequency (frequency of exchange), and intensity (strength of the ties among members) (Mitchell and Trickett 1980:30−31). Social networks include the family, friends, and colleagues with whom we interact on a daily basis. In describing them, we describe the functional structures in the social milieu that each of us uses in coping with illness and emotional burdens (Gottlieb 1985; Mitchell and Trickett 1980), reaching decisions about serious health problems (Berkman and Syme 1979), seeking help for personal or health-related problems (Neighbors 1984a; Neighbors 1984b), and reacting to new ideas (Rogers 1982). Social networks provide support for the establishment and maintenance of a sense of control over the circumstances of our lives (Minkler 1981) and for the management of major transitional life events (Banerjee 1983).

It is not difficult to understand the concept of social networks, but many of their functions may be far more sophisticated than we realize. A nine-year study of social networks, host resistance, and mortality, found that persons with poorly developed social support networks were more likely to die than those with extensive social networks; this association was independent of self-reported health status, socioeconomic status, health practices (such as smoking, drinking alcohol, weight control, and exercise), and year of death (Berkman and Syme 1979:186).

Whether minority status dervies from shared racial/ethnic characteristics, shared practices within the context of a subculture (for example, that of iv drug users), or shared sexual preferences, the experience of minority status gives rise to social networks that are often dense, homogeneous, and durable. Social networks are not unique to minorities, but because of the characteristics described above, they often play a major role in the day-to-day lives of individuals in minority groups.

Much of the published work on social networks and minority status has concentrated on their importance within the African-American community. Among African-Americans, for example, social networks are frequently used as "alternatives to formal help seeking as well as a supplement to professional help utilization" (Neighbors 1984b:630). Because of physical barriers (paucity of easily accessible primary health care facilities in low-income neighborhoods) and cultural barriers (mistrust of majority/government-run establishments) to professional health services, many African-Americans utilize informal social networks for coping with personal problems rather than seek out professional resources (Martineau 1977; Neighbors 1984b:563). Social network solutions to personal problems may be "more congruent with black norms, beliefs, or life-styles"—especially for those with limited economic resources (Neighbors 1984a:564). Minority groups involved in clandestine activities, such as homosexually active men or intravenous drug users, also have highly developed social networks made up of peers who share similar orientations and values. These social networks have developed into efficient and effective routes of information transfer in the shadow of a society that is often hostile and averse to the norms and circumstances of these groups.

Although the importance of networks among minorities is undoubtedly modulated by circumstances of socioeconomic class, it is apparent from the preceeding discussion that they are multifunctional, and by virtue of their structure, represent a valuable resource for efforts to disseminate information about AIDS prevention. Perhaps of greater consequence, they are a means of influencing the manner in which a target group acts upon the information it receives. Whether we are encouraging treatment for addictive drug use, discouraging the practice of needle sharing among intravenous drug users, or advocating the use of condoms as a means of preventing HIV transmission, many of the specific objectives of AIDS-prevention programs will be strongly influenced by prevailing group norms. If we have access to a social structure that can not only transmit information about AIDS prevention but that also has the capability to endorse such information as valuable and consequential to its members, we have a potent means of introducing normative

change into a target population. Social networks remind us that although we generally speak of health behavior change at an individual level, it is often a change in prevailing group norms and attitudes
about a behavior that results in social reinforcement and eventual
widespread adoption of healthier behaviors. As an example, cigarette smoking is far more prevalent in an environment where smoking confers status and is socially acceptable than in an environment
where it is seen as dangerous and socially unacceptable.

Using social networks to promote health is not new or unique.
Social network interventions have been developed for a number of
target populations, including inner-city residential hotel occupants
in midtown Manhattan (Cohen and Adler 1986) and the elderly
(Minkler 1981). The employment of Hispanic adolescents as inter-
viewers to learn more about barriers to service utilization and to
perform a community needs assessment in a Hispanic neighborhood
(Delgado 1981) is an example of gaining access to a social network
to learn more about its members. In many ways, our recognition of
the importance of social networks in the process of AIDS prevention compliments the concept of social marketing. Both of these
constructs recognize the necessity of actively involving the target
population in the process of promoting behavioral change: social
marketing, by attending to the population's needs in the creation of
a "product" that people will perceive as beneficial, and social networks, by recognizing that the social milieu of the target population
is a legitimate and valuable resource for the dissemination of information about AIDS prevention and a means of inducing normative
change within the group at risk.

This chapter has emphasized the importance of understanding
the various groups of individuals who are at risk for HIV infection as
a necessary prelude to the development of AIDS-prevention programs. Although the diversity of the groups is noteworthy, the fact
that many can be categorized as subcultures that share minority status of one sort or another, results in a commonality of approach—at
least at a theoretical level. As with any health-promotion endeavor,
a central tenet of AIDS prevention is the necessity for programs to be
reflective of the "characteristics, needs, and preferences" of the individuals for whom they are designed (Ad Hoc Work Group . . . 1987:
90). To minimize the importance of this concept is to run the risk of
developing services that are ineffectively promoted and inefficiently
used. By recognizing and addressing the specific circumstances of
the target group, we affirm the influence of group norms on health-
related behaviors, present ourselves in a supportive rather than an

intrusive posture, and increase the likelihood that our efforts will be successful.

REFERENCES

Ad Hoc Work Group of the American Public Health Association. 1987. "Criteria for the Development of Health Promotion and Education Programs." *American Journal of Public Health* 77(1):89–92.

Anderson, R., Underhill, G., Kenny, C., Shah, N., Burnell, R., Jeffries, D.J., and Harris, J.R.W. 1987. "AIDS Publicity Campaigns." *Lancet* i(8547): 1429–1430.

Bakeman, R., Lumb, J.R., Jackson, R.E., and Smith, D.W. 1986. "AIDS Risk-Group Profiles in Whites and Members of Minority Groups." *New England Journal of Medicine* 315(3):191–192.

Banerjee, B. 1983. "Social Networks in the Migration Process: Empirical Evidence on Chain Migration in India." *Journal of Developing Areas* 17:185–196.

Baumrind, D. 1985. "Familial Antecedents of Adolescent Drug Use: A Developmental Perspective." In C.L. Jones and R.J. Battjes (Eds.), *Etiology of Drug Abuse: Implications for Prevention.* National Institute on Drug Abuse Research Monograph 56. Rockville, Md.: U.S. Department of Health and Human Services.

Ben-Sira, Z. 1982. "The Health Promoting Function of Mass Media and Reference Groups: Motivating or Reinforcing of Behavior Change." *Social Science and Medicine* 16:825–834.

Berkman, L.F., and Syme, S.L. 1979. "Social Networks, Host Resistance, and Mortality: A Nine-Year Follow-Up Study of Alameda County Residents." *American Journal of Epidemiology* 109:186–204.

Black, J.L., Dolan, M.P., De Ford, H.A., Rubenstein, J.A., Penk, W.E., Robinowitz, R., and Skinner, J.R. 1986. "Sharing of Needles Among Users of Intravenous Drugs." *New England Journal of Medicine* 314(7):446–447.

Bloom, P.N., and Novelli, W.D. 1981. "Problems and Challenges in Social Marketing." *Journal of Marketing* 45:79–88.

Boffey, P.M. 1988. "AIDS Panel Calls for Major Effort on Drug Abuse and Health Care." *New York Times* February 25, A1 and B7.

Booth, W. 1988. "AIDS and Drug Abuse: No Quick Fix." *Science* 239:717–719.

Brody, J.E. 1988. "Trip Across Adolescence Is Just as Risky as Ever." *New York Times* March 3, B6.

Brown, L.S., Murphy, D.L., and Primm, B.J. 1987. "Needle Sharing and AIDS in Minorities." *Journal of the American Medical Association* 258(11):1474–1475.

Brunswick, A.F. 1980. "Social Meanings and Developmental Needs: Perspectives on Black Youth's Drug Abuse." *Youth and Society* 11(4): 449–473.

Carlson, G.A., and McClellan, T.A. 1987. "The Voluntary Acceptance of HIV Antibody Screening by Intravenous Drug Users." *Public Health Reports* 102:391–394.

Carpi, J. 1987. "Treating IV Drug Users—A Difficult Task or Staff." *AIDS Patient Care* 1(3):21–23.

Carrier, J.M. 1980. "Homosexual Behavior in Cross-Cultural Perspective," In J. Marmor (Ed.), *Homosexual Behavior: A Modern Reappraisal.* New York: Basic Books.

Centers for Disease Control. 1986. "Acquired Immunodeficiency Syndrome (AIDS) Among Blacks and Hispanics—United States." *Morbidity and Mortality Weekly Review* 35(42):655–666.

Chaisson, R.E., Osmond, D., Moss, A.R., Feldman, H.W., and Bernacki, P. 1987. "HIV, Bleach, and Needle Sharing." *Lancet* i(8547):1430.

Chambers, C.D., and Moffett, A.D. 1970. "Negro Opiate Addiction." In J.C. Ball and C.D. Chambers (Eds.), *The Epidemiology of Opiate Addiction in the United States.* Springfield, Ill.: Charles C. Thomas.

Clayton, R.R., and Ritter, C. 1985. "The Epidemiology of Alcohol and Drug Abuse Among Adolescents." In B. Stimmel (Ed.), *Alcohol and Substance Abuse in Adolescence.* New York: Haworth Press.

Cohen, C.I., and Adler, A. 1986. "Assessing the Role of Social Network Interventions with an Inner-City Population." *American Journal of Orthopsychiatry* 56(2):278–288.

Cook, C.C.H. 1987. "Syringe Exchange." *Lancet* i(8538):920–921.

Dan, B.B. 1987. "The National AIDS Information Campaign: Once Upon a Time in America." *Journal of the American Medical Association* 258(14):1942.

Dank, B.M. 1971. "Coming Out in the Gay World." *Psychiatry* 34:180–197.

Delgado, M. 1981. "Using Hispanic Adolescents to Assess Community Needs." *Journal of Contemporary Social Work* 62(10):607–613.

Des Jarlais, D.C., and Friedman, S.R. 1987a. "HIV Infection Among Intravenous Drug Users: Epidemiology and Risk Reduction." *AIDS* 1:67–76.

Des Jarlais, D.C., and Friedman, S.R. 1987b. "Target Groups for Preventing AIDS Among Intravenous Drug Users." *Journal of Applied Social Psychology* 17(3)251–268.

Des Jarlais, D.C., and Hopkins, W. 1985. " 'Free' Needles for Intravenous Drug Users at Risk for AIDS: Current Developments in New York City." *New England Journal of Medicine* 313(23):1476.

Desmond, D.P., and Maddux, J.F. 1984. "Mexican-American Heroin Addicts." *American Journal of Drug and Alcohol Abuse* 10(3):317–346.

Drucker, E. 1986. "AIDS and Addiction in New York City." *American Journal of Drug and Alcohol Abuse* 12 (1 and 2):165–181.

Faria, G., Barrett, E., and Meany-Goodman, L. 1985. "Women and Abortion: Attitudes, Social Networks and Decision Making." *Social Work in Health Care* 11(1):85–99.

Flay, B.R. 1987. "Mass Media and Smoking Cessation: A Critical Review." *American Journal of Public Health* 77:153–160.

Flay, B.R., DiTecco, D., and Schlegel, R.P. 1980. "Mass Media in Health Promotion: An Analysis Using an Extended Information-Processing Model." *Health Education Quarterly* 7(2):127–147.

Fox, K.F.A., and Kotler, P. 1980. "The Marketing of Social Causes: The First Ten Years." *Journal of Marketing* 44:24–33.

Friedman, S.R., Des Jarlais, D.C., and Sotheran, J.L. 1986. "AIDS Health Education for Intravenous Drug Users." *Health Education Quarterly* 13(4):383–393.

Friedman, S.R., Des Jarlais, D.C., and Sotheran, J.L. 1988. "AIDS Health Education for Intravenous Drug Users." In R.P. Galea, B.F. Lewis, and L.A. Baker (Eds.), *AIDS and IV Drug Abusers*. Owings Mills, Md.: National Health Publishing.

Froner, G. 1987. "Disinfection of Hypodermic Syringes by IV Drug Users." *AIDS* 1(2):133–134.

Gayle, J.A. 1987. "AIDS Education in Black America." *Health Education Journal* 46(2):77–78.

Ghodse, A.H., Tregenza, G., and Li, M. 1987. "Effect of Fear of AIDS on Sharing of Injection Equipment Among Drug Abusers." *British Medical Journal* 295:698–699.

Ginzburg, H.M. 1984. "Intravenous Drug Users and the Acquired Immune Deficiency Syndrome." *Public Health Reports* 99:206–212.

Ginzburg, H.M., French J., Jackson, J., Hartsock, P.I., MacDonald, M.G., and Weiss, S.H. 1988. "Health Education and Knowledge Assessment of HIV Diseases Among Intravenous Drug Users." In R.P. Galea, B.F. Lewis, and L.A. Baker (Eds.), *AIDS and IV Drug Abusers*. Owings Mills, Md.: National Health Publishing.

Goleman, D. 1987. "Teenage Risk Taking: Rise in Deaths Prompts New Research Effort." *New York Times* November 24, 13 and 16.

Gottlieb, B.H. 1985. "Social Networks and Social Support: An Overview of Research, Practice, and Policy Implications." *Health Education Quarterly* 12(1):5–22.

Guinan, M.E., and Hardy, A. 1987. "Epidemiology of AIDS in Women in the United States, 1981 Through 1986." *Journal of the American Medical Association* 257(15):2039–2042.

Handford, H.A., and Strickler, E.M. 1982. "Psychosocial Programs." In M.W. Hilgartner (Ed.), *Hemophilia in the Child and Adult*. New York: Masson.

Hanley-Hackenbruck, P. 1988. "'Coming Out' and Psychotherapy." *Psychiatric Annals* 18:29–32.

Hastings, G.B., and Scott, A.C. 1987. "AIDS Publicity: Pointers to Development." *Health Education Journal* 46(2):58–59.

Hays, W.C., and Mindel, C.H. 1973. "Extended Kinship Relations in Black and White Families." *Journal of Marriage and Family* 35:51–57.

Heaven, P.C.L. 1987. "Beliefs About the Spread of the Acquired Immunodeficiency Syndrome." *Medical Journal of Australia* 147(6):272–274.

Hofferth, S.L., Kahn, J.R., and Baldwin, W. 1987. "Premarital Sexual Activity Among U.S. Teenage Women over the Past Three Decades." *Family Planning Perspectives* 19:46–53.

Hogan, M.A. 1988. "In San Francisco, TV Battles on the Front Lines Against AIDS." *New York Times* February 21, H31 and H37.

Holman, C.D.J., Bucens, M.R., and Sesnan, T.M.K. 1987. "AIDS and the Grim Reaper Campaign." *Medical Journal of Australia* 147(6):306.

Horowitz, R. 1981. "Passion, Submission, and Motherhood: The Negotiation of Identify by Unmarried Inner-City Chicanos." *Sociological Quarterly* 22:241–252.

Howard, J., and Borges, P. 1970. "Needle Sharing in the Haight: Some Social and Psychological Functions." *Journal of Health and Social Behavior* 11:220–223.

Humphreys, L. 1970. *Tearoom Trade: Impersonal Sex in Public Places.* Chicago: Aldine.

Isay, R.A. 1988. "Homosexuaity in Heterosexual and Homosexual Men." *Psychiatric Annals* 18(1):43–46.

Job, R.F.S. 1988. "Effective and Ineffective Use of Fear in Health Promotion Campaigns." *American Journal of Public Health* 78:163–167.

Jones, E.F., Forrest, J.D., Goldman, N., Henshaw, S.K., Lincoln, R., Rosoff, J.I., Westoff, C.F., and Wulf, D. 1985. "Teenage Pregnancy in Developed Countries: Determinants and Policy Implications." *Family Planning Perspectives* 17(2):53–63.

Judson, F.N., Miller, K.G., and Schaffnit, T.R. 1977. "Screening for Gonorrhea and Syphilis in the Gay Baths—Denver, Colorado." *American Journal of Public Health* 67:740–742.

Kalman, T.P., Kalman, C.M., and Douglas, C.J. 1987. "Homophobia Among Physicians and Nurses Treating AIDS Patients." *American Journal of Psychiatry* 144(11):1514–1515.

Kandel, D.B. 1985. "On Processes of Peer Influences in Adolescent Drug Use: A Developmental Perspective." B. Stimmel (Ed.), *Alcohol and Substance Abuse in Adolescence.* New York: Haworth Press.

Kandel, D.B., and Logan, J.A. 1984. "Patterns of Drug Use from Adolescence to Young Adulthood: I. Periods of Risk for Initiation, Continued Use, and Discontinuation." *American Journal of Public Health* 74:660–666.

Karlen, A. 1980. "Homosexuality in History." In J. Marmor (Ed.), *Homosexual Behavior: A Modern Reappraisal.* New York: Basic Books.

Kelly, J.A., St. Lawrence, J.S., Smith, S., Jr., Hood, H.V., and Cook, D.J. 1987. "Medical Students' Attitudes Toward AIDS and Homosexual Patients." *Journal of Medical Education* 62:549–556.

Kerr, P. 1988. "Experts Find Fault in New AIDS Plan." *New York Times* Februry 7, 7.

Kingsley, L.A., Kaslow, R.A., Rinaldo, C.R., Detre, K., Odaka, N., Van Raden, M., Detels, R., Polk, B.F., Chmiel, J., Kelsey, S.F., Ostrow, D.G., and Visscher, B. 1987. "Risk Factors for Seroconversion to Human Immunodeficiency Virus Among Male Homosexuals." *Lancet* i(8529):345–349.

Kolata, G. 1988. "Perplexed Counselors and the Facts of Life." *New York Times* May 16, A13.

Kotler, P. 1984. "Social Marketing of Health Behavior." In L.W. Frederiksen, L.J. Solomon, and K.A. Brehony (Eds.), *Marketing Health Behavior.* New York: Plenum.

Kotler, P., and Levy, S. 1969. "Broadening the Concept of Marketing." *Journal of Marketing* 33:10–15.

Landrum, S., Beck-Saque, C., and Kraus, S. 1988. "Racial Trends in Syphilis Among Men with Same-Sex Partners in Atlanta, Georgia." *American Journal of Public Health* 78:66–67.

Leary, W.E. 1988. "Young Adults Show Drop in Cocaine Use." *New York Times* January 14, A24.

Leventhal, H., Safer, M.A., Panagis, D.M. 1983. "The Impact of Communications on the Self-Regulation of Health Beliefs, Decisions, and Behavior." *Health Education Quarterly* 10(1):3–31.

Levy, N., Carlson, J.R., Hinrichs, S., Lerche, N., and Schenker, M. 1986. "The Prevalence of HTLV-III/LAV Antibodies Among Intravenous Drug Users Attending Treatment Progarms in California: A Preliminary Report." *New England Journal of Medicine* 314(7):446.

Lewis, B.F., and Galea, R.P. 1988. "A Survey of the Perceptions of Drug Abusers Concerning the Acquired Immunodeficiency Syndrome (AIDS)." In R.P. Galea, B.F. Lewis, and L.A. Baker (Eds), *AIDS and IV Drug Abusers.* Owings Mills, Md.: National Health Publishing.

Lewis, C.E., and Lewis, M.A. 1984. "Peer Pressure and Risk-Taking Behaviors in Children." *American Journal of Public Health* 74(6):580–584.

Lohr, S. 1988. "There's No Preaching, Just the Clean Needles." *New York Times* Februry 29, A4.

McKusick, L., Conant, M.A., and Coates, T.J. 1985. "The AIDS Epidemic: A Model for Developing Intervention Strategies for Reducing High-Risk Behavior in Gay Men." *Sexually Transmitted Diseases* 12(4):229–233.

Malyon, A.K. 1981. "The Homosexual Adolescent: Developmental Issues and Social Bias." *Child Welfare* 60(5):321–330.

Manoff, R.K. 1985a. "Designing the Social Marketing Message." In R.K. Manoff, *Social Marketing: New Imperative for Public Health.* New York: Praeger.

Manoff, R.K. 1985b. "Mass Media: Social Marketing's Primary Tool." In R.K. Manoff, *Social Marketing: New Imperative for Public Health.* New York: Praeger.

Marmor, J. 1980. "Overview: The Multiple Roots of Homosexual Behavior." In J. Marmor (Ed.), *Homosexual Behavior: A Modern Reappraisal.* New York: Basic Books.

Martineau, W.H. 1977. "Informal Social Ties Among Urban Black Americans." *Journal of Black Studies* 8(1):83–104.

Mays, V.M., and Cochran, S.D. 1987. "Acquired Immunodeficiency Syndrome and Black Americans: Special Psychosocial Issues." *Public Health Reports* 102:224–231.

Mendelsohn, H. 1973. "Some Reasons Why Information Campaigns Can Succeed." *Public Opinion Quarterly* 37:50–61.

Minkler, M. 1981. "Applications of Social Support Theory to Health Education: Implications for Work with the Elderly." *Health Education Quarterly* 8:147–165.

Mitchell, R.E., and Trickett, E.J. 1980. "Task Force Report: Social Networks as Mediators of Social Support. An Analysis of the Effects and Determinants of Social Networks." *Community Mental Health Journal* 16:27–44.

Morlet, A., Guinan, J.J., Diefenthaler, I. Gold, J. 1988. "The Impact of the 'Grim Reaper' National AIDS Educational Campaign on the Albion Street (AIDS) Centre and the AIDS Hotline." *Medical Journal of Australia* 148:282–286.

Murphy, P.E. 1984. "Analyzing Markets." In L.W. Frederiksen, L.J. Solomon, and K.A. Brehony (Eds.), *Marketing Health Behavior*. New York: Plenum.

Murray, D.M., and Perry, C.L. 1985. "The Prevention of Adolescent Drug Abuse: Implications of Etiological, Developmental, Behaviorial, and Environmental Models." In C.L. Jones and R.J. Battjes (Eds.), *Etiology of Drug Abuse: Implications for Prevention*. National Institute on Drug Abuse Research Monograph 56. Rockville, Md.: U.S. Department of Health and Human Services.

National AIDS Network. 1987. *AIDS Education and Support Services to Minorities: A Survey of Community-Based AIDS Service Providers*. Washington, D.C.: National AIDS Network.

National Institute on Drug Abuse. 1982. "National Drug Abuse Treatment Utilization Survey." National Institute on Drug Abuse Statistical Series F, Number 10.

National Network of Runaway and Youth Services. 1985. *To Whom Do They Belong?* Washington, D.C.: National Network of Runaway and Youth Services.

Neighbors, H.W. 1984a. "Professional Help Use Among Black Americans: Implications for Unmet Need." *American Journal of Community Psychology* 12(5):551–566.

Neighbors, H.W. 1984b. "The Use of Informal and Formal Help: Four Patterns of Illness Behavior in the Black Community." *American Journal of Community Psychology* 12(6):629–644.

Newcombe, M.D., Maddahian, E., and Bentler, P.M., 1986. "Risk Factors for Drug Use Among Adolescents: Concurrent and Longitudinal Analyses." *American Journal of Public Health* 76:525–531.

Newman, R.G. 1987. "Methadone Treatment: Defining and Evaluating Success." *New England Journal of Medicine* 317(7):447–450.

Randolph, L.A., and Gersche, M. 1986. "Black Adolescent Pregnancy: Prevention and Management." *Journal of Community Health* 11:10–18.

Raveis, V.H., and Kandel, D.B. 1987. "Changes in Drug Behavior from the Middle to Late Twenties: Initiation, Persistance, and Cessation of Use." *American Journal of Public Health* 77:607–611.

Remafedi, G. 1987a. "Adolescent Homosexuality: Psychosocial and Medical Implications." *Pediatrics* 79(3):337.

Remafedi, G. 1987b. "Homosexual Youth: A Challenge to Contemporary Society." *Journal of the American Medical Association* 258(2): 222–225.

Remafedi, G. 1987c. "Male Homosexuality: The Adolescent's Perspective." *Pediatrics* 79(3):326–330.

Rivara, F.P., Sweeney, P.J., and Henderson, B.F. 1987. "Risk of Fatherhood Among Black Teenage Males." *American Journal of Public Health* 77:203–205.

Robbins, C., Kaplan, H.B., and Martin, S.S. 1985. "Antecedents of Pregnancy Among Unmarried Adolescents." *Journal of Marriage and the Family* 47:567–583.

Rogers, E.M., 1982. *Diffusion of Innovations.* New York: The Free Press.

Ross, M.W. 1985. "Psychosocial Factors in Admitting to Homosexuality in Sexually Transmitted Disease Clinics." *Sexually Transmitted Diseases* 12(2):83–87.

Ross, M.W. 1987. "Illness Behavior Among Patients Attending a Sexually Transmitted Disease Clinic." *Sexually Transmitted Diseases* 14(3): 174–179.

Saghir, M.T., Robins, E., and Walbran, B. 1969. "Homosexuality: Sexual Behavior of the Male Homosexual." *Archives of General Psychiatry* 21:219–229.

Schmalz, J. 1988. "Addicts to Get Needles in Plan to Curb AIDS." *New York Times* January 31, 1 and 12.

Scott, J.W. 1983. "The Sentiments of Love and Aspirations for Marriage and Their Association with Teenage Sexual Activity and Pregnancy." *Adolescence* 18(72):889–897.

Selwyn, P.A., Feiner, C., Cox, C.P., Lipshutz, C., and Cohen, R.L. 1987. "Knowledge About AIDS and High-Risk Behavior Among Intravenous Drug Users in New York City." *AIDS* 1(4):247–254.

Senft, K.R., Eyster, M.E., Haverstick, J., and Bartlett, G.S., 1981. "Risk-Taking and the Adolescent Hemophiliac." *Journal of Adolescent Health Care* 2(2):87–91.

Sherr, L. 1987. "An Evaluation of the U.K. Government Health Education Campaign on AIDS." *Psychology and Health* 1:61–72.

Silvestre, A., Lyter, D.W., Rinaldo, C.R., Kingsley, L.A., Forrester, R., and Huggins, J. 1986. "Marketing Strategies for Recruiting Gay Men into AIDS Research and Education Projects." *Journal of Community Health* 11(4):222–232.

Simon, R. 1982. "Family Perspectives in Chronic Illness." In M.W. Hilgartner (Ed.), *Hemophilia in the Child and Adult.* New York: Masson.

Smith, G.L. 1987. "Bisexuality: A Risk Factor for HIV Infection in Military Men." *Lancet* i(8572):1402–1403.

128   Identifying Targets of AIDS Prevention

Temoshok, L., Sweet, D.M., and Zich, J. 1987. "A Three-City Comparison of the Public's Knowledge and Attitudes About AIDS." *Psychology and Health* 1:43–60.

Troiden, R.R. 1979. "Becoming Homosexual: A Model of Gay Identity Acquisition." *Psychiatry* 42:362–373.

Warren, C. 1980. "Homosexuality and Stigma." In J. Marmor (Ed.), *Homosexual Behavior: A Modern Reappraisal.* New York: Basic Books.

Watney, S. 1987. "People's Perceptions of the Risk of AIDS and the Role of the Mass Media." *Health Education Journal* 46(2):62–65.

Weinberg, D.S., and Murray, H.W. 1987. "Coping with AIDS: The Special Problems of New York City." *New England Journal of Medicine* 317(23):1469–1473.

Wilkerson, I. 1988. "Two Decades of Decline Chronicled by Kerner Follow-Up Report." *New York Times* March 1, A12.

Williams, L.S. 1986. "AIDS Risk Reduction: A Community Health Education Intervention for Minority High-Risk Group Members." *Health Education Quarterly* 13(4):407–421.

Worden, J.K., Costanza, M.C., Foster, R.S., Jr., Lang, S.P., and Tidd, C.A. 1983. "Content and Context in Health Education: Persuading Women to Perform Breast Self-Examination." *Preventive Medicine* 12:331–339.

Yamaguchi, K., and Kandel, D.B. 1984. "Patterns of Drug Use from Adolescence to Young Adulthood: III. Predictors for Progression." *American Journal of Public Health* 74:673–681.

Zelnick, M., and Kantner, J.F. 1979. "Reasons for Nonuse of Contraception by Sexually Active Women Aged 15–19." *Family Planning Perspectives* 11:289–296.

Zeltzer, L., Kellerman, J., Ellenberg, L., Dash, J., and Rigler, D. 1980. "Psychologic Effects of Illness in Adolescence: II. Impact of Illness in Adolescents—Crucial Issues and Coping Styles." *Journal of Pediatrics* 97(1):132–138.

Chapter 5

Planning and Implementing
AIDS-Prevention Programs:
A Case Study Approach

Many of the same variables that are important for success in target group identification and outreach are equally important in the actual design of prevention programs. This fact, perhaps more than any other, emphasizes the significance and interrelatedness of all of the components of a prevention program and reminds us that prevention programs are more than the actual intervention or services provided to a target population. Instead, they encompass the manner in which target populations are identified and approached with information about the program; the design of the program, including specific recommendations about preventive behaviors; the manner in which the information is presented; the setting in which the services are delivered; the ease of access with which members of the target population can participate in the program; the relationships, both formal and informal, that the program maintains with other community resources; and the manner in which the efficacy of the program is evaluated.

This chapter will discuss a variety of American organizations that are involved in some aspect of AIDS prevention at the time of this writing (refer to Appendixes 1 and 2). They include the following: Association for Drug Abuse Prevention and Treatment (ADAPT), Brooklyn, New York; AIDS Lifeline, KPIX-TV, San Francisco; AIDS Prevention Project, Dallas County Health Department, Texas; AIDS Prevention Project, University of Pittsburgh, Pennsylvania; AIDS Resource Center, Dallas, Texas; Blacks Educating Blacks About Sexual Health Issues (BEBASHI), Philadelphia, Pennsylvania; Beth Israel's Methadone Maintenance Treatment Program, New York, New York; Gay Men's Health Crisis, New York, New York; Health Crisis Network, Dade County, Florida; Health Education and Risk Reduction Program, Dade County, Florida; Hemophilia Center of

Western Pennsylvania, Pittsburgh, Pennsylvania; New Jersey State Department of Health, Division of Narcotics and Drug Abuse Control, East Orange, New Jersey; and the San Francisco AIDS Foundation (SFAF), San Francisco, California. Some of these organizations are devoted exclusively to the prevention of HIV infection. Others provide services related to HIV prevention as part of a larger program (only their HIV-prevention services will be considered in this discussion). The intent of this chapter is not to present a compendium of American AIDS prevention services nor is it to evaluate programs identified in this analysis. Instead, the intent is to use specific examples from each program to illustrate fundamental concepts in the design and development of effective AIDS risk reduction programs.

We concur with the American Public Health Association (APHA) that health promotion represents a "wide variety of individual and community efforts to encourage or support health behavior" and that it may include "educational, organizational, economic, and environmental interventions" (Ad Hoc Work Group . . . 1987:89). We will also adopt their definition of the term "health education" as "learning experiences designed to assist individuals, groups, or communities in the voluntary control of their own health, as they define it" (p. 89).

Although the American Public Health Association's "Criteria for the Development of Health Promotion and Education Programs" (1987) were developed as guidelines "for establishing the feasibility and/or the appropriateness" of prevention programs (p. 89), for our purposes they will be used as generic standards by which program planners can guide their efforts (Appendix 3). Each of the five criteria will be presented sequentially, and their applications to the specific goal of preventing HIV infection will be discussed using examples from the organizations listed above.

Criterion 1: "A HEALTH PROMOTION PROGRAM SHOULD ADDRESS ONE OR MORE RISK FACTORS WHICH ARE CAREFULLY DEFINED, MEASURABLE, MODIFIABLE, AND PREVALENT AMONG THE MEMBERS OF A CHOSEN TARGET GROUP, FACTORS WHICH CONSTITUTE A THREAT TO THE HEALTH STATUS AND THE QUALITY OF LIFE OF TARGET GROUP MEMBERS" (Ad Hoc Work Group . . . 1987:89).

Almost everyone would agree that HIV infection is a threat to both the health status and quality of life of target group members, and scientists are in agreement about the behaviors that transmit this virus. Yet there may be a lack of consensus as to the identification of "risk factors," that is, behaviors that place an individual at increased risk for infection with HIV, and their relative importance in the process of prioritizing risk. The way an organization defines risk for HIV infection will influence the way it attempts to modify that risk, so this becomes one of the first issues to be resolved in the process of program development.

When we consider the sexual transmission of HIV, for example, just what is riskful behavior? Is it sexual intercourse with a person who is infected with HIV or at risk for infection, or is it a specific sexual act that is considered to carry a significant risk of infection? The former definition requires that individuals have accurate information about their partners' past behaviors and be aware of the HIV serostatus of all of their partners in order to reduce or eliminate their own risk of infection. The latter definition implies that persons should avoid specific sexual practices that carry a high risk of infection, and that they need not be aware of their partners' serostatus in order to protect themselves.

If we define risk in terms of specific sexual practices that are particularly effective in transmitting this virus, we must decide whether to advise *elimination* of those behaviors from the sexual repertoire, or *modification*, so that the risk is minimized to an acceptable level. If we advise eliminating certain behaviors altogether, we assume that individuals have no preferences regarding various sexual activities, and would be willing to substitute one behavior (which is low risk) for another (which is high risk). We also assume that an approach that is primarily informational (that is, "don't do this because it is dangerous to your health") will be persuasive enough to change behavior. Neither of these assumptions is supported by existing data or theory (see Chapter Three).

In actuality, there is no single sexual risk reduction message that is relevant to everyone, and all of the options listed above should be offered as strategies to reduce the risk of sexually acquired HIV infection. Celibacy is the safest and surest way to prevent infection with a sexually acquired pathogen. But, since it is unlikely that everyone will comply with such advice, it is included as one of several options. The philosophy of AIDS prevention should recognize the importance of reducing risk, even when it cannot be completely eliminated.

Risk-reduction interventions must include a range of choices that recognize and accommodate the various circumstances of the persons for whom they are intended. A married couple in which the husband is a young HIV-infected hemophiliac may not be willing to eliminate vaginal intercourse from their relationship, but may be quite amenable to using condoms and nonoxynol-9. A gay man who is not in a monogamous relationship may be willing to exclude anal intercourse from casual sexual encounters, but that same man, after becoming emotionally involved with a new partner, may wish to engage in condom-protected anal intercourse. A single college-age male may be aware of the possibility of HIV infection, but unwilling to remain celibate because he believes his risk of infection is minimal. These few examples emphasize the variability that can attend the definition and perception of risk for both program planners and the intended audience of the prevention program.

A consistent observation among the programs listed above was the importance of offering options to the clients in terms of reducing their risk of sexually acquired HIV infection. While many of these programs identified monogamy with an uninfected partner as an ideal adaptation to the AIDS epidemic, none limited their prevention message to this single recommendation. Nor did they unilaterally advise the complete elimination of specific sexual acts. Instead, they endorsed the modification of high-risk sexual behaviors in ways that would substantially reduce or negate the degree of risk. Prevention programs for gay and bisexual men uniformly stressed the danger of engaging in anal intercourse, especially for the receptive partner, and tended to offer clients the following two options: either eliminate this behavior or reduce its potential danger by the proper and consistent use of condoms and spermicides. In Beth Israel's methadone maintenance program, men and women who are being treated for heroin addiction are counseled about the risks of sexual and perinatal transmission of HIV, and are urged to use condoms with their sexual partners; they are not counseled to stop having sexual intercourse.

The offering of prevention options other than monogamy or celibacy is sometimes labeled as counterproductive, especially by groups that consider mutually monogamous, heterosexual intercourse within the confines of marriage as the only acceptable form of sexual expression (Steinfels 1988). Others may criticize the practice of offering options that carry any degree of risk, such as condom-protected intercourse—which can be associated with both product and user failure (Centers for Disease Control 1988a:134). Issues such as these are not uncommon in discussions of sexual risk reduction and should be addressed from the perspective that if risk behavior cannot be eliminated, it must be modified to decrease the chances of infection.

In the most specific sense, persons who use intravenous drugs are not at risk for HIV infection because of their drug use but rather because of the practices of sharing needles or using improperly cleaned syringes that are contaminated with HIV-laden blood. Eliminating the need to inject intravenous drugs by treating the underlying substance abuse problem is a logical step in reducing the risk of HIV infection. However, limiting AIDS-prevention initiatives among intravenous drug users to recruitment into treatment programs assumes that all drug users would be immediately willing to cease their drug use and that there are adequate treatment facilities available to accommodate them after they have made their decision to quit. It also assumes that once persons decide to stop using intravenous drugs, they will never again inject these substances. All of these assumptions are fallacious.

Many of the clinicians who were interviewed for this chapter agreed that, ultimately, most substance abusers want to enter treatment, but they cautioned that this does not usually happen until after the user becomes disenchanted with the drug and can no longer cope with the demands of the addiction. There is a general consensus that existing facilities for the treatment of intravenous drug users are inadequate, and according to the Presidential Commission on the Human Immunodeficiency Virus Epidemic, "the lack of treatment capacity has produced long waiting lists for treatment, in some cases up to six months" (Watkins et al. 1988:96). Although the number of available treatment facilities is expected to increase in the near future (Boffey 1988a), even drug users in treatment exhibit recidivism. Furthermore, treatment may not be an appropriate option from the perspective of occasional users who are not addicted to the drugs they inject but who are still at risk for HIV infection because they share contaminated needles and syringes. Finally, for certain drugs that can be injected, such as cocaine, there are no replacement therapies equivalent to methadone maintenance for heroin addiction. Therefore, if the HIV risk reduction message to intravenous drug users is limited to "stop injecting drugs," it will pass unheeded by many active and occasional users. As with sexual risk reduction, it is necessary to offer a variety of options.

In all of the programs visited, the primary message was to seek treatment to end drug-using behavior, but this was followed by a message that urged people who continue to inject drugs not to share needles and syringes. Or, if they do so, to first clean the needle and syringe with household bleach. This hierarchy of advice can sometimes precipitate the charge that these programs are encouraging drug use. Such accusations represent a misunderstanding of the programs' intentions. The primary objective of AIDS-prevention programs for IV drug users is to interrupt the transmission of HIV. Eliminating the need to inject drugs is one of the means of achieving this goal, but it should not be the only one, since it fails to accommodate persons who are unwilling to enter treatment or who might relapse either during or after treatment.

Because AIDS is an outcome of HIV infection and not sexual intercourse or IV drug use per se, there are ultimately no sexual or needle-use behaviors that can lead to HIV infection if they are limited to persons who are not infected. In view of this, there are those who believe that risk should be defined by testing for the presence of HIV infection. They reason that with widespread testing, risk can be consistently defined as HIV seropositivity rather than as the ability of a particular behavior to transmit the virus.

However, there are dangers in categorizing risk exclusively on the basis of HIV seropositivity. In some cases of sexually acquired HIV infection, a person may be infected, yet fail to react positively to the HIV antibody test for as long as six to fourteen months after exposure (Ranki et al. 1987:589). This observation is consistent with earlier work that documented that the virus can be recovered by culture from persons who are asymptomatic and antibody negative (Groopman et al. 1985; Salahuddin et al. 1984). Even among individuals who do not exhibit a long latency period between infection and seroconversion, antibodies to HIV that are detectable by commercially available tests may take, on average, thirty-one to fifty-eight days to develop (Cooper et al. 1987:1115). Therefore, it is possible for an individual to be infected with HIV and capable of transmitting the virus to sexual and needle-sharing partners, even in the presence of a negative antibody test. Repeated testing over time is one potential solution to this problem, but it will result in additional expense, especially if it is implemented on a large scale.

Sivak and Wormser (1986) have demonstrated that the prevalence of HIV infection within a population has an impact on the positive and negative predictive values of the test, that is, how likely a positive test is to identify infected individuals and how likely a negative test is to identify persons who are truly free of infection. Sivak and Wormser estimated that "in the general population" (those people who do not belong to groups having a recognized increased risk of

HIV infection) the positive predictive value of a screening test for antibodies to HIV was between .6 percent and 2.7 percent, meaning
that "more than 97 percent of positive tests will be falsely positive"
(p. 702). The negative predictive value of the test among persons
from the general population, however, is "exceedingly high" (p.
702), meaning that a person who tests negative and has no history of
riskful behaviors is almost certainly uninfected.

Another potential pitfall in defining risk solely on the basis of HIV
serostatus, rather than on the potential for a behavior to result in
transmission, is the unpleasant reality that not all human interac-
tions are characterized by honesty or mutual respect. Individuals
might misrepresent their HIV serostatus to their sexual or needle-
sharing partners, for reasons of personality, circumstance, malice, or
sheer inability to communicate this information accurately. Because they realize that their sexual or drug-use opportunities could
be adversely affected, or terminated, should they volunteer this
information, they may be loath to supply it. A disheartening manifestation of the desire to define risk solely on the basis of HIV serostatus, is the rise of commercial enterprises that sell "seronegative
cards" to uninfected individuals as a means of "ensuring" safe sexual encounters. At best such ventures are naive, at worst they are
potentially negligent.

Undoubtedly, counseling and testing for HIV infection will become more widespread, especially as monies for these activites are
increased and as legislation that protects the confidentiality of test
results and prohibits discrimination against HIV-infected persons is
enacted. The achievement of these circumstances notwithstanding,
it is important to realize that not everyone will want to be tested.
Testing for HIV infection is associated with a number of potent psychological and sociological issues. For example, some people may be
hesitant to submit to testing because they fear they would be unable
to "cope" with a positive test result (Lyter et al. 1987:471). Several
clinicians interviewed for this chapter were concerned that individuals currently in treatment for addictive intravenous drug use might
suffer relapse upon receiving a positive HIV antibody test.

These observations are not meant to minimize the importance of
HIV counseling and testing but to caution against relying solely on
test results in defining risk for HIV infection and the need for information about AIDS prevention. Informing people of their HIV serostatus does not guarantee that they will modify their behaviors in
the direction of AIDS risk reduction, nor is it necessary for them to
know their HIV serostatus in order to reduce their risk of acquiring

or transmitting HIV. In none of the programs visited was knowledge of HIV serostatus a prerequisite for a client to receive or to act upon risk-reduction information.

Most of the programs tended to categorize HIV counseling and testing as important tools in the approach to preventing HIV infection, but all emphasized changed behavior rather than testing as the most important product of their service. Programs within state or local health departments were inclined to emphasize testing more than those within community-based organizations; this is a manifestation of the traditional public health practice of screening large numbers of individuals for the early identification of persons at risk for a health problem or in need of treatment. However, the therapeutic options we can offer HIV-infected individuals are currently limited; this strategy may be far more effective when we can offer HIV-infected persons immediate treatment.

Although this criterion addresses risk as a definable, quantifiable, and modifiable fact, the persons for whom we are planning prevention programs may not perceive risk in a similar way. Among both heterosexuals (Siegel and Gibson 1988:67) and homosexuals (Jones et al. 1987; Valdiserri et al. 1988b) a major barrier to sexual behavior change may be the failure to perceive or fully accept how their own personal circumstances contribute to their risk of HIV infection. It is not just in the area of sexually transmitted diseases that we encounter this resistance. A review of published investigations based on the Health Belief Model (HBM) found "susceptibility" (feelings of personal vulnerability to a condition) to be significantly associated with the preventive health behaviors in 81 percent of the studies reviewed (Janz 1984:41).

Risks can be misjudged because of "difficulties in understanding probabilistic processes, biased media coverage, misleading personal experiences, and the anxieties generated by life's gambles" (Slovic 1987:281). Strong initial views of a subject influence the way subsequent information is processed (Slovic 1987:281), so individuals who initially learned about AIDS as a disease of highly promiscuous, urban, gay men and intravenous drug users may have difficulty appreciating their own risk of infection if they do not fit into either category—even though more recent information has expanded our understanding that HIV infection can be transmitted by heterosexual intercourse and that it may not require sexual activity with multiple partners.

Criterion 2: "A HEALTH PROMOTION PROGRAM SHOULD RE-
FLECT A CONSIDERATION OF THE SPECIAL CHARACTERISTICS,

NEEDS, AND PREFERENCES OF ITS TARGET GROUP(S)" (Ad Hoc Work Group . . . 1987:90).

This criterion was first introduced in Chapter Four, when the point was made that health-promotion programs must be acceptable to the individuals for whom they are planned. Although this advice is eminently rational, it belies the complex, at times murky, process by which behavior actually changes. While psychologically based theories stress the individual variables that influence the adoption of new behaviors, the more sociologically anchored theories of behavior change emphasize the process by which group norms influence individual patterns of behavior. The interplay between individual and group motives as they pertain to behavioral change is intricate and at times overlapping.

It sometimes seems as if the distinction between individual and group change is an arbitrary one, and most theoreticians recognize elements of both in the process of health-behavior change. For example, it is likely that individuals who are receptive to change are aided in the process if their peer groups uphold the changed behavior as a desirable group norm. It is also well known that utilizing group-specific sources of information that the target population views as "credible," whether these sources are community leaders or specific forms of media, can help to facilitate change at an individual level (Nelkin 1987:982; Solomon and DeJong 1986:306). Therefore, when dealing with a health problem such as HIV infection, in which groups that are disproportionately at risk of exposure (generally because of high background seroprevalence among their members) can also be categorized as minorities or subcultures, it is essential that we attend to the dynamics of the change process for the entire group and not limit our interest to change at an individual level.

Behavioral changes necessary to prevent HIV transmission can be considered as innovations. Studies on the diffusion of innovation emphasize the importance of communication of new ideas "through certain channels, over time, among the members of a social system" (Rogers and Shoemaker 1971:18). As Rogers and Shoemaker explain in their work on the diffusion of innovations, the most effective communication occurs when both the source and the receiver of a message are from similar backgrounds, a characteristic that they refer to as "homophily" (p. 14). They also emphasize that the social structure of a group can have significant effects on the behavior of individuals within that group. Referring to "system effects" that are mediated by group norms, practices, and social status within a group, Rogers and Shoemaker explain that the social structure actually influences the behavior of individuals within that system and that it can impede or facilitate the rate of diffusion and adoption of new ideas or practices (p. 29).

For example, if a group norm, such as needle sharing, has traditionally been associated with feelings of fraternity and bonding, it may be difficult for intravenous drug users to eliminate that behavior with close friends and sexual partners. Among ethnic groups who condone premarital sexual activity only when it is the consequence of unbridled passion, the use of condoms to prevent HIV infection will be rejected because it implies premeditation of sexual intercourse, which is antithetical to group beliefs.

Our earlier discussion of social networks presaged the significance of social systems in the transmission of innovations, in this instance, behavioral innovations that can reduce the likelihood of HIV infection. How individuals within a specific group communicate with one another, what values they commonly uphold, and how various behaviors are viewed by members of that group all have practical implications for the planning of targeted AIDS-prevention programs.

On the basis of these theoretical considerations, it is important to assess the role of the target group itself in disseminating information about AIDS risk reduction. As a specific example, the Centers for Disease Control report decreasing incidence of new HIV infection among homosexual men (1987a:13). This is probably owing, in part, to the response by gay men as a group to the threat of HIV infection and to their social systems and networks being used increasingly to support and amplify the message that modification of sexual behavior can prevent HIV infection. Conversely, among groups that do not see AIDS as a threat, whose social systems are not being used to spread and reinforce messages about behavioral change, we would expect to see a slower diffusion of innovations relating to behavioral change.

If program planners believe that behavioral change takes place in a unidimensional mode—that is, that information about the danger of certain behaviors will directly result in behavioral change—they may consider target group participation in program planning and implementation to be unnecessary. They may assume that using media channels to transmit information about behaviors that are associated with an increased risk of HIV infection would be sufficient to bring about the desired behavioral changes, and not appreciate that interpersonal channels of communication "are more effective in forming and changing attitudes toward the new idea" (Rogers and Shoemaker 1971:39), that is, in persuading persons to act on the information they have received by adopting new behaviors. They might also underestimate the importance of tailoring the program so that the innovation (the changed behavior) is viewed as compatible with group norms (p. 22). They may fail to appreciate the fact that while the individual may be the actual agent in whom the behavioral change is manifest, the group is the entity that promotes and reinforces this change.

State and local departments of health will be "held responsible for surveillance and control of the HIV epidemic" (Judson and Vernon 1988:387), and their prevention efforts are likely to emphasize client education, information dissemination, and HIV antibody testing and counseling. Although these are important functions in the campaign against AIDS, these activities, by themselves, are probably inadequate for reinforcing individuals' behavioral change through the process of influencing group norms. It is unlikely that these organizations will have the expertise, the authority (within the target groups), or perhaps, even the inclination to become directly involved in the kinds of activities that are necessary to change norms within the groups they need to reach. Client services at most departments of health are usually structured as a system of clinics to which individuals present for a distinct service. Such a structure is not well suited to the task of modulating behavioral norms, an activity that, by definition, is often carried out in locations where the behaviors are actually taking place.

AIDS education and condom distribution programs in gay bars and movie houses, workshops that attempt to eroticize safer sex, condom distribution programs for prostitutes on the streets, education about HIV transmission in juvenile detention centers where youth may be engaging in homosexual activities (although they are not self-identified as "gay"), and health education about the dangers of needle sharing and the need to clean needles and syringes with bleach in neighborhoods where the use of intravenous drugs is especially prevalent are examples of the kinds of activities that are capable of changing behavioral norms but that are impossible to conduct in a structured clinic setting.

In many instances, intensive promotion and long-term maintenance of behavioral change will devolve to the target community itself. Planners need to envision this development and work toward empowering target groups to successfully carry out this responsibility. Empowerment will often take the form of subcontract funding to community-based organizations that offer prevention services to clients who are at increased risk of HIV infection. Departments of health in many states, including California, Florida, New Jersey, New York, and Texas, have followed this route.

Individuals at increased risk for HIV infection often belong to socially disenfranchised segments of society. Many are economically disadvantaged as well. For these individuals, the subject of preventing HIV infection may be difficult to extricate from other concerns they harbor as minority group members. People who are beset with economic, social, psychological, or medical problems, may see AIDS as "simply another risk" (Goldsmith 1988:642), and this attitude can influence the manner in which they respond to organized initiatives to combat its spread. Gay men, for example, were widely suspicious of initial attempts to advocate changes in sexual behavior, "even those promulgated by their own advocacy organizations," because they perceived them as attempts to "undermine sexual identity" (Solomon and DeJong 1986:308). African-Americans had difficulties accepting their risk of HIV infection early in the epidemic, when much of the publicity centered on homosexuals (Mays and Cochran 1987), because they did not want to add to their already stigmatized status. Hispanics were also initially loath to address the problem of epidemic HIV infection because of its strong association with intravenous drug use and homosexuality (Friedman et al. 1987). Groups whose behaviors routinely place them in conflict with the legal system, such as prostitutes and intravenous drug users, are suspicious of risk-reduction initiatives that come from the establishment because of their past, usually negative, experiences with that sector.

It may also be difficult for program planners themselves to extricate their own feelings about a particular target group from the process of planning a targeted AIDS risk reduction program. Even if they understand the logic of an approach that incorporates target group norms and values, they may face tremendous resistance from outside agencies and other interested parties. Ambivalence and conflicting motives are apparent in the ongoing debate that characterizes the promotion of sexual risk reduction among homosexual men as an "endorsement" of the "gay life-style" (Booth 1987:1036), and in discussions that equate education on needle cleaning and sterile needle distribution programs with the facilitation of IV drug use (Fineberg 1988:595). The subject of AIDS prevention among sexually active adolescents is no less controversial and has revived the long-standing argument that educating youth about the prevention of sexually transmitted diseases is tantamount to encouraging premarital sexual activity (Kroger and Wiesner 1981).

Differences between minority and majority perspectives are unlikely to dissolve in the face of AIDS. Despite the lack of widespread endorsement for certain minority positions, cooperation of target groups is nonetheless widely recognized as necessary for the success of AIDS-prevention initiatives. All of the programs mentioned in this chapter have incorporated some mechanism, either formal or informal, that permits feedback from the target group.

The Association for Drug Abuse Prevention and Treatment (ADAPT) involves ex-drug users as both volunteers and board members. Paid outreach workers who visit "shooting galleries" to educate active drug users about the availability of treatment for their addiction, how to clean their "works", and how to use condoms, are encouraged to become intimately familiar with the subculture of intravenous drug users—short of injecting drugs themselves. Their familiarity with the mores of this group—often derived from their own past experience—enables them to anticipate many of the objections to preventive behaviors expressed by active users and to empathize with the difficulties their clients face in adapting to the threat of AIDS. From a social science perspective, their homophily makes it possible for them to gain access to the social system of IV drug users for the purpose of disseminating information about innovative behaviors. This strategy is also employed by the New Jersey State Health Department, where former intravenous drug users are hired as outreach workers to distribute coupons that entitle the bearer (active intravenous drug users who have not been in any form of drug treatment for the previous twelve months) to free heroin detoxification (Winerip 1988).

In group sessions, clinical staff members in Beth Israel's Methadone Maintenance Treatment Program have learned that among their clients' most important needs is information about how to discuss condoms—especially with partners who may be unaware of the client's history of intravenous drug use. Once this need was recognized, the staff created workshops in which clients could develop the communication and negotiation skills they needed to adopt condom use.

The Health Crisis Network (HCN) of Miami has an extensive system of advisory committees for a variety of target groups, including women, native-born African-Americans, Haitian blacks, Hispanic blacks, gay and bisexual men, teenagers, and people addicted to intravenous drugs. On the advice of these groups, HCN has been able to develop materials and programs that are culturally and ethnically sensitive. For example, an educational session on HIV infection targeted to Hispanic men did not refer to AIDS in the title because doing so often dissuades people from attending; instead it was entitled "How to Have an Affair Safer." Similarly, in designing AIDS-prevention programs for high school students, HCN plans to train one or two representatives from area high schools in the basics of HIV infection and prevention. These students will act as local resources in their schools. The active participation of adolescent advisors will help to ensure that issues relevant to adolescents will be a focus of the prevention work.

Program staff of south Florida's Health Education and Risk Reduction Program have learned that Haitian women have a strong cultural tradition of fatalism. Even after being told they are infected with HIV, they may not be willing to prevent conception because they believe that the outcome of the pregnancy (for example, whether they will have a healthy or infected baby) is determined by "fate" and is God's decision rather than their own. Efforts to prevent vertical transmission in this group must identify equally compelling cultural rationalizations for preventing perinatal infection. This will require guidance from the Haitian community.

The AIDS Prevention Project at the University of Pittsburgh evaluated a risk-reduction intervention designed to increase communication skills that would facilitate the negotiation of safer sexual practices among gay and bisexual men. The responsibility for developing this training module was subcontracted to a local community-based counseling agency that specialized in psychological and support services for sexual minority group members. The agency personnel's experience with sexual minorities greatly facilitated both their ability to develop this intervention and to gain its acceptance by the gay and bisexual men enrolled in this evaluation.

Gay Men's Health Crisis of New York has pioneered the development of workshop techniques that promote the acceptance of safer sexual behavior among gay men by eroticizing these practices. The organization itself was founded by members of the gay community in response to the burgeoning AIDS epidemic. Because their approach addresses homosexuality in an affirmative manner, it is considered controversial, especially by those who believe that homosexuality is immoral (Booth 1987:1036). Controversy notwithstanding, their interventions are based upon firsthand knowledge of the gay community and a realization of unmet needs within that community.

BEBASHI uses focus groups of black teenagers for feedback on the design and promotion of AIDS-prevention messages, and has found this approach to be especially effective in uncovering deficits in specific AIDS-prevention skills. For example, information from focus groups indicates that many people need to learn the "skill" of bringing up the subject of condoms with a new sexual partner. Information from the focus group is then incorporated into ongoing program development, so that this deficit can be corrected.

The San Francisco AIDS Foundation uses marketing campaigns as a major tool for educating target populations about preventing HIV infection. This group has consistently relied on preliminary market research, not only to uncover deficits in information but also to suggest approaches that would reflect the concerns and sensitivities of their intended audience. Their initial probability sample of urban male homosexuals suggested that "campaign messages emphasizing the social acceptability of safe sex may be more effective than messages that stress only the risks of unsafe practices" (Research and Decisions Corporation 1984:16). A subsequent study of heterosexuals with multiple or high-risk partners revealed that less than one-third of the sample felt personally threatened by AIDS and that the epidemic has had little impact on the frequency of unprotected vaginal intercourse (Research and Decisions Corporation 1986:2). The survey further revealed that heterosexual men were more likely than women to minimize the importance of AIDS risk reduction (Research and Decisions Corporation 1986:4). This information resulted in an AIDS-prevention campaign targeted to heterosexual women.

These examples illustrate the value of attending to the needs of target groups in the design of AIDS-prevention programs. Certainly this goal is facilitated within organizations whose mission is to provide some form of service to the target group. Clinical staff from regional hemophilia treatment centers are aware of the needs of their clients after years of caring for them. Doctors and nurses working at a primary health care facility in a low-income African-American neighborhood understand and can anticipate patient reactions to frank discussions of AIDS and its prevention. Organizations that specialize in the treatment of intravenous drug use appreciate the array of economic, medical, and psychosocial problems confronting the active user, and will address these issues in the design of AIDS-prevention programs. Social service agencies for homeless youth realize that prostitution is a means of survival for their clients and will develop AIDS-prevention programs that have a programatic component enabling homeless youth to support themselves in ways other than prostitution. Because of their knowledge of the populations they serve, these organizations are positioned to develop AIDS-prevention programs that are attuned to clients' needs. Of course, this experience must be melded to comparable AIDS-specific expertise and to economic support for this expansion of mission. The AIDS expertise can come from the public health establishment or from other community-based organizations whose mission is to provide services to HIV-infected clients.

Another way to create programs that are acceptable to a specific target population is to hire members of the targeted racial, ethnic, or sexual minority group to work either as full-time program staff or as consultants to the program. Although this strategy enhances the effectiveness of outreach activities, using target group members to promote or deliver a service is not the same as giving them a voice in program design, and does not, by itself, ensure that the second APHA criterion will be achieved. Furthermore, it is unrealistic to expect one person from a minority group to represent all of the diverse elements of that group. Therefore, to increase the likelihood that AIDS-prevention programs will reflect the special characteristics of their intended target groups, planners should work with individuals and organizations who have prior programmatic experience with the target group and who can base their advice on professional knowledge rather than merely on a particular personal attribute, such as skin color or shared sexual preference.

Building the target group's "characteristics, needs, and preferences" (Ad Hoc Work Group . . . 1987:90) into a risk-reduction program is, as any marketing strategist will recognize, only the first step in "selling" the program to a community. After making sure the product is appropriate to the customer's needs, the marketer has to advertise the product, distribute it, and price it to permit a reasonable exchange between buyer and seller (Assael 1985:3). Although, historically, health-related programs have not been marketed with the same intensity as commercial ventures, that situation is clearly changing for health care in general and for AIDS risk reduction programs in particular.

It is very useful to look at AIDS-prevention programs as a problem in "social marketing" (Kotler and Levy 1969), subject to the same general principles as commercial marketing. The concept of social marketing applies directly to the task of identifying the target population and to the larger job of developing and "selling" a risk-reduction product to a particular group.

In the commercial sense, advertising is a promotional activity that stimulates the consumption of a product, and the direction that advertising campaigns take is often dictated by the needs of the consumers for whom the product is intended (Assael 1985:131). In the social marketing of AIDS-prevention programs, advertising includes any activity that will encourage people to participate in the program. Based on their knowledge of the target group, planners should develop promotional messages that captialize on a group attribute. These messages can be conveyed by mass media or word of mouth, but to ensure a high degree of penetration into the social system or network of the target population, the means of transmission and the message must be compatible with target group norms. Messages that are too difficult to understand, perceived as judgmental, alien to the norms of the target group, threatening, or hostile will not be effective.

In commerce, "distribution" refers to the placement of a product in order to optimize its consumption. In the social marketing of AIDS-prevention programs, it is often necessary to decentralize prevention services in order to reach persons engaging in high-risk behaviors who would not otherwise be accessible. Planners should, therefore, expect that many of their services will be delivered off-site. AIDS-prevention services may be offered in locales as diverse as "shooting galleries," prisons and correctional facilities, classrooms, gay bars, bathhouses, and movie houses, welfare offices, topless bars, massage parlors, adult cinemas, housing projects, and street corners. In order to successfully "distribute" AIDS-prevention programs in these locales, program planners must be entirely familiar with their target populations. In many instances they will need to rely on target group representatives to disseminate prevention information in these settings.

Although "price" in commercial marketing generally refers to the money charged for the product, in the social marketing of AIDS prevention, materials and services are often distributed free of charge. However, this does not mean that there is no cost to the consumer. Client cooperation involves the expenditure of time and effort, and other intangibles may be involved in program participation; these should be considered to be real costs (Alexander and McCullough 1981:216–217). A bisexual man who fears disclosure of his homosexual activities may be hesitant to attend an educational meeting on AIDS in his community. The cost of participation for him is the fear and discomfort he experiences in risking disclosure. For a young homosexual who is ambivalent about his sexual preference, participation in an AIDS-prevention program may provoke anxiety related to unresolved conflict about his sexuality. Intravenous drug users who, for whatever reasons, are not ready to enter treatment, may consider AIDS-prevention programs that stress elimination of drug-using behaviors as too "costly" to participate in. Hemophiliac adolescents are likely to resent the additional burden that HIV infection places on their sociosexual development. Recognizing their infectious state requires more than just submitting to HIV counseling and testing; they must also accept the fact that they are capable of transmitting infection to sexual partners — and this is likely to result in significant emotional costs. Prostitutes may be hesitant to participate in AIDS-prevention programs that are closely linked with the criminal justice system because they fear self-incrimination. If program planners are unaware of these nonmonetary costs, they may have unrealistic expectations about the acceptability of their programs.

For a number of different reasons, therefore, it is essential that programs be designed with the needs of the target group as a fundamental consideration. This goal can only be achieved by communicating with target groups and incorporating their perceptions into product design and implementation. Whether it is through the use of probability sample surveys (for example, San Francisco AIDS Foundation), focus groups to review and refine AIDS-prevention messages (as is done by the Dallas County Health Department and BEBASHI), active advisory boards (Health Crisis Network), feedback from clients (Beth Israel Methadone Maintenance Program), or feedback from program staff and consultants who are members of the target group (AIDS Prevention Project, University of Pittsburgh, ADAPT, and New Jersey State Department of Health), a clear channel of communication between the planners and the planned-for is indispensable.

Criterion 3: "HEALTH PROMOTION PROGRAMS SHOULD INCLUDE INTERVENTIONS WHICH WILL CLEARLY AND EFFECTIVELY REDUCE A TARGETED RISK FACTOR AND ARE APPROPRIATE FOR A PARTICULAR SETTING" (Ad Hoc Work Group 1987:90).

In discussions of AIDS prevention, whether at a professional or lay level, this third criterion is usually of primary interest. Everyone would like to know what, exactly, will induce people to change their behaviors. At the outset, it must be clearly understood that there is no single answer to this question — either for HIV infection or for other health problems, such as cigarette smoking, teenage drug use, or unplanned pregnancy. In addressing the topic of human behavioral change, we must be willing to accept the premise that voluntary health-related behaviors can change for a variety of reasons, which may vary from person to person. We must also realize that we are somewhat limited by the paucity of published evaluations that deal specifically with HIV prevention. Therefore, much of our discussion of this third criterion will be based on the health theory outlined in Chapter Three, illustrated by specific programmatic examples. We will consider two broad categories of behavior in terms of their risk of transmitting HIV: sexual behavior and drug using behavior.

Although epidemic venereal infections have occurred prior to AIDS, the public health response to them has emphasized case identification and treatment rather than intensive efforts to educate clients about prevention of future episodes. The use of this medical model in efforts to control sexually transmissible diseases makes sense when the infections are treatable with conventional antibiotics or are preventable through vaccination (for example, hepatitis B virus). Because we have had affordable and accessible treatments available, we have not found it necessary to develop extensive behavioral interventions in responding to sexually transmissible infections. Furthermore, when curative therapy for HIV infection is identified, it is unlikely that we will persist in a behavioral response to prevention, not only because of our society's penchant for technologic solutions to problems but also because programs that emphasize behavioral rather than pharmacological solutions to sexually transmitted infections are relatively more expensive (because they are labor intensive) and are generally fraught with controversy over what behavioral modifications are most appropriate to advocate.

Among gay and bisexual men, it is apparent that changes in sexual behavior have occurred, and are continuing to occur, in response to the AIDS epidemic (Joseph et al. 1987; McKusick 1985b; McKusick 1985c; Martin 1987; Valdiserri 1989b; Winkelstein et al. 1987). Becker and Joseph (1988), in their review of AIDS and behavioral change, noted that "celibacy is not the preferred strategy of homosexual/bisexual men for dealing with the risk of AIDS" (p. 407), and that most men appeared to be "differentially reducing their number of sexual contacts outside of a primary relationship" and "eliminating or modifying anal intercourse by use of condoms" (p. 408). In areas of the country where the epidemic was first manifest, there is little doubt that changing sexual behaviors among gay men (Centers for Disease Control 1985; Centers for Disease Control 1987b) are reflective of changing sexual mores. In New York City and San Francisco, it is likely that the catastrophic number of deaths among gay men has accelerated normative change in this community. As early as 1985, McKusick and colleagues reported that "reduction from many to few partners was more likely to occur among those men who could remember the visual image of someone in the advanced stages of AIDS deterioration" (1985c:627).

Although behavioral risk reduction among gay men has been widespread, "it is certainly not complete" (Becker and Joseph 1988: 408). In communities where the incidence of AIDS is low, homosexual men may minimize their risk of HIV infection and continue to engage in unprotected receptive anal intercourse, a sexual practice placing them at great risk for infection (Jones et al. 1987, Valdiserri et al. 1988b). Because the seroprevalence of HIV infection in these areas may be many times greater than the actual incidence of symptomatic disease, these men run a substantial risk of becoming infected with HIV infection as a result of their behaviors (Fleming et al. 1987).

Even in areas where the incidence of AIDS is great, and one would expect profound behavioral change, there is evidence suggesting that behavioral modification is selective, and that men who are monogamous show "little reduction in suspected high-risk sexual activities, possibly because they feel protected by their monogamy" (McKusick et al. 1985b: 495). In a cross-sectional survey of 1,384 gay and bisexual men from southwestern Pennsylvania, enrolled in a prospective study of HIV infection, it was found that "men who reported multiple and/or anonymous partners within the past six months were more likely to use condoms than those reporting a single nonanonymous partner" (Valdiserri et al. 1988b:802). The authors believed that this finding might represent the minimization of HIV infection risk that can accompany a monogamous state. Bauman and Siegel, reporting on a cohort of 160 gay men in New York who were surveyed in 1985, suggested that "gay men tend to underestimate the riskiness of their sexual practices" because of "defensive posturing and cognitive distortion" (1987:343-344).

Even men who have modified their sexual practices in response to the AIDS epidemic may have episodes of recidivism, often associated with the use of alcohol and other drugs prior to or during sex (Stall et al. 1986). Condom use, in particular, is often adversely affected by the use of alcohol or drugs prior to sex. Ernst and Houts (1985) reported an association between alcohol abuse and the frequency of episodes of gonorrhea and syphilis among gay men, and Hart (1974:71) found that alcohol was cited by nearly a third of his sample of four hundred Australian soldiers in Vietnam as having an influence on their sexual behaviors, particularly regarding condom use. In the same cohort of gay and bisexual men referred to above, men who reported being "high" on alcohol and/or drugs during sex, with more than half of all of their partners in the past six months, were half as likely (their odds ratio was .5) to use condoms for insertive anal intercourse as compared to men who weren't "high" with any of their partners (Valdiserri et al. 1988b:802).

It is not unreasonable to assume that sexual behavioral change among gay men will continue, proportionally, in response to the severity of the AIDS epidemic, but such an approach does not adequately address individuals who are unsuccessful in achieving risk-reduction behavioral goals (Becker and Joseph 1988:408), nor does it make allowances for those persons who are only intermittently successful in maintaining risk-reduction behavior. It also does not address the circumstances of young sexually active men who are just beginning to explore their homosexuality. There may also be a tendency to inappropriately generalize epidemiologic findings from high-incidence areas to low-incidence areas. In San Francisco and New York, for example, the rate of new infections among homosexual men is estimated to be one percent or less (Boffey 1988d:22; McGann 1987:14), but these data may not accurately describe the transmission of the virus in other areas of the country, especially within communities of gay men where the incidence of AIDS is presently low. Therefore, to assume that the degree of behavioral change that has already occurred within the gay community is adequate minimizes the exigency that should characterize the public health response to an incurable infectious disease with a high mortality rate.

For the reasons listed above, there is still a great need to encourage and maintain behavioral risk reduction within the male homosexual population. Reviewing examples of programs that provide prevention services to gay men will enable us to identify standards that can be applied, with appropriate modifications, elsewhere, to other gay clients.

Early in the course of the epidemic, the San Francisco AIDS Foundation (SFAF), with funding support from the San Francisco Department of Public Health, commissioned a marketing firm to conduct a random probability sample telephone survey of self-identified gay and bisexual male residents of San Francisco (Research and Decisions Corporation 1984). This survey was designed to provide baseline demographic and sexual behavior measurements, measure the perceived impact of AIDS on gay sexual behaviors, document future behavioral intentions, and identify appropriate prevention messages and channels of communication.

The survey found an overall "attitudinal predisposition to successful AIDS adaptation," although there was some resistance to condom use for anal intercourse (Research and Decisions Corporation 1984: 13). It documented a variety of AIDS adaptation strategies, including celibacy, monogamy, and limitation of sexual activities to ones that do not result in the exchange of body fluids. Men who were less likely to report a change from unsafe to safe sexual practices tended to be older, less educated, have lower annual incomes, not know someone with AIDS, and not perceive the AIDS epidemic as a personal threat. The survey also documented that "one barrier to safe sex adaptation is the fact that certain unsafe sex practices are perceived as being highly enjoyable" (Research and Decisions Corporation 1984:15). In conclusion it was recommended that prevention campaign messages should "emphasize the social acceptability of safe sex" rather than stressing "only the risks of unsafe practices" (Research and Decisions Corporation 1984:16). The report also suggested that messages about the "pleasurability of safe sex alternatives" might decrease the frequency of unsafe practices (Research and Decisions Corporation 1984). Finally, the report suggested that newspapers and pamphlets were the media of choice for most gay and bisexual men who wanted to learn more about AIDS prevention.

The results of this survey were used to design a media campaign that stressed the efficacy of safer sex as a means of reducing the risk of HIV transmission and the concept "that safe sex has become a legitimate social norm" (Research and Decisions Corporation 1985: ii). These themes and subsequent ones, refined on the basis of ongoing market research (Research and Decisions Corporation 1985) and input from focus groups, resulted in a number of specific prevention messages that were disseminated through public forums, ads in the gay press, a local AIDS hotline, and group meetings (Research and Decisions Corporation 1985:2). Generally, these messages tended to emphasize the fact that AIDS was a sexually transmitted disease and that, although a cure was not likely in the immediate future, researchers did know which specific behaviors could transmit this infection. It also emphasized personal responsibility in avoiding the transmission of HIV, safer sex as an important way to reduce the risk of transmission, that most gay men in San Francisco had altered high-risk sexual activities in response to AIDS, and that practicing unsafe sex increased one's chances of contracting AIDS (Research and Decisions Corporation 1985:59).

In a follow-up probability sample conducted in April 1985, correlational analysis demonstrated an association between acceptance of the concepts of "safe sex efficacy" and "safe sex legitimacy" and a "decline in unsafe sex with secondary partners" (Research and Decisions Corporation 1985:ii). This, together with the observations that 85 percent of the respondents "reported reading one or more gay identified publications" in the month preceeding the interview, and that "74 percent could recall advertising containing AIDS prevention messages," suggested that the health promotion campaign had been effective (Research and Decisions Corporation 1985:ii).

The description of this media-based prevention campaign illustrates many of the standards that should be followed by other organizations planning similar ventures. The success of group-targeted, media-based campaigns to promote health behaviors is dependent on the proper identification of the target audience, sensitivity to cultural considerations, and identification of areas of resistance to the campaign message prior to delivery of that message (Manoff 1985). It should involve "preparatory stages of concept testing and consumer knowledge and attitude probing" prior to message design (Manoff 1985:74). All of these standards are apparent in our accounting of this prevention campaign.

Although we should not minimize the achievement of the SFAF in mounting this health-promotion campaign, the format of which has been applied to other at-risk populations, it is likely that part of its success has to do with the environment in which the message was received. The perception of the threat of AIDS experienced by gay men in San Francisco is certainly substantial, given the large number of AIDS cases and their widespread distribution within the gay community. According to the San Francisco Health Department, as many as half of the gay men in the city may be infected with HIV (Boffey 1988d:22). Also, the gay community in San Francisco, even prior to the AIDS epidemic, was well organized, and had a highly evolved infrastructure, including a widely circulated gay-specific press. Therefore, it is not certain whether such a campaign would be equally effective in an area where the gay community is not as severely affected by AIDS, is not as highly organized, and does not have the minority-specific media resources that are available to gay men in San Francisco. One possible implication is that in order for AIDS-prevention media campaigns to be equally effective within other gay communities, it may be necessary to support those communities in the development of their own specific resources, including service organizations and group-specific media.

The philosophy of promoting risk reduction as a socially acceptable and legitimate response to AIDS in order to change group norms
about specific riskful behaviors and to induce subsequent behavioral
change, has been maintained by the Foundation and repeated for a
number of different target groups, including women, intravenous
drug users, Hispanics, and African-Americans.

Another approach to AIDS prevention for gay men is based on the
same standard of accelerating behavioral change by promoting its
acceptance within the group, but this approach does not rely on the
media. Instead, it utilizes group process.

The Gay Men's Health Crisis (GMHC) in New York has developed
a unique workshop format for safer sex, which has been replicated in
several cities across the country (Palacios-Jimenez and Shernoff
1986). In the structure of a supportive group, men are encouraged to
talk about the impact AIDS has had on their lives, particularly regarding their sexual practices. Negative reactions to safer sex are addressed in a positive and caring manner, and the group focuses on
the erotic elements of safer sex. Using conventional psychotherapeutic group techniques, men are able to enact episodes that focus
on the negotiation of safer sexual encounters. The workshop is not
informational in content, that is, it is not a forum for defining what
is considered to be safe sex and what is not. Instead, the assumption
is that all of the participants have basic information about HIV transmission and prevention. The working definition of safe sex for the
groups is "on me, not in me, unless you're in me with a condom"
(Palacios-Jimenez and Shernoff 1986:15).

In its attempt to promote the widespread and rapid acceptance of
safer sex, GMHC has extended its approach to include erotic films
that depict safer sex practices and erotic comic books. The comic
books created an intense controversy at the federal legislative level
when they were criticized for promoting homosexuality (Booth
1987). Despite the conflict that such an approach is bound to generate, especially in segments of the population that question the
propriety of homosexuality per se, preliminary results indicate that
it may be effective in achieving the desired level of behavioral
change. A study that randomized 619 men into four groups (one
group viewed an erotic film, one group was given erotic printed materials that described safer sex, one group attended a session conducted by a man with AIDS, and a control group was given written
information but did not participate in a group discussion), revealed
that the greatest change toward safer sexual behaviors occurred in
the group that had seen the film (Kolata 1987:18).

It is not inappropriate to question GMHC's choice of this format

as a means to promote the acceptance of safer sex within particular segments of the gay community. Certainly, the thought of discussing intimate aspects of sexuality, with the intent of making
safer sexual behaviors appear to be more erotic, and therefore more
acceptable, is difficult for many people to accept, even within the
gay community. However, one way to understand this approach is
to return to the subject of innovation diffusion.

In considering how change occurs among a group of people, social scientists recognize the importance of "supporting" people, or
building "support systems" to facilitate the process of change; that
is, they tap into existing systems of communication and use them to
encourage new ideas or behaviors (Nelkin 1987). The functions of
"support" in the change process are to help people overcome moti-
vational barriers, to affirm the worth and importance of the target
society, and to overcome apathy and despair (Bennis et al. 1976).
This theoretical approach is consistent with our earlier discussion
of the diffusion of innovations, which emphasized a primary role of
the group itself as a means of transmitting new ideas (Rogers and
Shoemaker 1971).

Diffusion can be considered a "special type of communication"
by which new ideas and behaviors "spread to the members of a
social system" (Rogers and Shoemaker 1971:12). Just as health theorists distinguish among changes in knowledge, attitude, and behavior, social scientists also realize that it is possible for people to know
about an innovation (such as safer sex), and even to believe that it is
worthwhile or sensible, yet not adopt it (p. 108). Apropos of our
specific example of sexual risk reduction among gay men, accurate
knowledge of safer sex guidelines is not necessarily related to subsequent sexual behavior (Joseph et al. 1987; McKusick 1985b; Valdiserri 1987b).

Programs that promote the erotic qualities of safer sex are attempting to accelerate the acceptance of the innovation by influencing what Rogers and Shoemaker describe as the "persuasion
function" (1971:109). As individuals decide about any new idea, at
some stage they form "a favorable or unfavorable attitude toward
the innovation" (p. 109). The persuasion function occurs after an individual has learned about an innovation (note that the GMHC safer
sex workshop is not informational in content). This stage has been
described as a "vicarious trial," during which the individual "feels a
need for reinforcement of his attitudes toward the new idea" (p.
109). In seeking out this reinforcement, he is most likely to communicate with peers to compare his perceptions of the innovation with
theirs (p. 109). The safer sex workshop format can thus be seen as a

re-creation of the persuasion stage, under controlled conditions, which allows the facilitator to reinforce the perception that the sexual behaviors that gay men need to adopt in order to reduce their risk of HIV infection are just as satisfying emotionally and physically as unsafe practices.

This theoretical explanation of the eroticization of safer sex will not convince everyone of its necessity. Why not stress personal responsibility as a motivation for changing sexual behavior or, for that matter, even survival? Why is it even necessary to convince someone to modify his sexual behavior or run the risk of contracting a disease that is currently incurable? Many gay men have, in fact, successfully changed their sexual behaviors for precisely these reasons—without having to be convinced that safer sex is just as satisfying as high-risk sex. However, there are others who cannot successfully initiate or maintain safer sexual behaviors, and they are the target population for the safer sex workshops.

Unlike the two community- based organizations discussed above, the AIDS Prevention Project at the University of Pittsburgh was a randomized trial conducted in a university setting. The primary question posed by this research was whether or not gay and bisexual men who received skills training in the area of discussing safer sex, including the use of condoms, would manifest more pronounced changes in the direction of safer sexual behavior compared to men who had attended a small-group lecture about safer sex that did not incorporate skills training.

The skills-training session employed a variety of conventional psychotherapeutic techniques, including role playing, psychodrama, and group process. In the session, men were able to discuss the importance of sex in their lives, to consider the impact of HIV testing on future sexual behavior, and to role play the discussion of safer sex with a new sexual partner. The facilitator of the session stressed the social acceptability and legitimacy of safer sex and helped the group develop adaptation strategies for confronting barriers to safer sexual practice.

From March 1986 through March 1987, 584 men were randomized into this study and were followed for approximately twelve months after their intervention. Men who received the skills training demonstrated a statistically significant increase in condom use for insertive anal intercourse compared to their peers who had not received such instruction. In fact, in sessions providing skills training, condom use for insertive anal intercourse increased, on average, 44 percent, compared to only 11 percent, on average, in sessions that did not provide skills training (Valdiserri et al. 1989b).

The men who participated in this trial were not representative of the entire gay community. The fact that they were willing to self-identify as "gay" and participate in research (in fact, many were recruited directly from the Pittsburgh component of the Multicenter AIDS Cohort Study), means that the findings may not be generalizable to all segments of the gay population. However, studies of this nature suggest that for certain groups of gay men, the frequency of condom use for insertive anal intercourse can be increased by providing skills training that teaches men how to negotiate safer sexual enounters and that allows them to rehearse such encounters. The potential contribution of skills training to the adoption of safer sexual behaviors is especially significant given our awareness that knowing about the risk of unsafe behaviors, by itself, may be inadequate to modify or eliminate those behaviors. In a study from Finland, among 235 homosexual men who were given repeated information about safer sexual practices, 57 percent still continued to engage in anal intercourse—42 percent of them without condoms (Valle 1988).

Emphasis on the social acceptability of sexual risk reduction for gay men was a consistent theme among all of the programs visited. Another consistent theme was the absence of fear-based messages. As described in Chapter Three, fear-based communications can be effective in creating "more favorable attitudes" about a risk reduction behavior, but fear alone is considered inadequate to motivate specific protective action (Leventhal et al. 1983:3). While fear-based messages may have a place among groups who remain unconvinced that AIDS is a real threat, they must always be presented in conjunction with specific behavioral recommendations for reducing risk.

Although all of the prevention programs for gay and bisexual men described in this chapter provide clients with information about HIV counseling and testing services, none considered HIV testing a necessary prerequisite for behavioral change or made disclosure of HIV antibody status a requirement for participation. This lack of emphasis on HIV testing may be due, in part, to the lack of expert consensus on the effects of HIV testing on subsequent behavior. It may also relate to the fact that a significant percentage of the urban gay population is already HIV infected (Centers for Disease Control 1987a). Knowing the hopelessness that can afflict people who know they are infected with HIV, some caregivers may be hesitant to emphasize testing prior to the advent of available treatment for the asymptomatic HIV-infected client.

The importance of learning one's HIV serostatus (that is, whether one is infected or not) in the overall process of behavioral change remains under study. At this point, we can only say that for some people, learning their test results will probably contribute significantly to future preventive behaviors, while for others, the test results may have no effect, or perhaps even a negative one. Legislative changes protecting the confidentiality of HIV test results and prohibiting discrimination against HIV-infected persons are likely to make counseling and testing more attractive options for some clients. In a study conducted in Oregon comparing client response to confidential versus anonymous testing, it was found that the availability of anonymous testing increased overall demand for testing by 125 percent among gay and bisexual clients (Fehrs et al. 1988).

Before considering programs that promote sexual risk reduction among heterosexuals, we must address several issues that are relevant to the approaches currently being undertaken. First, the number of cases of heterosexually transmitted AIDS in this country is small in comparison to the number of cases that can be linked to homosexual transmission or to needle sharing among intravenous drug users. Between March 1987 and March 1988, the Centers for Disease Control reported that among adults with AIDS, only 4 percent of diagnosed cases were attributable to heterosexual transmission (1988b:224).

Between 1981 and 1986, 1,819 adult women were diagnosed with AIDS in America. This number represented nearly 7 percent of the total number of adult AIDS cases, and approximately 25 percent of adult AIDS cases excluding homosexual and bisexual men (Guinan and Hardy 1987:2040). The majority of these women (52 percent) were intravenous drug users, 14 percent had become infected as a result of sexual intercourse with a drug-using partner, and 2 percent were infected through sexual relations with a bisexual partner (Guinan and Hardy 1987:2040).

When we consider the entire heterosexual population of the United States, the actual risk of HIV infection is quite low, because of the large size of the denominator and the small size of the numerator. Despite intermittent reports that HIV infection is spreading rampantly among the heterosexual population (Boffey 1988c), all current studies indicate that in the absence of other known risks for infection, such as intravenous drug use, bisexuality, or hemophilia, the "national prevalence of HIV infection among such persons remains very low compared to persons with specific risk behavior or known sexual exposure to persons at increased risk" (Centers for Disease Control 1987a:11). Current estimates of HIV seroprevalence in the "general population" are .021 percent among military recruits and .006 percent for blood donors (Centers for Disease Control 1987a:12).

Therefore, the risk of HIV infection secondary to heterosexual intercourse is greatly influenced by the social and sexual histories of the persons involved. If one of the partners is an intravenous drug user, a prostitute, a hemophiliac, a bisexual man, or has received a blood transfusion prior to 1985, we consider the potential for HIV infection to be much greater than when neither of the partners has a history of behaviors that might indicate prior HIV infection.

On the basis of existing seroprevalence studies it appears that infection with HIV is more evenly distributed within the gay community than it is within the heterosexual community. Since it has been suggested that "heterosexual transmission is most likely to occur in areas with the highest rates of AIDS and HIV infection among intravenous drug users" (Centers for Disease Control 1987a:11), the unequal heterosexual distribution reflects the disparate levels of HIV infection among various IV drug using communities. Rates of infection are extremely high on the eastern seaboard, but currently much lower in other American cities (Centers for Disease Control 1987a:2).

These findings suggest a significant barrier confronting program planners who are developing AIDS-prevention initiatives for heterosexual clients. Namely, how to present accurate information that explains that HIV infection is not as widespread in the heterosexual population as other sexually acquired infections, such as syphilis, without minimizing the real threat to persons who are at increased risk. To make matters worse, several reports document that a single episode of heterosexual intercourse, even with an infected partner, may not result in infection (Hearst and Hulley 1988; Padian et al. 1987). Hearst and Hulley estimate that the risk of HIV infection from a single episode of penile-vaginal intercourse with ejaculation, where condoms are not used and where one of the partners is infected with the virus and the other is not, is approximately 1 in 500 (Hearst and Hulley 1988:2429). It is hardly surprising that "perceptions of low vulnerability" and "confusion regarding the magnitude of the threat" remain major barriers to sexual behavior modification among heterosexuals (Siegel and Gibson 1988).

In a random probability sample of four hundred heterosexuals with multiple and/or high-risk partners, conducted in San Francisco in 1986, concern about AIDS "was considerably below" levels of concern expressed by gay and bisexual men (Research and Decisions Corporation 1986:1). Less than one-third of the sample reported that they felt "personally threatened" by AIDS, and although many of the sample reported that they had reduced their number of sex partners, there was little evidence that these concerns had any impact on the frequency of unprotected vaginal intercourse (no use of condoms) (Research and Decisions Corporation 1986:2).

Attempting to address this risk differential, a majority of the programs highlighted in this chapter have focused on the heterosexual partners of so-called high-risk individuals, especially intravenous drug users, rather than attempting to reach every heterosexually active person. This strategy is different from the one employed for gay men, where, because of the high level of HIV infection within that population, the risk of contracting HIV is more evenly distributed and most gay men are considered to be at substantial risk of infection.

For example, the Dallas County Health Department's AIDS Prevention Project sends outreach workers into low-income Hispanic and African-American communities to educate intravenous drug users and their partners about the risks of HIV infection that accompany unprotected sexual intercourse and needle sharing. Volunteers from ADAPT inform male intravenous drug users about the dangers of HIV transmission to their sexual partners and offspring, and they routinely distribute condoms along with bleach kits for sterilization of "works." Clinical staff from the Methadone Maintenance Treatment Program of the Beth Israel Hospital in New York City hold group sessions for the female sexual partners of men in their program to educate these women about the sexual and perinatal transmission of HIV. The Hemophilia Center of Western Pennsylvania provides HIV antibody counseling and testing for both male hemophiliacs and their female sexual partners; as part of their counseling they discuss the importance of condom use as a means of preventing HIV transmission.

Women who support themselves or supplement their income by prostitution are considered to be at increased risk for HIV infection both because of their repeated heterosexual exposures to multiple male clients and also because many are intravenous drug users. In fact, the "HIV antibody prevalence is three to four times higher among prostitutes who acknowledge IV drug use than among those who do not" (Centers for Disease Control 1987a:8).

In Dallas, the County Health Department's community demonstration project (AIDS Prevention Project) sends an outreach worker to topless bars, massage parlors, and modeling studios to educate the women employed there about the manner in which HIV is transmitted. The outreach worker plans her visits to coincide with times when women are not busy with clients, and in brief sessions, focuses on the use of condoms for oral, anal, and vaginal intercourse as well as on the dangers of perinatal viral transmission.

The San Francisco AIDS Foundation collaborates with the Mid-City Consortium to provide risk-reduction education to prostitutes, usually in a hotel somewhere in the "Tenderloin" district of the city. In order to promote their intervention, they offer one hundred dollars in cash or one hundred free condoms to the prostitute who gets the highest score on their safe sex quiz. In addition to the transmission of HIV, the workshop addresses the negotiation of safer sex with clients and other partners, and ways to make safer sex more acceptable by eroticizing it. Prostitutes who use intravenous drugs are also instructed about cleaning their "works" with bleach. The educators stress that HIV infection is preventable and do not make moral judgments about the social circumstances of their workshop participants.

Identifying persons who are at increased risk of HIV infection as a result of heterosexual intercourse with high-risk partners, is an appropriate and logical approach to AIDS prevention—although it is not always an easy one. For the female partners of bisexual men, it may be especially difficult. Many of the health educators who were interviewed for this chapter indicated that women are not usually aware that their partners are bisexual. A survey of 433 women attending two contraceptive care clinics in Pittsburgh, Pennsylvania, revealed that nearly 4 percent of the women reported sex with a bisexual man within the past five years, while 11 percent suspected that a partner may have been bisexual but were not sure (Valdiserri et al. 1988a). Many bisexual men do not share information about their homosexual activities with female partners and often go outside their communities to engage in these sexual activities clandestinely.

The majority of male intravenous drug users have female partners who are not IV drug users themselves (Friedman et al. 1986:388), and clinical staff from the Beth Israel Methadone Maintenance Treatment Program indicated that it is not unusual for these men to have female sexual partners who are unaware of their drug use behaviors. Likewise, most women may not be able to determine whether a male partner has a history of sexual relations with prostitutes, nor are sexually active adolescent hemophiliacs eager to share the details of their disease with female partners (like other adolescents, they do not want to appear different from their peers).

Although intensive efforts to prevent heterosexually acquired HIV infection should target persons at increased risk, basic information about HIV transmission and prevention must be provided to all sexually active persons. This approach is dictated both by prudence and also in recognition of the fact that "few individuals are likely to possess" accurate information about the past or current high-risk behaviors of their prospective partners (Siegel and Gibson 1988:67). Perhaps the most important point to stress when providing education to the general heterosexual population is that sexual intercourse with partners whose past behaviors are unknown can be very dangerous. Prevention campaigns should (a) emphasize the necessity of talking with potential partners about their past behaviors and should (b) discourage unprotected intercourse with individuals who are recent acquaintances or strangers. This combined message is likely to have a greater "yield" than one that focuses on AIDS as a sexually transmitted disease (which is already known to many Americans) or one that advises celibacy prior to marriage (which is unpopular with many adolescents and adults).

At the programmatic level, there is an increasing awareness that heterosexuals must overcome a number of barriers in order to translate accurate AIDS information into behavioral action. More than one of the health educators interviewed felt that among many Hispanic, black, and adolescent heterosexuals, AIDS is still viewed as a "gay white disease", and that even in the presence of accurate information about HIV transmission, clients may not act on risk-reduction recommendations. These observations relate to our earlier discussion of risk perception and are consistent with psychological studies on risk-taking behavior that indicate that "risk-seeking preferences are common when people must choose between a sure loss and a substantial probability of a larger loss" (Kahneman and Tversky 1982:160). In other words, most people, when confronted with the choice between the sure loss of an opportunity for sexual intercourse (because of the risk of potential HIV infection), compared to the probability (which is not a certainty) of the larger loss of becoming infected with HIV, will take a risk and choose the latter because it is not a "sure loss."

In a sample of sexually active adolescents from San Francisco who were surveyed over a one-year period to determine their knowledge, attitudes, and frequency of condom use, respondents were aware of the ability of condoms to prevent AIDS and placed high value on the use of condoms to prevent AIDS, but these perceptions were "neither reflected in increased intentions to use condoms nor in increased use" (Kegeles et al. 1988:460). Kegeles and her colleagues suggest that this discrepancy is secondary to the fact that adolescents "may not feel personally vulnerable to contracting diseases from their sex partners" (p. 461). As described earlier, "perceived susceptibility" is one of the significant dimensions of the Health Belief Model of health-related behaviors (Janz and Becker 1984).

Several of the programs cited in this chapter are attempting to increase the personal identification and acceptance of risk for HIV infection among heterosexuals. The community demonstration project in Dallas, Texas, funded by the Centers for Disease Control, has worked with commercial marketers to develop a series of AIDS-prevention posters intended for young adults. These posters present a series of stark black-and-white photographic images associated with death: a tombstone; a hearse containing a casket; and a body on a stretcher, covered by a shroud. The photograph is accompanied by a slogan that relates to the image and a brief narrative that personalizes the risk of HIV infection for adolescents. Along with the anxiety-provoking images, there are specific instructions about how the risk of AIDS can be minimized. The primary message is to say no to sex and drugs, followed by instructions, for those who do choose sexual activity, to limit themselves to a single partner and to always use condoms. The posters stress that AIDS is incurable but that it is preventable.

This particular poster campaign has not been evaluated, but it is based on information obtained from a precampaign focus group which indicated that increasing perceptions of risk by adolescents would increase personal identification with the threat of AIDS. Although fear-based campaigns have not been well accepted among gay men (McKusick 1985a), they may play an important role in heightening perceived susceptibility among persons who have difficulties recognizing their risk of infection. However, it is important to reiterate that fear alone is inadequate to change behavior (Leventhal et al. 1983), and that fear is most effective in health-promotion campaigns "if the campaign allows for the desired behavior to be reinforced by a reduction in the level of fear" (Job 1988:163).

Another way to make individuals recognize and accept their risk of HIV infection is by designing interventions that personalize the threat of AIDS. In San Francisco, volunteers with AIDS and ARC (AIDS-related complex) visit high schools and talk to students about how their lives have changed as a result of AIDS. The intent is not to frighten students into recognizing their risks, but to forge an identification with the person who is infected, at an individual level, which will enable students to accept and act on risk-reduction information. Similar approaches have been taken in teen pregnancy prevention programs where a doll or animal is "adopted" by a "couple" who are responsible for caring for it. As a result of their experiences and reactions to this responsibility, they gain insight into the negative consequences of unplanned pregnancy—insights that would not develop if students are merely instructed that premarital sexual intercourse is "dangerous" because it can result in pregnancy.

A final avenue for increasing the perception of HIV infection risk is through HIV antibody testing. A positive test for HIV antibody may be the only thing that will bring some heterosexuals to accept AIDS as a real threat to their well-being. The knowledge that they are already infected may enable them to avoid reinfection with other HIV strains and to prevent the spread of the virus to their sexual partners. However, relying only on HIV antibody testing as a means of making the threat of AIDS real to heterosexual clients does have an inherent liability. Namely, persons who test negative may continue to engage in high-risk activities, such as unprotected sexual intercourse, because they interpret the negative test to mean that their past behaviors have been safe.

Even if heterosexual clients are willing to accept their risk of HIV infection, there may be other barriers to the practice of safer sex, especially with respect to the use of condoms. The reasons condoms are not used more often, for either disease prophylaxis or prevention of pregnancy, have been the subject of various studies and commentaries (Bergman 1980; Darrow 1975; Felman and Santora 1981; Free and Alexander 1976; Hart 1974; Hinman 1976; Siegel and Gibson 1988). Research on the factors that dissuade people from using condoms have revealed three broad categories of barriers: objective, situational, and subjective.

Of the objective barriers, perhaps the most significant is the lack of access to a readily available supply of condoms. In a study that examined the feasibility of offering condoms to heterosexual adolescent males, primarily for contraception, Arnold and Cogswell suggested that commercial distribution through such outlets as barbershops, restaurants, pool halls, grocery stores, and gas stations, could greatly increase the use of condoms (1971). Many of the prevention programs identified in this chapter distribute free condoms to intravenous drug users, their sexual partners, and prostitutes.

Health educators routinely carry a generous supply of condoms, which they offer to clients as part of their outreach education in neighborhoods or business establishments where unsafe sexual practices are likely to take place or where "high-risk" persons are likely to congregate. Similar outreach activities are common for gay and bisexual men.

Of the situational variables, the two most important are the failure to plan in advance for sexual intercourse, so that condoms are often unavailable, and the use of alcohol and/or drugs prior to or during sex, which can lead to the improper use of condoms or worse, failure to use them altogether (Hart 1974). Premeditation of sexual intercourse is especially difficult for adolescents, who often feel that unless sex is spontaneous it is not "romantic" (Stark 1986). Studies exploring the reasons sexually active teenagers fail to use contraceptives often find that "a teenager's desire for completely spontaneous sex is tied to the belief that being 'swept off your feet' or 'carried away' is forgivable, but having premeditated sex is not" —and condom use requires premeditation (Stark 1986:28). Compared to adults, teenagers have difficulty appreciating the consequences of their actions (Goleman 1987), and this too contributes to their underutilization of condoms as a means of preventing both pregnancy and sexually transmitted diseases, such as HIV infection. However, it is not only adolescents who are remiss in their use of condoms for preventing the untoward consequences of sexual intercourse. In a survey of 864 patients attending a venereal disease clinic in metropolitan New York, which included adolescent as well as adult clients, 64 percent of the respondents reported that they "seldom" or "never" used condoms (Felman and Santora 1981:334).

Perhaps the most frequently cited reasons for the failure to use condoms—whether for pregnancy prevention, sexually transmissible disease prophylaxis, or both—are related to subjective opinions. Beliefs that condoms interfere with sexual pleasure (Felman and Santora 1981; Hinman 1976; Valdiserri 1989a), that they are unnatural (Felman and Santora 1981; Hinman 1976), that condoms would be offensive to one's partner (Arnold 1972; Curjel 1964), that condoms are unacceptable because of their association with sexual promiscuity and prostitution (Valdiserri 1988), or that purchasing them would be too embarrassing (Yarber and Williams 1975), have all been cited as reasons for not using them.

Programs designed to prevent the sexual transmission of HIV should give serious consideration to the reasons for failure to use condoms. Certainly, health educators must ensure that clients have adequate information about condoms, including what kinds to buy, how to put them on, why they should only be lubricated with water-based preparations, and how to ensure that they will not slip off after a male partner has lost his erection. But, this is only the beginning of any condom promotion initiative. Condom promotion programs must not only provide information about the mechanics of condom use, they must incorporate approaches to remove or modify barriers to use.

In attempting to modify barriers to condom use, two basic issues must be addressed: the first relates to the "image" of the condom. In consumer research, one school of thought holds that much of "consumption behavior is actually social behavior" (Solomon 1983:319). This construct recognizes that products have a symbolic value in addition to their utilitarian one, and that consumption of a product often serves to reinforce the consumer's self-image and the image the consumer wants to project to others. People dress in certain ways, live in specific neighborhoods, or drive a special kind of automobile because they want to present a particular image of themselves, an image that is predetermined by a consumer and reinforced by the product. This perspective assumes that product image is defined by the product user, not necessarily by the objective worth of the product (Sirgy 1982), and that consumption of a product is often influenced by the symbols attached to that product (Sirgy 1982).

When we consider condoms as a product, it is apparent that they have a long-standing history of negative associations. Their connection with extramarital sexual activity, their ability to prevent conception, and their characterization, at times, as an emblem of sexual incontinence have undoubtedly influenced the way that we react to them (Valdiserri 1988). In this country, it is sobering to realize that prior to 1971, when contraception was removed from the prohibitions of the Comstock Act, information about the contraceptive capabilities of condoms was not permitted to be sent by mail because it was classified as obscene (Reed 1978:102). In 1973, a survey of state laws relating to condom distribution and sales revealed that "twelve states still restricted the advertising of condoms as contraceptives, nine states prohibited their display, nine states restricted sales to pharmacies and physicians, and twelve states prohibited their sale from vending machines" (Free and Alexander 1976:442).

The negative symbolism associated with condoms remains strong in our society; premarital sexual activity and contraception continue to generate public debate. Granted, the AIDS epidemic has propelled condoms into the public conciousness and into the realm of "quasi-polite" conversation. It has also fueled the growth of the condom industry, as well as related opportunistic enterprises whose products include items such as condom earrings, key chains, bumper stickers, posters, and sportswear. But increased awareness of AIDS notwithstanding, the condom is still a product capable of generating controversy.

In Traverse City, Michigan, in 1987, a bitter debate ensued after a local businessman asked the city commission's permission to sell condoms in vending machines (Wilkerson 1987). Issues raised during the debate extended from "the use of condoms to AIDS to homosexuality, promiscuity, immorality, and the effects all this will have on children and the town's image as a tourist haven" (Wilkerson 1987:8). This example is not raised to highlight the political turmoil experienced by a small rural community, nor to claim that condoms cannot be obtained in locations other than pharmacies (in many places, they can). Instead, it supports our assertion that many people still view condoms with a substantial degree of trepidation. As a product, they are often judged from a moral perspective as contributing to unfettered sexual expression and immorality, rather than from a health perspective that recognizes their ability to serve a number of positive health-related functions.

When the administrative board of the United States Catholic Conference, which represents the nation's three hundred Catholic bishops, issued a report on AIDS in America which suggested that teaching about condoms as a means of preventing transmission of HIV might be appropriate in certain circumstances "if grounded in the broader moral vision" (Goldman 1987b:17), it ignited immediate criticism from more conservative bishops (Goldman 1987a), who opposed it vigorously.

It is still difficult to advertise contraceptives on most national television and radio networks, and commercials urging the use of condoms to prevent the spread of HIV have not been widespread in this country (Lader 1987; Lipman 1987).

The continuing perception that condoms are controversial and somehow immoral can, not surprisingly, have an adverse effect on their actual use. Even the condom's ability to prevent the transmission of sexual pathogens, which is a positive feature from a health perspective, could be viewed symbolically as indicating that one of the partners in a sexual relationship is diseased or unclean. Five percent of 759 sexually active women from western Pennsylvania indicated that "they would be insulted" if a male partner wanted to use a condom with them; 9 percent weren't sure how they would react (Valdiserri 1989a). Although the majority of women surveyed disagreed with this statement, there remain those whose attitudes suggest that negative reactions to product symbolism may be an impediment to their using condoms for disease prevention.

In 1976, a survey designed to assess knowledge, attitudes, and behaviors regarding prophylaxis for sexually transmitted diseases was conducted on two hundred sexually active adolescent girls from Indianapolis, Indiana. Although the girls rated the condom as an effective preventive measure, "less than one-fifth of the population who stated they would have intercourse in the future indicated that they planned to use the device" (Yarber 1977:139). Questionnaire items designed to assess the girls' attitudes about condoms revealed only a partial acceptance, and Yarber concluded that the findings supported the need for "further education, particularly for the development of a positive attitude towards the condom" (Yarber 1977: 139).

To combat negative attitudes about condom use, many prevention programs attempt to densensitize potential users by presenting the condom in a nonthreatening and, at times, even humorous way. Although such an approach may seem to minimize the gravity of relationships involving sexual expression, the underlying motive is to get people to view the condom as an integral, nonthreatening, and symbolically neutral component of sexual activity. Extrapolating from consumer theory (Solomon 1983; Sirgy 1982), replacing the negative image of the condom with one that is associated with prudency, responsibility, and caring for one's partner, will increase its use by providing a positive self-image for its users.

An essential part of encouraging the use of condoms is helping people find ways to talk about them without being overwhelmed by embarrassment or shame. The second of the two issues referred to earlier has to do with teaching clients the communication skills necessary to discuss the use of condoms with a sexual partner and to overcome a partner's resistance to their use. Women especially, may be unsure of how to introduce the subject of condoms with a new sexual partner, or even with a current partner with whom condoms have not been previously used (Valdiserri 1989b). In fact, health educators from several programs suggested that the widespread popularity of oral contraceptives, which do not require male participation or cooperation, has resulted in women becoming experienced sexually but relatively inexperienced in discussing reproductive health issues with their partners. Skills training to promote condom use is a specific example of the safer sex negotiation skills that should be provided in any AIDS-prevention program. The need to develop these skills was universally recognized by all of the programs visited, although some have made more progress than others toward achieving this goal.

When female partners of men enrolled in Beth Israel's Methadone Maintenance Treatment Program are invited to attend group sessions on the risk of sexually transmitted HIV infection, they participate in role playing as a means of understanding and anticipating their male partner's possible reactions to the suggestion of condom use. A variety of hypothetical situations permit women to rehearse possible responses to negative reactions, such as "you don't trust me" or "we've never used them before." These skills are no less critical for male intravenous drug users, who often have difficulties verbalizing their feelings and may be quite adept at denial.

A survey of heterosexuals with multiple and/or high-risk partners, conducted in 1986 by the San Francisco AIDS Foundation (SFAF), revealed that within the month prior to the telephone survey respondents reported an average of nearly eleven episodes of vaginal intercourse without a condom with their primary partners; the monthly frequency for episodes of vaginal intercourse with a condom averaged less than two (Research and Decisions Corporation 1986:63). The frequency of condom use for vaginal intercourse with secondary partners was even lower. The survey concluded that although there is an "attitudinal openness to condom usage," the actual behavior "lags far behind" (Research and Decisions Corporation 1986:119). Similar findings were reported from a separate 1987 survey of contraceptive use practices among 10,000 sexually active American women between the ages of fifteen and forty-four. Namely, "although 60 percent of the women said they had a favorable attitude toward condoms," only 16 percent of unmarried women reported using them as a method of contraception (Kolata 1988:B7).

In 1988, in response to these findings and feedback from ongoing focus groups, the SFAF printed a brochure entitled "Condoms for Couples." In addition to depicting the basic mechanics of condom use, this brochure addresses many of the psychological and social barriers that would be discussed in a skills training session. The brochure offers suggestions about how to introduce the subject of condoms with a partner and lists responses that can be employed to diffuse or counter five common objections to condom use, such as "they're not romantic," "you don't trust me," "I don't use condoms," "we've already had sex without them," and "we don't need them because I love you" (San Francisco AIDS Foundation 1988).

Focus group research conducted by Blacks Educating Blacks About

Sexual Health Issues (BEBASHI) in Philadelphia, Pennsylvania, also indicated that sexually active women often lack the communication skills necessary to discuss the subject of condoms with a sexual partner. To foster the development of these skills, BEBASHI holds "home parties," where one woman hosts a party for her female friends and colleagues, to preview and purchase a variety of lingerie. Condom use is introduced as part of this presentation, and women are given information about condoms, as well as pointers on how to bring up the subject with a male sexual partner. To assist in the development of the skills necessary for consistent and correct condom use, women role play a variety of situations relating to condom use. The facilitator of the party guides the women through their enactments, and through the medium of group process, the women share their own ideas, feelings, attitudes, and suggestions about promoting the use of condoms.

Gay men report many of the same barriers to consistent condom use as do heterosexual men and women (Valdiserri 1988b). Therefore, encouraging condom use for both heterosexual and homosexual clients must go beyond merely providing information about the "do's and don'ts" of condoms, to encompass specific skills training that will enable clients to translate this knowledge into action.

Although the task of developing programs to prevent the sexual transmission of HIV may seem overwhelming, when we consider designing interventions that will "clearly and effectively" (Ad Hoc Work Group . . . 1987:90) stop the transmission of HIV by ending the practices of drug injection and needle sharing among intravenous drug users, we are confronted with an even greater challenge. While the promotion of safer sexual behavior may require intensive and innovative interventions to initiate and support people through the process of behavioral change, interventions targeted to drug users have two obstacles to overcome: the inherent obstacle of promoting behavioral change and the added burden of dealing with addictive drug use.

Interrupting the transmission of human immunodeficiency virus among IV drug users is clearly one of the most pressing priorities among AIDS-prevention programs. Epidemiologic evidence indicates that intravenous drug users are the major reservoir of infection in the heterosexual population (Centers for Disease Control 1987a). At the same time, HIV seroprevalence data suggest that in communities with a low prevalence of HIV infection among IV drug users "a window of opportunity exists where prompt, vigorous, and aggressive efforts at prevention" could have a major impact in preventing the "catastrophic spread" of virus that has been seen elsewhere (Lange et al. 1988:443).

A multitude of published reports suggest that intravenous drug users, especially those from communities with a high incidence of AIDS, have already manifested behavioral changes in response to the threat of AIDS. These changes include an "increased demand" for un-used sterile needles and syringes (Des Jarlais et al. 1985; Des Jarlais and Hopkins 1985; Ginzburg et al. 1986); self-reported decreases in the sharing of injection equipment (Friedman et al. 1986; Ghodse et al. 1987; Selwyn et al. 1987; Skidmore et al. 1988); cleaning of nee-dles and syringes with a bleach solution (Chaisson 1987; Friedman et al. 1986; Froner 1987; Moss et al. 1988); and termination of intra-venous drug use altogether (Conviser and Rutledge 1988; Ghodse et al. 1987; Selwyn et al. 1987). Among IV drug users in New Jersey "fear of AIDS" has been cited by nearly half of the clients as "one of their reasons for entering treatment" (Des Jarlais and Friedman 1987a:71).

It would appear that many intravenous drug users, like many gay men, have recognized and accepted the threat of AIDS as a real one. Some estimates suggest that as many as one-third of all addicts have modified their behavior in response to AIDS (Booth 1988:718). But, the job of AIDS-prevention programs is to ensure that this behavioral modification is extended, accelerated, and maintained. This is espe-cially critical in communities where the seroprevalence of HIV in-fection is currently low, and where prevention programs have an op-portunity to maintain this low rate of infection (Lange 1988).

In addition to efforts that attempt to avert the sexual transmis-sion of HIV from drug users to their partners, there are two major approaches to AIDS prevention in this population: interrupting the transmission of the virus by discouraging needle sharing or the use of contaminated needles and terminating the need to inject intrave-nous drugs by treating the subject's dependency problem. Although both approaches are often simultaneously employed, they target two different subgroups: those users who do not wish to end their drug use, and those who do.

Interrupting the transmission of HIV from the use of shared drug injecting equipment is widely recognized as an important objective of AIDS prevention programs (Brunet et al. 1987; Des Jarlais and Friedman 1987a; Dougherty 1988; Friedman et al. 1986). Achieving this objective will not be an easy accomplishment, by anyone's reckoning, and will involve more than just disseminating infor-mation about the dangers of sharing needles. Because IV drug users rely on oral communication (Des Jarlais and Friedman 1987b), it is doubtful that a media campaign would be sufficient to extinguish needle sharing behavior, and Friedman and his colleagues have cautioned that "face-to-face education" is essential for prevention initiatives among this group (1986:391). This necessitates outreach efforts to locales where needle sharing behavior is occurring, most notably in "shooting galleries" (Serrano and Goldsmith 1988; Wiebel and Altman 1988).

Shooting galleries are described in gritty detail by Des Jarlais and his colleagues (1986:116–120), whose account depicts two such establishments in New York City. Intravenous users go to these places, usually after they have purchased their drug, to "shoot up" in privacy. The shooting gallery owner rents the user a set of "works" which may have been used by scores of persons beforehand, with only cursory cleaning between uses. Health educators and outreach workers who enter this sort of environment must be thoroughly familiar with it, lest they become more concerned about the disquieting ambience of the shooting gallery than they are about the risky behaviors taking place within.

One should not assume that IV drug users share needles only because they are unaware of the dangers of HIV transmission. Even after the recruitment and training of a health educator who is familiar with the drug-using subculture, and who is willing to enter the unpleasant world of the shooting gallery to educate users about the inherent dangers of sharing "works," other barriers may impede the translation of this information into behavioral change.

For many years, it has been well-recognized that needle sharing serves both social and psychological functions for the participants (Howard and Borges 1970). Along with the economic pragmatism of sharing a scarce and usually illegal commodity (needles and syringes are only available with a doctor's script in many states), needle sharing is a form of socialization for neophyte drug users and signifies camaraderie among users (Howard and Borges 1970). In a questionnaire survey of 240 active and recovering intravenous drug users, Connors and Galea found that 86 percent reported sharing needles, and 40 percent of these shared needles three or more times a week (1988:388). Based on her survey results and other ethnographic observations, she concluded that needle sharing is "deeply embedded" in the social and cultural fabric of the intravenous drug using society. Even when IV drug users have decreased their frequency of needle sharing, they may still continue to share needles with close friends, relatives and sexual partners (Friedman et al.

1986; Ghodse et al. 1987; Marmor et al. 1987; Selwyn et al. 1987). Finally, and perhaps most important, is the recognition that addictive behavior is not always rational, and that a user who is experiencing withdrawal symptoms may opt to share a needle rather than forego self-administration of drug, because of the exigencies of his addiction (Friedman et al. 1986:385).

The Association for Drug Abuse Prevention and Treatment (ADAPT) in Brooklyn, New York, employs volunteers, many of them ex-drug users, to go into neighborhoods where IV drug use is common, often into shooting galleries (Morgan 1988), to teach drug users about HIV transmission and how to clean their "works" with bleach. ADAPT volunteers distribute "prevention kits," which contain a vial of 5.25 percent bleach solution, a vial of water, cotton wool, a bottle cap (the "cooker" used to heat and dissolve the drug prior to injection), a condom, and a pamphlet that stresses the importance of terminating drug use but describes the procedure for cleaning drug equipment if the recipient is still using drugs.

Before entering these neighborhoods, outreach workers make sure that their activities are known to the official and unofficial authorities in the community. For example, if they plan on setting up an information table in a housing project where IV drug use is a problem, they inform the superintendent of the building about their organization and the materials they will be distributing. When they work in shooting galleries, they inform the police, the drug dealer, the drug pusher, and the "lookouts" about their educational activities before they begin. These actions help ensure adequate cooperation and safeguard volunteers from becoming caught up in any police activity or criminal action related to the selling or distribution of drugs. Outreach workers from ADAPT never enter a neighborhood surreptitiously and they do not begin their prevention education until they have the cooperation of all of the significant "players" in the drug subculture within that setting. The fact that many outreach workers are familiar with these "players" and their roles, as a result of past drug use, helps to facilitate this interchange.

Prevention programs in New Jersey (New Jersey State Health Department), Texas (Dallas County Health Department, AIDS Prevention Project), and San Francisco (Mid-City Consortium in collaboration with the San Francisco AIDS Foundation) also employ outreach workers who seek out active intravenous drug users to educate them about the dangers of needle sharing and the sexual transmission of HIV. Some of these programs provide education only; others provide education in addition to bleach sterilization kits.

All of the programs identified in this discussion recognized the importance of entering into the drug user's environment to promote AIDS risk reduction, and to achieve this, many employ recovering drug users to serve as outreach workers. This practice exemplifies the necessity of understanding target subcultures in order to promote behavioral change within them. Although these practices do not necessarily guarantee that the intervention will be successful (that is, that the outreach worker will be able to convince drug users to stop injecting drugs or to discontinue the practice of needle sharing), they do offer a high degree of certainty that the message will not be blocked because of resistance to the transmitter. Whether we choose to explain this as a manifestation of the concept of homophily (see discussion of diffusion of innovation), or from a pragmatic perspective that appreciates the value of outreach workers who are thoroughly familiar with the drug subculture, the practice of using a "representative" from the target population to deliver a risk reduction intervention is common (Schmidt 1988).

Using former addicts as health educators may also serve another function: they can influence the self-efficacy of their clients. The concept of self-efficacy was developed and promoted by Bandura (1977) as a means of explaining how "future behavior is based on one's present perception of ability to perform that behavior" (Lorig 1985:232). It postulates that individuals' perceptions of their capabilities affects how motivated they will be to change their behavior, what behaviors they will attempt to change, how much effort they will devote to the task, and how long they will persevere in this change once they encounter difficulties (O'Leary 1985:438). Studies on behaviors as diverse as cigarette smoking, weight control, contraception, alcohol use and exercise find "strong relationships between self-efficacy and healthy behavior change and maintenance" (Strecher 1986:73). These studies suggest that when self-efficacy is enhanced, it can result in subsequent behavioral change, and that "self-efficacy appears to be a consistent predictor of short- and long-term success" with regard to behavioral change and maintenance (Strecher et al. 1986:75).

Efficacy expectations are learned from four major sources: personal experience, vicarious experience through observation of events and others, verbal persuasion from an outside source, and physiological state (Strecher 1986:75). An intravenous drug user may doubt his ability to avoid needle sharing (that is, he has low self-efficacy in reference to preventing this behavior) because he has been unsuccessful at such attempts in the past (personal experience), because none of his peers seem to be able to stop sharing needles (vicarious experience), and because when a "fix" is presented to him in "works" that someone else has already used, his craving for the drug overwhelms his intention to not share needles (physiological state). However, exposing active drug users to outreach workers who are former addicts may raise their perceptions of self-efficacy vicariously, by the observation of models who have successfully mastered addiction and through verbal persuasion (outreach workers encourage clients and tell them that they are capable of preventing HIV infection and stopping their use of drugs).

Just as efforts to prevent the sexual transmission of HIV among gay men should address the broader social circumstances of minority sexual preference, and AIDS-prevention programs within the schools must confront the public debate on adolescent sexuality, AIDS-prevention programs targeted to intravenous drug users must consider the larger societal issues of drug use and drug abuse treatment.

America is currently reevaluating its position on the problem of drug use, and the outcome of this national debate is certain to influence both how we deal with the drug problem as a society and also how we deal with the individual drug user. A 1988 State Department report indicated that the production of coca, marijuana, and opium poppy crops has increased substantially in most countries, and that drug production and trafficking "remain big business" (Sciolino 1988:1). While the reasons for this increase in production are relatively simplistic from an economic point of view, solutions to the problem are not as easy to identify, and must address global economic issues, international law, diplomatic relations, corruption in foreign governments, and foreign banking regulations (Sciolino 1988). Because the drug problem in America is part of a larger global concern, attempts to redress it through legislation and national policy formulation often uncover conflicting political agendas and priorities (Sciolino and Engelberg 1988). Proposed legislation to permit America's military to combat the distribution of illegal drugs in this country underscores the "growing antidrug fervor" in the United States Congress (Rasky 1988:1), as does the Senate's 1988 approval of an additional 2.6 billion dollars to anti-drug programs, bringing the total 1989 allocation to 6.6 billion dollars (Fuerbringer 1988).

Programs implemented to stem the importation and distribution of drugs are distinct from programs designed to interrupt the cycle of addictive drug use. Nonetheless, they do influence one another. Political and legislative antecedents are largely responsible for popular perceptions about drug use in America (see Chapter Two) and have influenced attitudes about the treatment of drug abuse. Central to the public conception of drug addiction is a long-standing question which has yet to be resolved: is drug addiction an illness or a criminal activity? Certainly, it contains elements of both, and while most practitioners view it as a medical problem, law makers and the general public are more likely to regard it as a crime. The fact that many addicts support their habits through illegal activities, such as prostitution or theft, further clouds the distinction.

Debate on this question is likely to intensify as funding increases to fuel America's "war on drugs." These observations are not meant to minimize the importance of a strong, well-funded, and centrally coordinated effort to stop drug trafficking. However, such an effort does position the public to view "drugs" as an absolute evil, and secondarily to consider addicts as wrongdoers rather than as sick, dependent individuals.

The consequences of viewing drug addiction as simultaneously a medical and legal problem are most apparent in the controversy surrounding AIDS-prevention programs that advocate the distribution of sterile needles and syringes to prevent the further spread of HIV. An experiment to test the impact of distributing free hypodermic needles and syringes to intravenous drug users in New York City (Lambert 1988c) was criticized for lending "legitimacy to drug use" (Marriott 1989:12). The experiment was designed to compare the frequency of drug use and needle sharing and the rate of HIV infection between users who were given sterile injection equipment while waiting for drug treatment, and those who were not. Two months into the experiment, it had to be modified because of a "failure to reach out to drug users" (Marriott 1989:12). Confinement of the project to a government office building by pressure from neighborhood groups also had a significant effect on enrollment in the program (Gross 1989). Portland, Oregon (Lambert 1988a), and Boston, Massachusetts (Gold 1988b), are also considering the implementation of pilot programs for sterile needle and syringe exchange. These programs have been resisted by officials and citizens who believe that such programs simply encourage drug using behavior (Lambert 1988b) and that making sterile injection equipment available "would put government in the position of assisting addicts with their habits" (Kerr 1988:7). One opponent in Boston argued that such a plan "has got nothing to do with AIDS," and that taxpayers would be paying for the habits of addicts (Gold 1988b:A22). Reservations about these pilot programs are not inappropriate, and some intravenous drug users themselves are unsure whether providing sterile needles and syringes "would encourage noninjectors to start injecting" (Ghodse et al. 1987:699). However, intransigent resistance to considering this option generally reflects the persistent view of addiction as a criminal activity rather than an illness (Barron 1988).

Sterile needle and syringe distribution has been employed in several European countries including Denmark, England, Ireland, Italy, the Netherlands, Scotland, and Switzerland (Brunet et al. 1987; Des Jarlais 1987a; Hart et al. 1988; Lefton 1988; Lohr 1988; Marks and Perry 1987). In 1987, the Netherlands distributed approximately 700,000 sterile needles and syringes, and indicated that only 25 percent of the addicts in their program reported needle sharing: a reduction of nearly 50 percent from 1985 figures (Lefton 1988:41). Also of note, there has been "no decrease in demand for either methadone or drug free treatment," nor has there been a reported increase in intravenous drug use as a result of this intervention (Des Jarlais and Friedman 1987a:72). Like most of these programs, participants are required to return used needles in order to obtain clean ones. Buning found that drug users who participated in the program (known as "exchangers"), were likely to be older, have a longer history of intravenous drug use, and share needles significantly less often compared to drug users who did not participate in the exchange (Buning et al. 1988).

A pilot needle and syringe exchange program in Sydney, Australia, incorporated testing of the returned equipment for the presence of antibody to HIV (Wodak et al. 1987). Wodak and his colleagues were not able to comment on the efficacy of this pilot study in terms of reducing needle sharing, but they did believe that the testing of the used equipment was an effective "means to evaluate measures that are designed to reduce the transmission of HIV among intravenous drug abusers" (Wodak et al. 1987:275). In Lund, Sweden, sterile equipment for injection has been provided to intravenous drug users since November 1986. After a medical examination and education about the parenteral and sexual transmission of HIV, addicts receive two to four syringes, needles, and condoms. Participants are required to exchange used injection equipment in order to get new, sterile supplies. Clients are also given information about HIV counseling, testing facilities, and treatment opportunities. Ljungberg and colleagues report that through this program they have provided services to nearly 500 addicts, representing one-sixth of the estimated population of intravenous drug users in their community (Ljungberg et al. 1988). Commenting on the effects of their program, they noted that "only a handful of new HIV cases have been found" and that "no serious negative effects have emerged so far." They also reported that less than 50 percent of the persons enrolled had any prior contact with treatment programs, and that, as a result of their efforts, "many previously unknown drug abusers" have been brought into contact with treatment programs (Ljungberg et al. 1988:387). A similar observation has been made in London, England, where 65 percent of 300 drug users enrolled in a syringe exchange program "were not in contact with any other agency" (Mulleady et al. 1988:388). The ability of needle and syringe exchange programs to identify users who have no prior contact with health care or drug abuse treatment systems has important long-range implications for prevention programs and may come to be recognized as an effective way of identifying users for enrollment into treatment programs.

Many who criticize the distribution of sterile needles and syringes as a means of AIDS prevention point to Italy, where, despite the availability of needles and syringes, HIV infection rates have continued to increase among IV drug users, "rising from 5 percent to 50 percent in two or three years" among addicts in Milan (Moss 1987: 389). However, at least one report indicates that although needles and syringes are available without prescription in Italy, most pharmacists will not sell them to drug users (Tirelli et al. 1988).

Unfortunately, these limited observations do not permit conclusive evaluation of the efficacy of this prevention strategy—especially since "almost no data have been systematically collected about the relationships between the legal availability of sterile equipment and levels of IV drug use prior to the AIDS epidemic" (Des Jarlais and Friedman 1987a:72). However, there is enough secondary information to suggest that it should not be discounted as an option. In *Confronting AIDS: Update 1988*, the Institute of Medicine and National Academy of Sciences endorse the belief that "evaluation of the effectiveness of providing sterile needles and injection equipment to drug abusers in certain circumstances is an essential part of planning a prevention strategy" (Institute of Medicine and National Academy of Sciences 1988:86). As the HIV epidemic intensifies, it is likely that a number of American cities will try needle and syringe distribution and exchange programs. We cannot predict the outcome of these efforts, but we can guess that they will be accompanied by controversy because of the different perspectives that attend the complicated phenomenon of intravenous drug use.

Terminating dependency on drugs is the other major strategy of

AIDS-prevention programs targeted to intravenous drug users. Although to many, terminating drug use would seem to be the ideal solution to AIDS prevention among this group, it is, like so many of our responses to AIDS, neither easily implemented nor universally acceptable to all the individuals at risk. Merely making treatment opportunities available will not ensure that all addicts will enter treatment. Although the fear of AIDS is likely to promote the addict's desire to terminate drug use, (Conviser and Rutledge 1988; Des Jarlais and Friedman 1987a), this variable must be considered in conjunction with data indicating that the mean interval between first daily opiate use and first voluntary treatment may be as long as eight years (Desmond and Maddox 1984:330).

In Jorquez's retrospective study of "retirement" from heroin use in twenty-nine former heroin addicts, he reported that the crucial turning point in their heroin-using careers "was often associated with a profoundly moving cognitive/emotional experience which invariably occured during crisis episodes" (Jorquez 1983:343). In the early stages of this process, former addicts begin to actively extricate themselves from the social relationships they have developed within the heroin-using world (Jorquez 1983:343). Jorquez describes this process as one that takes tremendous physical and emotional energy and cautions that the retiring addict must struggle "on a daily basis" to remain abstinent (Jorquez 1983:355). It is important to realize that quitting drugs also means abandoning a society of which the IV drug user has been a member, often for several years. To the outsider unfamiliar with the drug-using subculture, relationships embedded within destructive behavior and addictive despair would seem to be easily and eagerly discarded. But, for the addict who has defined self and companionship on the basis of these relationships, separating from them is not made any less painful by society's value judgments about their worth. Furthermore, many drug addicts, especially if they are poor, may lack the social, emotional, or financial resources to identify alternatives to an environment where drug use is a daily reality. Therefore, optimism about the effect of increasing treatment opportunities must be tempered by an awareness that basic social issues in the client's environment are likely to moderate the outcome of treatment.

For example, a study of 1,174 heroin addicts who were relocated and interviewed six years after completing treatment for their drug use, found that the personal background and family circumstances of the individual were important contributors to predicting the impact of treatment at long-term follow-up. Those persons with "greater family resources" were more likely to have a favorable long-term outcome compared to those who lacked family support (Hater et al. 1984:39). The investigators concluded that "family and personal background variables made unique contributions to the prediction of a follow-up composite outcome (representing drug use, employment, and criminality) and a general well-being measure" (Hater et al. 1984:29)—again emphasizing the significance of the social milieu in moderating the outcome of treatment.

Another, more obvious, barrier to ending drug dependency is the current inability of drug treatment programs to accomodate clients in need. In New York City, where it is estimated that there may be as many as two hundred thousand intravenous drug users, only about thirty-three thousand were in treatment programs as of early 1988 (Schmalz 1988). According to Drucker, this situation is due, in part, to the relatively low level of funding of such programs" (1986: 176). Inadequate treatment resources in New York City have resulted in long waiting lists for both methadone maintenance programs and for residential ("drug-free") treatment programs (New York City Commission on Human Rights 1987; Selwyn et al. 1987; Weinberg and Murray 1987). At a national level it is estimated that there may be as many as 1.2 million intravenous drug users, and that only 148,000 of them are in treatment programs at any one time (Boffey 1988b:B7).

In response to this urgent need, both state and federal government agencies have announced their intention to expand funding to drug treatment facilities. In New York, state officials announced early in 1988 that they would increase funding to drug treatment programs to accommodate additional clients (Kerr 1988). The Presidential Commission on AIDS has also called for a multimillion dollar expansion of drug abuse treatment facilities by urging the hiring of "32,000 drug treatment specialists and setting up 3,300 drug centers" (Boffey 1988b:A1).

This expansion is likely to make a significant contribution to slowing the spread of HIV infection among intravenous drug users. In a three-year study of methadone maintenance programs in New York City, Philadelphia, and Baltimore, 71 percent of clients who remained in treatment for one or more years "had ceased IV drug use", while 82 percent of those who left treatment "rapidly relapsed" into using heroin (Ball et al. 1988:384), indicating that for heroin addiction, at lest, methadone maintenance can be an effective means of preventing further use of this drug and subsequent exposure to HIV. In both New York and Sweden, analysis of rates of HIV infection among intravenous drug users enrolled in methadone maintenance treatment programs revealed that those persons who entered prior to 1983 had a lower rate of HIV infection compared to persons who entered after this time (Blix and Gronbladh 1988; Hartel et al. 1988), again supporting the assertion that methadone maintenance can be an effective means of preventing heroin addicts from returning to injecting that drug.

However, it is important to recognize the limitations of drug abuse treatment, regardless of its promotion as a strategy to prevent HIV transmission. While it is "generally acknowledged that treatment works well while clients remain in a program," follow-up often reveals a dampening of long-term treatment effects (Hubbard et al. 1984:63).

The Treatment Outcome Prospective Study (TOPS), is a federally funded longitudinal evaluation of clients before, during, and after treatment for intravenous drug addiction in a variety of settings, including outpatient methadone maintenance programs, residential drug-free programs, outpatient drug-free programs, and outpatient detoxification programs (Hubbard et al. 1984). In reviewing the data from TOPS between the years of 1979 to 1981, Hubbard and his colleagues reported that after methadone treatment, daily or weekly use of heroin and other narcotics decreased by 70 percent for clients who remained in the program for three to twenty-four months. Over one-third of long-term residential drug-free clients reported no weekly use of any drug in the year after treatment, and one-fourth of long-term outpatient drug-free clients reported no weekly use of any drugs in the year after treatment (Hubbard et al. 1984:60). In general, clients who remained in treatment longer appeared to have more positive outcomes at follow-up (Hubbard et al. 1984:57). When client retention rates were examined, outpatient drug-free clients were found to be the most likely to leave treatment in a week or less. In residential drug-free programs, over one-fourth of the clients dropped out during the first month of treatment. The best retention rates were seen with methadone maintenance programs, where three months after intake, nearly 65 percent of the clients remained in treatment (Hubbard et al. 1984:55).

In conclusion, Hubbard and his colleagues found that in all of the treatment modalities "more than one-third of the clients report not using their pretreatment primary drug during the follow-up period"

(1984:60). To many, these "success" rates might seem slim. But this does not mean that increasing treatment opportunities for intravenous drug users is inappropriate or ill-advised—only that our expectations for the success of this strategy must be tempered by an awareness that treatment is not uniformly successful, and that outcomes can be influenced by many factors, including quality of the program and availability of supportive care (Ball et al. 1988).

The choice of a particular drug treatment modality is dependent upon clinical, psychological, and social factors, the discussion of which is beyond the scope of this book. The available data indicate that methadone maintenance is an appropriate and effective treatment for at least some heroin addicts. However, the expansion of methadone maintenance programs in response to AIDS is likely to bring forth critics who see this approach as the replacement of one addiction with another (Booth 1988). Methadone maintenance has been criticized because of the indeterminate length of time that many heroin addicts are on replacement, and because it does not "'cure' patients, or render them immune from such societal ills as unemployment, alcoholism, marijuana smoking, and criminality" (Newman 1987:448). The fact that methadone maintenance programs can be evaluated on a number of different parameters in addition to abstinence from heroin use (DeLeon 1984:69), only strengthens our assertion that drug use is a complex problem that requires comprehensive intervention at both medical and social levels; it is not amenable to a "quick fix" solution (Booth 1988).

Even when treatment leads to successful termination of addiction to one drug, such as heroin, participants may continue to inject other substances, such as cocaine (Drucker 1986:172; Hasin et al. 1988). Des Jarlais and Friedman report that over 83 percent of the heroin users in their studies have also injected cocaine (1988:1945). Chaisson and his colleagues found that 26 percent of 673 intravenous drug users on methadone maintenance therapy for heroin addiction "began injecting cocaine after entry into treatment" (Chaisson et al. 1988).

Treating persons who inject cocaine is especially difficult, since, unlike methadone maintenance for heroin addiction, there is no replacement therapy for IV cocaine use. Therapy of stimulant abuse typically entails "initiation of abstinence and relapse prevention" (Gawin and Ellinwood 1988:1177). Preventing relapse involves techniques such as "rehearsing avoidance strategies, altering life-style, developing drug-free socialization networks, extinguishing conditioned cues, and reducing external stress" (p. 1177). Successfully maintaining a state of abstinence usually requires "long-term group psychotherapy modeled after self-help groups such as Alcoholics Anonymous" (p. 1178). Although expanded drug treatment facilities may increase the number of persons who initiate abstinence from stimulants such as cocaine, they can not ensure continued abstinence, especially if the basic psychosocial needs of the client are not being addressed as part of the program.

Clients may leave treatment before program completion; may continue to inject drugs while they are in treatment, although perhaps at a reduced rate; or may return to drug use even after completion of a treatment program (Gold 1988a). These facts emphasize the importance of providing information early in the course of treatment about the dangers of needle sharing and the manner in which injection equipment can be disinfected. For clinical staff who have devoted their careers to preventing needle-injecting behaviors, this recommendation may be difficult to accept, and subsequently inadequately implemented. This dilemma is especially marked in drug-free residential communities, where staff concerns about the effect of needle-cleaning education on the process of addiction termination have been identified as significant barriers to the widespread implementation of AIDS-prevention programs in those settings (Gold 1988a).

Although expanding drug treatment facilities may not be a prevention panacea for HIV infection among IV drug users, there are many positive aspects of aligning AIDS-prevention with drug treatment programs. Because of the high seroprevalence of HIV infection among certain communities of IV drug users, especially those from the northeastern part of the United States (Lange et al. 1988), there is an urgent need to interrupt the transmission of HIV from infected drug users to their sexual partners and from women (infected through IV drug use or sexual contact with an IV drug user) to their children. Drug treatment programs can serve as a focal point for targeting not only the extinction of needle-transmitted HIV but also sexually and perinatally transmitted infection. These goals can be achieved even if the success of terminating IV drug use itself is not always a certainty.

Beth Israel's Methadone Maintenance Treatment Program (MMTP) is the largest drug treatment program in the United States and operates twenty-three community-based clinics within four boroughs of New York City. In Beth Israel's MMTP, clients are educated by the clinical staff regarding the dangers of needle sharing, the importance of disinfecting needles, and the manner in which HIV is sexually transmitted. Female partners of the male clients, many of whom are not IV drug users, are invited to attend (with the client's permission and in accordance with the strict confidentiality requirements of the organization) a group session conducted by a female clinical staff member. This session covers essential information about AIDS and includes a group discussion of condom use, complete with role playing and the formulation of strategies to encourage male partners to use condoms. Prior to implementing this program, the staff received special training in human sexuality counseling.

Like many of the programs cited in this chapter, HIV antibody counseling and testing is offered to clients who are interested in learning their HIV serostatus, but the clinical staff does not view this as a pre-requisite for the initiation or maintenance of behavioral change. Among IV drug users, in fact, caution has been advised lest the knowledge of a positive result eventuate in relapse to drug use (Gold 1988a).

The New Jersey State Department of Health has developed a unique approach to AIDS prevention under the aegis of drug treatment. Identifying economic constraints as a potential barrier to drug treatment (New Jersey does not provide free heroin detoxification), they employ ex-addict outreach workers to distribute coupons to active IV drug users, entitling them to free outpatient heroin detoxification. As part of the outreach and detoxification program, IV drug users are provided with basic information about AIDS prevention. This ingenious strategy incorporates several of the marketing principles previously described. This program identifies a "product" for which there is a consumer demand, advertises it in a nonthreatening way by employing ex-addict outreach workers, and "prices" it so that consumption is made more desirable.

Interventions that work toward making a drug-free condition more desirable than addiction are likely to increase demand for drug treatment. To achieve this goal, however, program planners and drug treatment specialists must be able to identify economic, social, and psychological incentives for addicts to remain in treatment after enrollment and to abstain from injecting drugs after the treatment program is completed. Such an approach will be costly and labor intensive, but is more likely to net the desired outcomes than one that views drug treatment as the mere extinction of physiological addiction. Certainly, "curing" the addiction is essential, but the complexity of the phenomenon of drug use calls for solutions that are comprehensive and multidimensional, and that address the social antecedents of the problem just as thoroughly as the medical ones.

In developing programs to prevent the transmission of HIV among intravenous drug users, the program planner must never lose sight of the fact that drug use is both a medical and a social problem.

Criterion 4: "A HEALTH PROMOTION PROGRAM SHOULD IDEN-TIFY AND IMPLEMENT INTERVENTIONS WHICH MAKE OPTIMUM USE OF AVAILABLE RESOURCES" (Ad Hoc Work Group . . . 1987: 91).

The fourth criterion for health-promotion programs could just as easily appear in a book on organizational management and planning. Essentially, it directs planners to identify pre-existing or potential resources within their environments that can be used to optimize the chances of a successful program outcome. Most management texts caution planners to perform a careful assessment of available resources (whether personnel, fiscal, or technical) at the outset of a project in order to accurately estimate unmet needs, project the costs of addressing those needs, calculate potential benefits, summarize the experience of others who have undertaken similar efforts, and utilize existing resources rather than develop new ones. Administrators of all types hate to reinvent the wheel; planners of AIDS-prevention programs are no exception.

To maximize the outcome of AIDS-prevention programs, it is desirable to define "available resources" in the broadest possible sense. This not only increases the number of opportunities to reach individuals with a risk-reduction message but also promotes reinforcement of the message: it will be heard from multiple sources in different contexts. Since the ultimate goal of all AIDS-prevention programs is behavioral change rather than information dissemination per se, reinforcement is essential.

Community-based organizations, social clubs, entertainment facilities, schools and college campuses, factories, prisons and correctional institutions, public welfare offices, church groups, health care providers, the media, and celebrity spokespersons are all examples of potential resources that are available to the person planning AIDS-prevention initiatives. In fact, any gathering of people or means to reach groups should be considered as potential resources. To the person planning health promotion programs, there is almost no such thing as an inappropriate forum for prevention education—although interventions must be tailored to the particular target audience and occasion.

Very often, the goal of effective resource utilization is addressed through the process of collaboration. Organizations with extensive experience in providing AIDS-related or other services to members of "high-risk" groups are called upon by other agencies to participate in the development and execution of AIDS-prevention programs. They may act as consultants, provide training and information, or function as subcontractors who are charged with carrying out specific program objectives.

Among the programs cited in this chapter, examples of collaboration are quite common. The San Francisco Health Department has a long-standing history of working with the San Francisco AIDS Foundation and has subcontracted with that organization to produce both print and video materials. BEBASHI serves as a training resource for the large number of community and social organizations with whom they network. Florida's Health Education and Risk Reduction Program, a federally funded initiative that targets "high-risk" populations in four counties in southern Florida, has subcontracted with the Health Crisis Network of Miami to conduct baseline AIDS-information and sexual-practice surveys among the gay and bisexual population of the greater Miami area. Gay Men's Health Crisis of New York has provided AIDS training for counselors from a variety of institutions, including detention facilities, public schools, and adolescent primary health care facilities. The Dallas County Health Department subcontracts with a community-based organization providing counseling services to persons with HIV infection. The New Jersey State Department of Health employs nearly thirty AIDS coordinators who are placed in community-based organizations offering drug treatment services; they act as on-site resources and as liaisons between the local organizations and the health department.

In addition to the obvious advantages of working with organizations that have experience with AIDS prevention, collaboration can promote the input of target group members into the implementation and service delivery phase of program development: When community-based organizations collaborate with public health departments, for example, they bring a unique perspective based on their experience of providing services to intravenous drug users, or gay men, or racial/ethnic minorities. That is not to say that departments of health have not provided services to these groups prior to the AIDS epidemic. However, because of their mission, most community-based organizations have a closer link with their clients, offer services that are usually "packaged" comprehensively, and are more dependent on the support of their constituents, and therefore, more sensitive to their needs. Health departments, in contrast, serve many different groups of clients; usually offer categorical services, often in different locales and in different programs; develop program services on the basis of legislative mandate; and must be responsive to the needs of numerous constituents comprising both the public at large and appropriate governmental authorities. By their very nature, community-based organizations are more directly aware of the needs of their clients than are governmentally funded organizations that are limited by their categorical approach and the large numbers of constituents they serve. Therefore, collaboration between the two kinds of organizations can promote the awareness of the "special characteristics, needs, and preferences" of target groups (Ad Hoc Work Group . . . 1987:90).

The permutations of collaboration that can and have occurred in response to AIDS are innumerable. Labor unions and professional organizations serve as facilitators and sponsors of AIDS-prevention initiatives for their members. Academicians are called upon by public health departments and community-based organizations to help design and evaluate risk-reduction interventions. Media representatives work with departments of public health to publicize information about AIDS prevention and to advertise existing prevention services. As the number of diagnosed AIDS cases grows larger, the impact of AIDS will diffuse throughout broader segments of society, and organizations of all kinds will respond to the epidemic by collaboration and coalition building with one other.

While the other criteria we have reviewed focused primarily on intervention design, this one addresses the process of implementation. Implementation is the mirror image of planning—it is the process that translates preparatory developmental work into a physical product. It encompasses all of the activities undertaken to make a program functional and is as critical for success as program design. The legislative arena is replete with examples of laws that were based on well-documented needs, but because of inadequate or faulty implementation, fell short of their goals. The same can happen to AIDS-prevention programs.

Even a well-funded, theoretically sound program will have only a limited impact if it is not properly implemented. In the broadest sense, implementation requires insight, not only into the special characteristics of the people for whom the program is being planned but also the environment into which the program is to be interposed and the existing constraints on resources. Political, policy, and organizational issues that have little to do with AIDS prevention in a technical sense can have a significant impact on the implementation of AIDS-prevention programs.

For example, a program might have as a specific goal the need to develop skills that would enable young, sexually active women to introduce the subject of condoms with a male sexual partner. Perhaps this goal is predicated on preliminary focus-group research indicating that women are often unsuccessful in convincing their male partners to use condoms. Although the provision of skills training is grounded in health theory and the need for such training has been documented by prior work, this program might encounter resistance if it were to be implemented in a high school setting— not because it is an inappropriate response to AIDS prevention, but because it conflicts with school policy or concerns parents who believe that it will promote premarital sexual activity.

Suppose, instead, that this same program is to be implemented in a family planning clinic setting, a natural location for such an activity. Successful implementation requires that the clinic's staff learn the negotiation and role playing skills they will be teaching to clients. If clinical staff feel inadequately prepared—because training sessions are poorly designed or because client education materials, or the time to perform the client education are lacking—they are apt to perform half-heartedly or decide that this additional responsibility is beyond their capabilities. Even with proper staff training, the program could fail because the planners did not look carefully at the flow of clients through the agency to determine how this new service might be integrated into existing services. Should the skills training be worked into the regular counseling routine? Should the client flow be changed to permit adequate time to conduct this training? Will this new service require additional staff? If these questions are not addressed during the implementation process, the specific prevention goals of the program may become lost in a muddle of poor scheduling, hurried staff, and disgruntled patients.

Implementation problems notwithstanding, the use of existing community resources to promote AIDS-prevention programming is an entirely logical strategy. It can accelerate implementation and service delivery by capitalizing on prior experience, and can decrease program costs by truncating the "learning curve" associated with program start-up. Training costs can be reduced appreciably by relying on individuals who are actively involved in dispensing AIDS-related health and social services. Broadening access to individuals at increased risk for HIV infection by formalizing linkages with organizations providing social, economic, or health-related services to those people will ensure that the intervention is delivered to a wide audience. Embedded within these potential benefits, however, is a risk. Resources are not infinite. They must be replenished, and this requires longitudinal rather than reactive planning.

Many of the organizations that provide prevention services to individuals at increased risk of HIV infection also provide social and support services to people who already have AIDS. These organizations are often heavily subsidized by private contributions and substantial volunteer effort. In the 1985 fiscal year, community-based AIDS organizations in San Francisco recorded over 130,000 hours of volunteer labor (Arno 1986:1325). Despite the admirable performance record of these community-based organizations in combatting the spread of AIDS, especially within the gay community, their continued ability to do so may be constrained by the large number of people who will develop symptomatic HIV disease within the next decade. The urgency of directing resources to sick persons in obvious need suggests that prevention activities may take a fiscal back seat to support programs, even within the same organization. In the gay community, many of the leaders and volunteers who support prevention efforts may themselves fall ill with HIV-related illness. Without the influx of additional resources, both human and financial, these community organizations will be hard-pressed to maintain AIDS-prevention services at the level required to minimize new infection. Although all of us anticipate the development of curative treatment for HIV infection, we must plan prevention programs under the assumption that they will be long-range services and that the next generation will require these services.

Resources must not only be replenished, they must also be targeted to organizations, groups, areas, and individuals with the greatest need. Although educating the general public about AIDS is necessary, it should not be undertaken at a level that would jeopardize funding to the groups in greatest need of prevention services. This is a very real problem, which will become increasingly apparent as the epidemic progresses and as anxiety levels about the risk of AIDS increase among groups whose risk of infection is actually quite small. It would be a mistake to put substantial resources into educating low-risk heterosexuals about HIV prevention while underfunding efforts that target heterosexuals whose risk is great because of IV drug use or sexual intercourse with IV drug users, hemophiliacs, and bisexual men. Likewise, prevention efforts that continue to emphasize the dissemination of information about AIDS rather than skills training that will enable clients to act on the information they already have, or programs that support individuals throughout the initiation and maintenance of behavioral change, would be a misapplication of resources. Funding for prevention services must not be limited to those with a single philosophy or to a single entity. It cannot be simple equity that dictates how resources should be distributed across a variety of organizations, it must be rational planning.

Finally, the ability of various "resources" to promote AIDS prevention is a relative, not an absolute, phenomenon. Modalities that are effective for one target group in a particular setting may not necessarily transpose to another group with equal success. Although there is a great need and interest in developing prevention models that can be duplicated on a larger scale, it is still necessary for program planners to tailor interventions to the circumstances and needs of their communities. By performing a preliminary assessment, either through survey or focus groups, informed judgements can be made about client needs and what resources would be most effective and appropriate in meeting those needs.

Few urban gay communities have a print media as extensive and well read as San Francisco's. Therefore, relying on San Francisco's success with this resource as a model for spreading information about AIDS in other gay communities (where media resources are limited) may prove to be ineffective. Even in San Francisco, it is possible that readers of the gay and general press are far less in need of prevention services than those who do not read the papers. African-American youth may be loath to learn about AIDS prevention by reading brochures but amenable to group discussions led by members of their own communities. A poster campaign that warns of the dangers of needle sharing may not reach intravenous drug users, whereas direct person-to-person contact would. Spanish-language radio programs about AIDS that have been successful in reaching the Cuban community in southern Florida may be less effective when applied to Hispanics in the southwestern United States.

It is worth taking a closer look at the use of electronic media, particularly television, in AIDS-prevention programs. Experience with television and AIDS underscores the importance of understanding the strengths and limitations of a particular resource prior to program design.

There are a number of reasons television is a seemingly attractive resource for AIDS prevention. It is a nearly ubiquitous medium. Almost every dwelling in the United States has a television, and in the average household, "sets are in use approximately seven hours per day" (Bryant and Gerner 1981:154). Also, it can reach children and teenagers before they start using drugs or having sex. On average, adolescents spend 17.25 hours per week watching television (Lawrence et al. 1986:431). This medium can be a source of health-related information. Twenty-four percent of nearly 600 teenagers who were surveyed on the sources of their information about contraception identified television "far more than any other source" (Pearl et al. 1982:13). And television does have the *potential* to influence behavior. Television can contribute to the viewers' "conceptions of social reality" (Pearl et al. 1982:62) and has been documented to "modify viewers' behavior in a prosocial direction" (Rushton 1982: 255). As a source of "observational learning experiences," television is able to deliver program messages that increase "generosity, helping, cooperation, friendliness, adhering to rules, delaying gratification, and a lack of fear" (Rushton 1982:255). Television also affects a child's sexual socialization, by acting as a "relatively secure environment from which to glean insights into the meaning of sexuality in adult life" (Roberts 1982:209).

Such impressive credentials are difficult to ignore, and it would seem ludicrous to not take full advantage of television as a resource. To do that, however, we must distinguish between television's ability to provide information about AIDS and reinforcement cues, and its ability to actually promote behavioral change.

As a means of providing the general public with information about AIDS, television is nonpareil. "AIDS Lifeline," an education and public service campaign produced by KPIX-TV in San Francisco (Hogan 1988) exemplifies this potential. Its series of five nationally syndicated specials dealt with basic information about AIDS, the heterosexual transmission of HIV, the impacts of AIDS on the health care system, a documentary on the Names Project Quilt (a national memorial to those who have died of AIDS), and children with AIDS. The campaign focused on nontargeted information for the general public rather than on specific risk-reduction messages targeted to high-risk groups. It was designed so that it could be adapted to each of the cities where it was broadcast through the use of local reporters, news anchors, and in-studio community experts, who answered viewer questions after each of the presentations. In addition to the programs, the campaign provided public service announcements, updated special reports, and a videotape that parents could use in their homes in discussions of AIDS with their children.

The AIDS Lifeline campaign demonstrates the capabilities of television in providing information about AIDS. However, whether television is actually capable of promoting and maintaining AIDS risk-reduction behavior is another matter—one that has not yet been resolved. Manoff explains that the impact of health-promotion campaigns delivered through mass media is often blunted by the "inadequacy" of the message design and failure to conduct "preparatory stages of concept testing and consumer knowledge and attitude probing" (1985:74). This theme is reiterated by Solomon, who, in a review of televised health campaigns, emphasized the necessity of a "thorough understanding of the relevant beliefs, information needs, knowledge levels, current behaviors, and blockages to change on the part of the target audience segments" (1982:318).

There is some evidence that mass media (including television) health-promotion campaigns can bring about behavioral change. In Flay's evaluation of forty mass media programs designed to influence cigarette smoking, he found that information campaigns were capable of producing changes in awareness, knowledge, and attitudes, and that "extensive national campaigns produced meaningful behavioral change" (1987:153). He noted that "intensive television and radio programming of high frequency, extended reach, and long duration can produce behavioral effects," and suggested that successful campaigns were characterized by a reinforcement of existing information and a supplementation of ongoing initiatives (Flay 1987:155). In Ben-Sira's study of Israeli adults who had been exposed to a televised smoking abstinence program, he observed that exposure among high-risk groups was lower than among median-risk groups, and that the main value of the television campaign appeared to be in reinforcing behavioral change among those who had already decided to quit smoking rather than in motivating behavioral change per se (1982:825).

Apropos of AIDS prevention, such experience suggests that to use television effectively to actually promote behavioral change, a planner would have to determine, first, which groups in need of specific prevention information about AIDS could be reached by television, what the best time would be to reach them, and, second, what sort of messages would be acceptable to the groups and would promote specific changes in sexual and drug-using behaviors.

A number of potential barriers come to mind regarding these objectives. Most significant is the issue of content. The behaviors that are responsible for the transmission of HIV are not as "public," as widely visible, or as well-understood by nonparticipants, as those pertaining to cigarette smoking. Although many of the strictures first encountered in discussing AIDS on prime-time television have been removed, human sexual behavior, which is globally, of course, the major mode of HIV transmission, remains a controversial and value-charged topic. In November 1987, "all three national networks rejected a thirty-second paid advertisement on birth control submitted by the Association of Reproductive Health Professionals" because of internal censorship guidelines (Lader 1987). Although this advertisement was in no way lurid, and despite the fact that millions of Americans both endorse and practice birth control, the subject matter was not considered appropriate for television viewing audiences. The implications for AIDS-prevention messages are clear. In most instances, those who judge the "appropriateness" of AIDS-prevention messages on television will not be the people who are at greatest risk for infection. This is in direct conflict with the second criterion of health-promotion programs discussed earlier in this chapter.

Censorship is an especially important consideration when we recognize the commercial nature of television in America. Although television has a variety of functions, including entertainment, information dissemination, and education, it is first and foremost a commercially driven enterprise. The commercial nature of television suggests that it will remain limited in its ability to develop messages that deal specifically with selling "products" such as condom-protected intercourse or needle-cleaning behavior. Because of these limitations, it is not likely that television will subsume the function of actually initiating behavioral change; the messages necessary to do so would have to deal explicitly with the behaviors responsible for transmission and are likely to encounter resistance from network censors.

While television may be limited in its ability to be used for potentially controversial public health messages targeted to persons who are at increased risk for HIV infection, it does have a role to play in influencing social norms that can contribute to AIDS prevention. Programming wields a great deal of influence in this regard. There is definite evidence that what we view on television has an impact on the way we perceive ourselves and our world, and on our subsequent behaviors. Perhaps the most widely known research finding on the behavioral effects of television is the association between aggressive behavior in children and adolescents and the viewing of violent television programs (Pearl et al. 1982:6). Another example is found in a recent review of childhood attitudes toward thinness and fatness. Feldman and his colleagues suggest that the ubiquitous media message that thinness equals beauty and "the good life" contributes to adolescent eating disorders (1988:190). More germane to our discussion is the research of Roberts, who believes that television is often used by children to fill gaps in their information about human sexuality (1982).

The Harvard Alcohol Project is an example of a health-promotion campaign designed to integrate a health message directly into television programming rather than limit the message to public service announcements. In order to dissuade people from driving while under the influence of alcohol, the project will place into television scripts dialogue relating to the concept of "designated drivers" (that is, persons who agree not to drink during social events so they can assume the responsibility of driving friends and family home) (Rothenberg 1988:E6). Although there is consensus that driving under the influence of alcohol is dangerous and the "designated driver" approach is a sound one, the campaign has been subject to criticism. Some people fear that is places too much power to dictate social norms into the hands of television networks, and others believe that such ventures "undermine the idea that the family is the place were morality should be taught" (Rothenberg 1988:E6).

Negative reactions to the Harvard Alcohol Project represent some of the attitudinal barriers obstructing the use of electronic media to promote any particular health behavior. Even if there is consensus that the behavior is dangerous and that the prevention message is sound, fear often remains that such ventures are manipulative and, therefore, unacceptable.

Controversy notwithstanding, this same approach could conceivably be used to promote responsible sexual behavior as a social norm. By modifying its practice of depicting sexual encounters as unplanned and generally free of untoward consequences, television could set the stage for the widespread endorsement of safer sexual practices. In this regard it would function as both a reinforcer and a cue, reminding viewers of the serious potential consequences of unplanned sexual intercourse and of the responsibilities associated with sexual behavior. Specific behaviors that constitute safer sex (for example, the use of condoms and spermicides during all episodes of penetrative intercourse) need not be described in such broadcasts, as long as information about them is available to viewers from other sources. This approach might be more palatable to the general public than an explicit series of public service announcements about sexual risk reduction. It might also be better received by adolescents, who would respond to it primarily as information about sexual behavior, rather than as a warning about AIDS.

Planners should recognize that television offers the immediate advantages of reaching large numbers of persons with nontargeted information about AIDS, of publicizing AIDS service organizations and sources of additional information about the illness and its prevention, and of validating the gravity and relevance of AIDS for everyone (Ross and Carson 1988). Although we recognize television's potential to promote AIDS risk reduction through programming that depicts responsible sexual behavior and demonstrates the negative consequences of drug use in a realistic and nonmoralistic way, the popularity of this approach and the subsequent degree to which it can affect the spread of HIV are currently unknown. The use of television as a tool for AIDS prevention is limited by the fact that not all viewers are equally vulnerable to infection, nor do they all agree on what constitutes appropriate risk reduction, or how information about risk reduction should be presented. A general limitation of using television for the modification of health behaviors is the belief that such attempts are overtly or covertly manipulative.

This brief discussion on the application of television to the objective of AIDS prevention is meant to underscore the need to recognize the strengths and limitations of each of the various resources available to planners of AIDS-prevention programs. Other resources (such as personnel, organizations, and media) should be similarly analyzed during the planning stages of program development. Whether we choose to describe it as prudent management or good public health practice, understanding the ways in which resources can be most appropriately applied to the problem of preventing HIV infection will help to ensure successful program outcomes.

Criterion 5: "FROM THE OUTSET, A HEALTH PROMOTION PROGRAM SHOULD BE ORGANIZED, PLANNED, AND IMPLEMENTED IN SUCH A WAY THAT ITS OPERATION AND EFFECTS CAN BE EVALUATED" (Ad Hoc Work Group . . . 1987:91).

Although the ultimate goal of any AIDS-prevention program is to eliminate or reduce the risk of HIV transmission, it is possible for prevention programs to accomplish any, all, or none of the following objectives: increase knowledge about HIV infection, transmission, and prevention; increase understanding about HIV antibody testing and results interpretation; change attitudes about specific behavioral modifications (such as condom use or needle and syringe cleaning); change the perception of HIV infection risk; and reduce, eliminate, or modify behaviors that increase the risk of HIV infection. Changed behavior is the most desirable goal of any prevention program because its benefits, in terms of interrupting viral transmission, are the greatest. The other outcomes are also desirable, however, especially because many theorists believe that persons must pass through stages of information assimilation and attitudinal change before they actually change their behaviors.

Evaluation allows program managers to determine whether their efforts have been translated into tangible outcomes and what those outcomes are. However, evaluation is not limited to a reckoning of changed behavior. It can also be used to describe those activities, referred to throughout this chapter, that are undertaken before or during the implementation process to "control, assure, or improve the quality of performance or delivery" (Green and Lewis 1986:362). Evaluators refer to these activities as process evaluation when measures are limited to the implementation phase of a program, and as formative evaluation when measures include both preprogram and implementation activities (Green and Lewis 1986:27). Examples of the kinds of preprogram activities that might be included in a formative evaluation are "pretesting, making pilot studies, and forming focus groups" (Green and Lewis 1986:27). Formative and process evaluation are best characterized as ways to obtain "short-loop diagnostic feedback" on the quality of the program (Green and Lewis 1986:27).

Even in terms of evaluating the effects of a program, we can distinguish between impact evaluation (short-term effects) and outcome evaluation (long-term consequences). Impact evaluation assesses the immediate effect of the intervention on such variables as "knowledge, attitudes, perceptions, skills, beliefs, access to resources, and social support" (Green and Lewis 1986:276). Outcome evaluation assesses the long-term effects of the program in terms of changes in health status among the participants. For most of the AIDS-prevention programs discussed in this chapter, formative and impact evaluations are appropriate activities to undertake. However, few programs have the resources to successfully complete outcome evaluation.

The subject of evaluating AIDS-prevention programs is discussed extensively in a later chapter. However, a few specific comments about the evaluation activities of the programs cited in this chapter are helpful as an introduction to the topic. In most of the organizations visited, evaluation strategies were not well developed, and when they were present, they tended to be limited to measures of program accountability; for example, how many people attended an educational session, how many persons were educated by outreach workers, how many brochures about AIDS prevention were distributed during a given period of time, or how many condoms were distributed to persons at risk for HIV infection. Several programs contained elements of impact evaluation, most notably through the use of a pretest measure of knowledge and attitudes followed by a posttest administered immediately after the intervention. Process evaluation, when present, tended to be informal, Documented outcome evaluation was noted only in an academic research setting (AIDS Prevention Project, University of Pittsburgh).

There are a number of reasons for the limited evaluation of AIDS-prevention programs, especially among community-based organizations. The most common is a lack of funding for such activities. Evaluation strategies often require the input of specialists, and when budgets are constrained, consultants are usually lacking. Also, the powerful sense of urgency that accompanies the inception and development of many AIDS-related community organizations often makes proactive planning difficult. Administrators are often pressed to respond quickly to unmet needs, which may well preclude planning services in an evaluable format. Furthermore, client suspicions about the use of personal information pertaining to sexual practices and drug use, which would have to be collected at periodic intervals in order to extend impact evaluation beyond the immediate posttest period, has remained an impediment to evaluation in most nonresearch settings. Finally, because evaluation is not in itself a client service, many program administrators are hesitant to spend substantial portions of their budgets on it.

However, as this criterion suggests, not every AIDS-prevention program needs to be evaluated, as long as it is designed and implemented so that it *could* be evaluated (Ad Hoc Work Group . . . 1987: 91). Although most AIDS-prevention programs will not have the resources to undertake outcome evaluations, the principles that guide formative, process, and impact evaluation are consistent with many of the standards we have previously discussed, especially those that stress the need to tailor prevention services so that they will be acceptable, understandable, and meaningful to the specific target group that is to receive them. Designing prevention programs so that they can be evaluated is another way of safeguarding the quality of those programs.

Nevertheless, the need for program evaluation may become acute as the focus of HIV prevention efforts shifts to smaller groups of individuals who are more difficult to identify, more refractory to behavioral change, and in need of more highly specialized and individualized prevention services. Still, it is unlikely that such information will be forthcoming unless funding agencies are willing to subsidize the costs involved, including the advisements of technical experts in the field of evaluation methodology.

Given the dynamic nature of the AIDS epidemic, it is unlikely that, at the time of this writing, all of the interventions that will be developed in response to HIV infection have yet been identified. In reviewing currently active prevention programs, our intent is not to present a catalogue of AIDS-prevention formulas as much as it is to heighten the reader's awareness of the complexity of AIDS-prevention programming, to suggest strategies that might be useful in confronting common barriers to behavioral change, to discuss the potential pitfalls in the design and implementation of these programs, and to illustrate these points through a series of specific program examples. These comments have been organized and presented under the rubric of five generic criteria that can be used as standards to guide the development of future initiatives (Valdiserri 1987a).

Nowhere is the dynamic nature of AIDS prevention more evident than in the subject of HIV testing. As the next chapter will explain, the ability to detect HIV infection by laboratory means is a tremendous achievement that has virtually eliminated transfusion as a mode of HIV transmission in this country and elsewhere in the industrial world. However, the impact of HIV testing at an individual level, especially in terms of behavioral change, is an unfolding story —and one that is likely to become more complex with changes in legislation pertaining to HIV testing, discrimination against HIV-infected persons, and confidentiality of test results. Advances in medical therapeutics enabling physicians to initiate treatment of HIV infection prior to major symptomatic consequences will also affect the way people at increased risk of HIV infection come to view the test. When planning AIDS-prevention programs, the HIV antibody test should be viewed as a heterogeneous "product" of prevention programs, whose value is influenced by personal perspective, time, and circumstance.

REFERENCES

Ad Hoc Work Group of the American Public Health Association. 1987. "Criteria for the Development of Health Promotion and Education Programs." *American Journal of Public Health* 77(1):89–92.

Alexander, K., and McCullough, J.M. 1981. "Application of Marketing Principles to Improve Participation in Public Health Programs." *Journal of Community Health* 6(3):216–222.

Arno, P.S. 1986. "The Nonprofit Sector's Response to the AIDS Epidemic: Community-Based Services in San Francisco." *American Journal of Public Health* 76(11):1325–1330.

Arnold, C.B. 1972. "The Sexual Behavior of Inner-City Adolescent Condom Users." *Journal of Sexual Research* 8:298–309.

Arnold, C.B., and Cogswell, B.E. 1971. "A Condom Distribution Program for Adolescents: The Findings of a Feasibility Study." *American Journal of Public Health* 61(4):739–750.

Assael, H. 1985. *Marketing Management: Strategy and Action.* Boston: Kent.

Ball, J.C., Lange, W.R., Myers, C.P., and Friedman, S.R. 1988. "The Effectiveness of Methadone Maintenance Treatment in Reducing IV Drug Use and Needle Sharing Among Heroin Addicts at Risk for AIDS." Abstract 8503, proceedings from the *IV International Conference on AIDS*, Book 2, page 384.

Bandura, A. 1977. *Social Learning Theory.* Englewood Cliffs, N.J.: Prentice-Hall.

Barron, J. 1988. "Health Chief Cautious on Needle Plan." *New York Times* March 15, B4.

Bauman, L.J., and Siegel, K. 1987. "Misperceptions Among Gay Men of the Risk for AIDS Associated with Their Sexual Behavior." *Journal of Applied Social Psychology* 17(3):329–350.

Becker, M.H., and Joseph, J.G. 1988. "AIDS and Behavioral Change to Reduce Risk: A Review." *American Journal of Public Health* 78(4):394–410.

Bennis, W.G., Benne, K.D., Chin, R., and Corey, K.E. (Eds.). 1976. *The Planning of Change.* 3rd ed. New York: Holt, Rinehart & Winston.

Ben-Sira, Z. 1982. "The Health Promoting Function of Mass Media and Reference Groups: Motivating or Reinforcing of Behavior Change." *Social Science Medicine* 16:825–834.

Bergman, A.B. 1980. "Condoms for Sexually Active Adolescents. *American Journal of Disease in Children* 134:247–249.

Blix, O., and Gronbladh, L. 1988. "AIDS and IV Heroin Addicts: The Preventive Effect of Methadone Maintenance in Sweden." Abstract 8548, proceedings from the *IV International Conference on AIDS*, Book 2, page 395.

Boffey, P.M. 1988a. "AIDS Panel Backs Wide Drive in U.S." *New York Times* March 3, B5.

Boffey, P.M. 1988b. "AIDS Panel Calls for Major Effort on Drug Abuse and Health Care." *New York Times* February 25, A1 and B7.

Boffey, P.M. 1988c. "Masters and Johnson Say AIDS Spread Is Rampant." *New York Times* March 6, 14.

Boffey, P.M. 1988d. "Spread of AIDS Abating, But Deaths Will Still Soar." *New York Times* February 14, 1 and 22.

Booth, W. 1987. "Another Muzzle for AIDS Education?" *Science* 238:1036.

Booth, W. 1988. "AIDS and Drug Abuse: No Quick Fix." *Science* 239:717–719.

Brunet, J.B., Des Jarlais, D.C., and Koch, M.A. 1987. "Report on the European Community Workshop on Epidemiology of HIV Infections:

Spread Among Intravenous Drug Abusers and the Heterosexual Population, Robert Koch Institute, Berlin, 12–14 November 1986." *AIDS*
1:59–61.

Bryant, W.K., and Gerner, J.L. 1981. "Television Use by Adults and Children: A Multivariate Analysis." *Journal of Consumer Research* 8:
154–161.

Buning, E.C., Hartgers, C., Verster, A.D., van Santen, G.W., and Coutinho,
R.A. 1988. "The Evaluation of the Needle/Syringe Exchange in Amsterdam." Abstract 8513, proceedings from the *IV International Conference on AIDS*, Book 2, page 387.

Centers for Disease Control. 1985. "Self-Reported Behavioral Change
Among Gay and Bisexual Men—San Francisco." *Morbidity and Mortality Weekly Report* 34:613–615.

Centers for Disease Control. 1987a. "Human Immunodeficiency Virus Infection in the United States: A Review of Current Knowledge." *Morbidity and Mortality Weekly Report* 36(S-6):1–48.

Centers for Disease Control. 1987b. "Self-Reported Changes in Sexual
Behaviors Among Homosexual and Bisexual Men from the San Francisco City Clinic." *Morbidity and Mortality Weekly Report* 36:187–
189.

Centers for Disease Control. 1988a. "Condoms for Prevention of Sexually
Transmitted Diseases." *Morbidity and Mortality Weekly Report*
37(9):133–137.

Centers for Disease Control. 1988b. "Quarterly Report to the Domestic Policy Council on the Prevalence and Rate of Spread of HIV and AIDS in
the United States." *Morbidity and Mortality Weekly Report* 37(14):
223–226.

Chaisson, R.E., Osmond, D., Moss, A.R., Feldman, H.W., and Bernacki, P.
1987. "HIV, Bleach, and Needle Sharing." *Lancet* i(8547):1430.

Chaisson, R.E., Osmond, D., Bacchetti, P., Brodie, B., Sande, M.A., and
Moss, A.R. 1988. "Cocaine, Race, and HIV Infection in IV Drug
Users." Abstract 8502, proceedings from the *IV International Confer-
ence on AIDS*, Book 2, page 384.

Connors, M.M., and Galea, R.P. 1988. "Anthropological Investigations of
the Meaning and Practices of Needle Use and Sharing Among Intravenous Drug Users (IVDUs)." Abstract 8518, proceedings from the *IV
International Conference on AIDS*, Book 2, page 388.

Conviser, R., and Rutledge, J.H. 1988. "The Need for Innovation to Halt
AIDS Among Intravenous Drug Users and Their Sexual Partners."
AIDS Public Policy Journal 3(1):43–50.

Cooper, D.A., Imrie, A.A., and Penny, R. 1987. "Antibody Response to Human Immunodeficiency Virus After Primary Infection." *Journal of Infectious Diseases* 155(6):1113–1118.

Culbert, S.A. 1976. "Consciousness Raising: A Five-Stage Model for Social
and Organizational Change." In W.G. Bennis, K.D. Benne, R. Chin
and K.E. Corey (Eds.), *The Planning of Change*. 3rd ed. New York:
Holt, Rinehart & Winston.

Curjel, H.E. 1964. "An Analysis of the Human Reasons Underlying the Failure to Use a Condom in 723 Cases of Venereal Disease." *Journal of the Royal Navy Medical Service* 50:203–209.

Darrow, W.W., and Wiesner, P.J. 1975. "Personal Prophylaxis for Venereal Diseases." *Journal of the American Medical Association* 233(5): 444–446.

DeLeon, G. 1984. "Program-Based Evaluation Research in Therapeutic Communities." In F.M. Tims and J.P. Ludford (Eds.), *Drug Abuse Treatment Evaluation: Strategies, Progress, and Prospects.* Rockville, Md.: National Institute of Drug Abuse Research Monograph 51, U.S. Department of Health and Human Services.

Des Jarlais, D.C., and Hopkins, W. 1985. "'Free' Needles for Intravenous Drug Users at Risk for AIDS: Current Developments in New York City." *New England Journal of Medicine* 313(23):1476.

Des Jarlais, D.C., Friedmann, S.R., and Hopkins, W. 1985. "Risk Reduction for the Acquired Immunodeficiency Syndrome Among Intravenous Drug Users." *Annals of Internal Medicine* 103:755–759.

Des Jarlais, D.C., Friedman, S.R., and Strug, D. 1986. "AIDS and Needle Sharing Within the IV Drug Use Subculture." D.A. Feldman and T.M. Johnson (Eds.), *The Social Dimensions of AIDS: Method and Theory.* New York: Praeger.

Des Jarlais, D.C., and Friedman, S.R. 1987a. "HIV Infection Among Intravenous Drug Users: Epidemiology and Risk Reduction." *AIDS* 1:67–76.

Des Jarlais, D.C., and Friedman, S.R. 1987b. "Target Groups for Preventing AIDS Among Intravenous Drug Users." *Journal of Applied Social Psychology* 17(3):251–268.

Des Jarlais, D.C., and Friedman, S.R. 1988. "Intravenous Cocaine, Crack, and HIV Infection." *Journal of the American Medical Association* 259(13):1945–1946.

Desmond, D.P., and Maddux, J.F. 1984. "Mexican-American Heroin Addicts." *American Journal of Drug and Alcohol Abuse* 10(3):317–346.

Doughery, J.A. 1988. "Prevention of HIV Transmission in IV Drug Users (IVDUs)." Abstract 8533, proceedings from the *IV International Conference on AIDS*, Book 2, page 392.

Drucker, E. 1986. "AIDS and Addiction in New York City." *American Journal of Drug and Alcohol Abuse* 12(1 and 2):165–181.

Ernst, R.S., and Houts, P.S. 1985. "Characteristics of Gay Persons with Sexually Transmitted Diseases." *Sexually Transmitted Diseases* 12(2):59–63.

Fehrs, L.J., Foster, L.R., Fox, V., Fleming, D., McAlister, R.O., Modesitt, S., and Conrad, R. 1988. "Trial of Anonymous Versus Confidential Human Immunodeficiency Virus Testing." *Lancet* ii(8607):379–381.

Feldman, W., Feldman, E., and Goodman, J.T. 1988. "Culture Versus Biology: Children's Attitudes Toward Thinness and Fatness." *Pediatrics* 81(2):190–194.

Felman, Y.M., and Santora, F.J. 1981. "The Use of Condoms by VD Clinic Patients: A Survey." *CUTIS* 27:330–336.

Fineberg, H.V. 1988. "Education to Prevent AIDS: Prospects and Obstacles," *Science* 239:592–596.

Flay, B.R. 1987. "Mass Media and Smoking Cessation: A Critical Review." *American Journal of Public Health* 77:153–160.

Fleming, D.W., Cochi, S.L., Steece, R.S., and Hull, H.F. 1987. "Acquired Immunodeficiency Syndrome in Low-Incidence Areas: How Safe Is Unsafe Sex?" *Journal of the American Medical Association* 258:785–787.

Free, M.J., and Alexander, N.J. 1976. "Male Contraception Without Prescription." *Public Health Report* 91(5):437–445.

Friedman, S.R., Des Jarlais, D.C., and Sotheran, J.L. 1986. "AIDS Health Education for Intravenous Drug Users." *Health Education Quarterly* 13(4):383–393.

Friedman, S.R., Sotheran, J.L., Abdul-Quader, A., Primm, B.J., Des Jarlais, D.C., Kleinman, P., Mauge, C., Goldsmith, D.S., El-Sadi, W., and Masfansky, R. 1987. "The AIDS Epidemic Among Blacks and Hispanics." *Milbank Quarterly* 65(2S):2–54.

Froner, G. 1987. "Disinfection of Hypodermic Syringes by IV Drug Users." *AIDS* 1(2):133–134.

Fuerbringer, J. 1988. "Senate Adds $2.6 Billion to Antidrug Programs." *New York Times* April 15, A19.

Gawin, F.H., and Ellinwood, E.H. 1988. "Cocaine and Other Stimulants: Actions, Abuse, and Treatment." *New England Journal of Medicine* 318(18):1173–1182.

Ghodse, A.H., Tregenza, G., and Li, M. 1987. "Effect of Fear of AIDS on Sharing of Injection Equipment Among Drug Abusers." *British Medical Journal* 295:698–699.

Ginzburg, H.M., French, J., Jackson, J., Hartsock, P.I., MacDonald, M.G., and Weiss, S.H. 1986. "Health Education and Knowledge Assessment of HTLV-III Diseases Among Intravenous Drug Users." *Health Education Quarterly* 13(4):373–382.

Gold, A.R. 1988a. "AIDS Crisis Spurs Shift in Program for Addicts. *New York Times* April 27, A16.

Gold, A.R. 1988b. "Boston City Council Backs Plan on Sterile Needles to Fight AIDS." *New York Times* April 28, A22.

Goldman, A.L. 1987a. "2 Divided Camps of Bishops Form over Catholic AIDS Policy Paper." *New York Times* December 17, 15.

Goldman, A.L. 1987b. "U.S. Bishops Offer Program to Fight Spreading of AIDS." *New York Times* December 11, 1 and 17.

Goldsmith, M.F. 1988. "Sex Experts and Medical Scientists Join Forces Against a Common Foe: AIDS." *Journal of the American Medical Association* 259(5):641–643.

Goleman, D. 1987. "Teenage Risk Taking: Rise in Deaths Prompts New Research Effort." *New York Times* November 24, 13 and 16.

Green, L.W., and Lewis, F.M. 1986. *Measurement and Evaluation in Health Education and Health Promotion*. Palo Alto, Calif.: Mayfield.

Groopman, J.E., Hartzband, P.I., Shulman, L., Salahuddin, S.Z., Sarngadharan, M.G., McLane, M.F., Essex, M., and Gallo, R. 1985. "Antibody Seronegative Human T-Lymphotropic Virus Type III (HTLV-III)-Infected Patients with Acquired Immunodeficiency Syndrome or Related Disorders." *Blood* 66:742–744.

Gross, J. 1989. "Needle Exchange for Addicts Wins Foothold Against AIDS in Tacoma." *New York Times* January 23, 8.

Guinan, M.E., and Hardy, A. 1987. "Epidemiology of AIDS in Women in the United States, 1981 Through 1986." *Journal of the American Medical Association* 257(15):2039–2042.

Hart, G. 1974. "Factors Influencing Venereal Infection in a War Environment." *British Journal of Venereal Diseases* 50:68–72.

Hart, G., Carvell, A., Johnson, A.M., Feinmann, C., Woodward, N., and Adler, M.W. 1988. "Needle Exchange in Central London." Abstract 8512, proceedings from the *IV International Conference on AIDS*, Book 2, page 386.

Hartel, D., Selwyn, P.A., Schoenbaum, E.E., Klein, R.S., and Friedland, G.H. 1988. "Methadone Maintenance Treatment (MMTP) and Reduced Risk of AIDS and AIDS-Specific Mortality in Intravenous Drug Users (IVDUs)." Abstract 8546, proceedings from the *IV International Conference on AIDS*, Book 2, page 395.

Hasin, D.S., Grant, B.F., Endicott, J., and Harford, T.C. 1988. "Cocaine and Heroin Dependence Compared in Poly-Drug Abusers." *American Journal of Public Health* 78(5):567–569.

Hater, J.J., Singh, B.K., and Simpson, D.D. 1984. "Influence of Family and Religion on Long-Term Outcomes Among Opioid Addicts." In B. Stimmel (Ed.), *Cultural and Sociological Aspects of Alcoholism and Substance Abuse.* New York: Haworth Press.

Hearst, N., and Hulley, S.B. 1988. "Preventing the Heterosexual Spread of AIDS." *Journal of the American Medical Association* 259(16): 2428–2432.

Hinman, A.R. 1976. "The Condom as Prophylactic." *Bulletin of the New York Academy of Medicine* 52(8):1004–1011.

Hogan, M.A. 1988. "In San Francisco, TV Battles on the Front Lines Against AIDS." *New York Times* February 21, H1–3.

Howard, J., and Borges, P. 1970. "Needle Sharing in the Haight: Some Social and Psychological Functions." *Journal of Health and Social Behavior* 11:220–223.

Hubbard, R.L., Rachal, J.V., Craddock, S.G., and Cavanaugh, E.R. 1984. "Treatment Outcome Prospective Study (TOPS): Client Characteristics and Behaviors Before, During, and After Treatment." In F.M. Tims and J.P. Ludford (Eds.), *Drug Abuse Treatment Evaluation: Strategies, Progress, and Prospects.* Rockville, Md.: National Institute on Drug Abuse Research Monograph 51, U.S. Department of Health and Human Services.

Institute of Medicine and National Academy of Sciences. 1988. "Confronting AIDS: Update 1988." Washington D.C.: National Academy Press.

Janz, N.K., and Becker, M.H. 1984. "The Health Belief Model: A Decade Later." *Health Education Quarterly* 11(1):1–47.

Job, R.F.S. 1988. "Effective and Ineffective Use of Fear in Health Promotion Campaigns." *American Journal of Public Health* 78:163–167.

Jones, C.C., Waskin, H., Gerety, B., Skipper, B.J., Hull, H.F., and Mertz, G.J. 1987. "Persistence of High-Risk Sexual Activity Among Homosexual Men in an Area of Low Incidence of the Acquired Immunodeficiency Syndrome." *Sexually Transmitted Diseases* 14(2):79–82.

Jorquez, J.S. 1983. "The Retirement Phase of Heroin Using Careers." *Journal of Drug Issues* 13:343–365.

Joseph, J.G., Montgomery, S.B., Emmons, C.A., Kessler, R.C., and Ostrow, D.G. 1987. "Magnitude and Determinants of Behavioral Risk Reduction: Longitudinal Analysis of a Cohort at Risk for AIDS." *Psychology and Health* 1:73–96.

Judson, F.N., and Vernon, T.M. 1988. "The Impact of AIDS on State and Local Health Departments: Issues and a Few Answers." *American Journal of Public Health* 78(4):387–393.

Kahneman, D., and Tversky, A. 1982. "The Psychology of Preferences." *Scientific American* 246:160–173.

Kegeles, S.M., Adler, N.E., and Irwin, C.E. 1988. "Sexually Active Adolescents and Condoms: Changes Over One Year in Knowledge, Attitudes, and Use." *American Journal of Public Health* 78(4):460–461.

Kerr, P. 1988. "Experts Find Fault in New AIDS Plan." *New York Times* February 7, 7.

Kolata, G. 1987. "Erotic Films in AIDS Study Cut Risky Behavior." *New York Times* November 3, 18.

Kolata, G. 1988. "Use of Condoms Lags, Survey of Women Finds." *New York Times* July 28, B7.

Kotler, P., and Levy, S. 1969. "Broadening the Concept of Marketing." *Journal of Marketing* 33:10–15.

Kroger, F., and Wiesner, P.J. 1981. "STD Education: Challenge for the 80s." *Journal of School Health* April, 242–246.

Lader, L. 1987. "The Networks Censor Health." *New York Times* November 17, 31.

Lambert, B. 1988a. "Addicts in Portland, Oregon, Will Get Free Hypodermic Needles." *New York Times* June 10, A13.

Lambert, B. 1988b. "Drug Group to Offer Free Needles in New York City to Combat AIDS. *New York Times* January 8, 1 and 11.

Lambert, B. 1988c. "New York to Begin Free-Needle Plan for Drug Addicts." *New York Times* August 12, A1 and B3.

Lange, W.R., Snyder, F.R., Lozovsky, D., Kaistha, V., Kaczaniuk, M.A., and Jaffe, J.H. 1988. "Geographic Distribution of Human Immunodeficiency Virus Markers in Parenteral Drug Abusers." *American Journal of Public Health* 78(4):443–446.

Lawrence, F.C., Tasker, G.E., Daly, C.T., Orhiel, A.L., and Wozniak, P.H.

1986. "Adolescent's Time Spent Viewing Television." *Adolescence* 21(82):431–436.

Lefton, D. 1988. "Nations Report on Needle Distribution." *American Medical Association News* March 4, 41–45.

Leventhal, H., Safer, M.A., and Panagis, D.M. 1983. "The Impact of Communications on the Self-Regulation of Health Beliefs, Decisions, and Behavior." *Health Education Quarterly* 10(1):3–31.

Lipman, J. 1987. "Censored Scenes: Why You Rarely See Some Things in Television Ads." *The Wall Street Journal* August 17, 23.

Ljungberg, B., Andersson, B., Christensson, B., Hugo-Persson, M., Tunving, K., and Ursing, B. 1988. "Distribution of Sterile Equipment to IV Drug Abusers as Part of an HIV Prevention Program." Abstract 8514, proceedings from the *IV International Conference on AIDS*, Book 2, page 387.

Lohr, S. 1988. "There's No Preaching, Just the Clean Needles." *New York Times* February 29, A4.

Lorig, K., and Laurin, J. 1985. "Some Notions About Assumptions Underlying Health Education." *Health Education Quarterly* 12(3):231–243.

Lyter, D.W., Valdiserri, R.O., Kingsley, L.A., Amoroso, W.P., and Rinaldo, C.R. 1987. "The HIV Antibody Test: Why Gay and Bisexual Men Want or Do Not Want to Know Their Results." *Public Health Reports* 102(5):468–474.

McGann, N. 1987. "HIV Infection Rate Down in San Francisco." *Sexual Health Reports* 8(4):14.

McKusick, L., Conant, M. A., and Coates, T.J. 1985a. "The AIDS Epidemic: A Model for Developing Intervention Strategies for Reducing High-Risk Behavior in Gay Men." *Sexually Transmitted Diseases* 12(4): 229–233.

McKusick, L., Horstman, W., and Coates, T.J. 1985b. "AIDS and Sexual Behavior Reported by Gay Men in San Francisco." *American Journal of Public Health* 75:493–496.

McKusick, L., Wiley, J.A., Coates, T.J., Stall, R., Saika, B., Morin, S., Charles, K., Hostman, W., and Conant, M.A. 1985c. "Reported Changes in the Sexual Behavior of Men at Risk for AIDS, San Francisco, 1982–1984: The AIDS Behavioral Research Project." *Public Health Reports* 100:622–629.

Manoff, R.K. 1985. "Mass Media: Social Marketing's Primary Tool." In R.K. Manoff, *Social Marketing: New Imperative for Public Health*. New York: Praeger.

Marks, J., and Parry, A. 1987. "Syringe Exchange Programme for Drug Addicts." *Lancet* i:691–692.

Marmor, M., Des Jarlais, D.C., Cohen, H., Friedman, S.R., Beatrice, S.T., Dubin, N., El-Sadr, W., Mildvan, D., Yancovitz, S., Mathur, U., and Holzman, R. 1987. "Risk Factors for Infection with Human Immunodeficiency Virus Among Intravenous Drug Abusers in New York City." *AIDS* 1:39–44.

Marriott, M. 1989. "Needle Plan is Revised to Attract Drug Addicts." *New York Times* January 30, 12.

Martin, J.L. 1987. "The Impact of AIDS on Gay Male Sexual Behavior Patterns in New York City." *American Journal of Public Health* 77: 578–581.

Mays, V.M., and Cochran, S.D. 1987. "Acquired Immunodeficiency Syndrome and Black Americans: Special Psychosocial Issues." *Public Health Reports* 102:224–231.

Morgan, T. 1988. "Inside a 'Shooting Gallery': New Front in the AIDS War." *New York Times* February 8, B1 and B5.

Moss, A.R. 1987. "AIDS and Intravenous Drug Use: The Real Heterosexual Epidemic." *British Medical Journal* 294:389–390.

Moss, A.R., Chaisson, R., Osmond, D., Bacchetti, P., and Meakin, R. 1988. "Control of HIV Infection in Intravenous Drug Users in San Francisco." Abstract 8530, proceedings from the *IV International Conference on AIDS,* Book 2, page 391.

Mulleady, G., Green, J., Flanagan, D., Burnyeat, S., Wade, B., Clarke, H., and Marten, R. 1988. "Evaluation of a Syringe-Exchange Scheme." Abstract 8519, proceedings from the *IV International Conference on AIDS,* Book 2, page 388.

Nelkin, D. 1987. "AIDS and the Social Sciences: Review of Useful Knowledge and Research Needs." *Reviews of Infectious Diseases* 9(5): 980–986.

Newman, R.G. 1987. "Methadone Treatment: Defining and Evaluating Success." *New England Journal of Medicine* 317(7):447–450.

New York City Commission on Human Rights, AIDS Discrimination Unit. 1987. "Aids and People of Color: The Discriminatory Impact." New York: City of New York Commission on Human Rights.

O'Leary, A. 1985. "Self-Efficacy and Health." *Behavioral Research Therapy* 23(4):437–451.

Padian, N., Marquis, L., Francis, D.P., Anderson, R.E., Rutherford, G.W., O'Malley, P.M., and Winkelstein, W. 1987. "Male-to-Female Transmission of Human Immunodeficiency Virus." *Journal of the American Medical Association* 258(6):788–790.

Palacios-Jimenez, L., and Shernoff, M. 1986. *Eroticizing Safer Sex.* New York: Gay Men's Health Crisis, Inc.

Pearl, D., Bouthilet, L., and Lazar, J. (Eds.). 1982. *Television and Behavior: Ten Years of Scientific Progress and Implications for the Eighties. Volume I: Summary Reports.* Rockville, Md.: U.S. Department of Health and Human Services.

Ranki, A., Krohn, M., Allain, J.P., Franchini, G., Valle, S.L., Antonen, J., Leuther, M., and Krohn, K. 1987. "Long Latency Precedes Overt Seroconversion in Sexually Transmitted Human Immunodeficiency Virus Infection." *Lancet* ii(8559):589–593.

Rasky, S.F. 1988. "Senate Factions Search for Way to Widen Military Role on Drugs." *New York Times* May 13, A1 and A15.

Reed, J. 1978. *From Private Vice to Public Virtue: The Birth Control Movement and American Society Since 1830.* New York: Basic Books.

Research and Decisions Corporation. 1984. *Designing an Effective AIDS Prevention Campaign Strategy for San Francisco: Results from the First Probability Sample of an Urban Gay Male Community.* San Francisco: Research and Decisions Corporation.

Research and Decisions Corporation. 1985. *Designing an Effective AIDS Prevention Campaign Strategy for San Francisco: Results from the Second Probability Sample of an Urban Gay Male Community.* San Francisco: Research and Decisions Corporation.

Research and Decisions Corporation. 1986. *Designing an Effective AIDS Prevention Campaign Strategy for San Francisco: Results from the First Probability Sample of Multiple/High-Risk Partner Heterosexual Adults.* San Francisco: Research and Decisions Corporation.

Rist, F., and Watzl, H. 1983. "Self-Assessment of Relapse Risk and Assertiveness in Relation to Treatment Outcome of Female Alcoholics." *Addictive Behavior* 8:121–127.

Roberts, E.J. 1982. "Television and Sexual Learning in Childhood." In D. Pearl, L. Bouthilet, and J. Lazar (Eds.), *Television and Behavior: Ten Years of Scientific Progress and Implications for the Eighties. Volume II: Technical Reviews.* Rockville, Md.: U.S. Department of Health and Human Services.

Rogers, E.M., and Shoemaker, F.F. 1971. *Communication of Innovations: A Cross-Cultural Approach.* 2nd Edition. New York: Free Press.

Ross, M.W., and Carson, J.A. 1988. "Effectiveness of Distribution of Information on AIDS: A National Study of Six Media in Australia." *New York State Journal of Medicine* 88:239–241.

Rothenberg, R. 1988. "This Time It's Clear: TV Has a Message for Us." *New York Times* September 4, E6.

Rushton, J.P. 1982. "Television and Prosocial Behavior." In D. Pearl, L. Bouthilet, and J. Lazar (Eds.), *Television and Behavior: Ten Years of Scientific Progress and Implications for the Eighties. Volume II: Technical Reviews.* Rockville, MD.: U.S. Department of Health and Human Services.

Salahuddin, S.Z., Markham, P.D., Redfield, R.R., Essex, M., Groopman, J.E., Sarngadharan, M.G., McLane, M.F., Sliski, A., and Gallo, R.C. 1984. "HTLV-III in Symptom-Free Seronegative Persons." *Lancet* ii(8417–8418):1418–1420.

San Francisco AIDS Foundation. 1988. "Condoms for Couples." San Francisco: San Francisco AIDS Foundation.

Schmalz, J. 1988. "Addicts to Get Needles in Plan to Curb AIDS." *New York Times* January 31, 1 and 12.

Schmidt, W.E. 1988. "In AIDS Battle, Hope for Addict Arises on Street." *New York Times* July 5, A14.

Sciolino, E. 1988. "U.S. Finds Output Of Drugs in World Growing Sharply." *New York Times* March 2, A1 and 6.

Sciolino, E., and Engelberg, S. 1988. "Narcotics Effort Foiled by U.S. Security Goals." *New York Times* April 10, 1 and 10.

Selwyn, P.A., Reiner, C., Cox, C.P., Lipshutz, C., and Cohen, R.L. 1987. "Knowledge About AIDS and High-Risk Behavior Among Intravenous Drug Users in New York City." *AIDS* 1:247-254.

Serrano, Y., and Goldsmith, D. 1988. "ADAPT: A Response to HIV Infection in Intravenous Drug Users in New York." Abstract 8538, proceedings from the *IV International Conference on AIDS*, Book 2, page 393.

Siegel, K., and Gibson, W.C. 1988. "Barriers to the Modification of Sexual Behavior Among Heterosexuals at Risk for Acquired Immunodeficiency Syndrome." *New York State Journal of Medicine* 88(2):66–70.

Sirgy, M.J. 1982. "Self-Concept in Consumer Behavior: A Critical Review." *Journal of Consumer Research* 9:287–300.

Sivak, S.L., and Wormser, G.P. 1986. "Predictive Value of a Screening Test for Antibodies to HTLV-III." *American Journal of Clinical Pathology* 85(6):700–703.

Skidmore, C.A., Robertson, J.R., Roberts, J.J.K., Foster, K., Smith, J.H., and Rhein, H. 1988. "HIV Infection in IVDA: A Follow-Up Study Indicating Changes in Risk Taking Behaviour." Abstract 8510, proceedings from the *IV International Conference on AIDS*, Book 2, page 386.

Slovic, P. 1987. "Perception of Risk." *Science* 236:280–285.

Solomon, D.S. 1982. "Health Campaigns on Television." In D. Pearl, L. Bouthilet, and J. Lazar (Eds.), *Television and Behavior: Ten Years of Scientific Progress and Implications for the Eighties. Volume II: Technical Reviews.* Rockville, Md.: U.S. Department of Health and Human Services.

Solomon, M.R. 1983. "The Role of Products as Social Stimuli: A Symbolic Interactionism Perspective." *Journal of Consumer Research* 10:319–329.

Solomon, M.Z., and DeJong, W. 1986. "Recent Sexually Transmitted Disease Prevention Efforts and Their Implications for AIDS Health Education." *Health Education Quarterly* 13(4):301–316.

Stall, R., McKusick, L., Wiley, J., Coates, T.J., and Ostrow, D.G. 1986. "Alcohol and Drug Use During Sexual Activity and Compliance with Safe Sex Guidelines for AIDS: The AIDS Behavioral Research Project." *Health Education Quarterly* 13(4):359–371.

Stark, E. 1986. "Young, Innocent, and Pregnant." *Psychology Today* 20(10): 28–30, 32–35.

Steinfels, P. 1988. "Southern Baptists Won't Give Out Surgeon General's Report on AIDS." *New York Times* September 23, B3.

Strecher, V.J., DeVellis, B.M., Becker, M.H., and Rosenstock, I.M. 1986. "The Role of Self-Efficacy in Achieving Health Behavior Change." *Health Education Quarterly* 13(1):73–91.

Tirelli, U., Vaccher, E., and Diodato, S. 1988. "Syringe Supply Among Intravenous Drug Users in Italy." *AIDS* 2(2):141.

Valdiserri, R.O., Lyter, D.W., Leviton, L.C., Stoner, K., and Silvestre, A. 1987a. "Applying the Criteria for the Development of Health Promotion and Education Programs to AIDS Risk Reduction Programs for Gay Men." *Journal of Community Health* 12(4):199–212.

Valdiserri, R.O., Lyter, D.W., Kingsley, L.A., Leviton, L.C., Schofield, J.N., Huggins, J., Ho, M., and Rinaldo, C.R. 1987b. "The Effect of Group Education on Improving Attitudes About AIDS Risk Reduction." *New York State Journal of Medicine* 87:272–278.

Valdiserri, R.O. 1988. "Cum Hastis Sic Clypeatis: The Turbulent History of the Condom." *Bulletin of the New York Academy of Medicine* 63(3): 237–245.

Valdiserri, R.O., Bonati, F.A., Proctor, D.M., and Glaser, D. 1988a. "HIV Antibody Testing in a Family Planning Clinic Setting." *New York State Journal of Medicine* 88:623–625.

Valdiserri, R.O., Lyter, D.W., Leviton, L.C., Callahan, C.M., Kingsley, L.A., and Rinaldo, C.R. 1988b. "Variables Influencing Condom Use in Gay and Bisexual Men." *American Journal of Public Health* 78:801–805.

Valdiserri, R.O., Arena, V., Proctor, D.M., and Bonati, F.A. 1989a. "The Relationship Between Women's Attitudes About Condoms and Their Use: Implications for Condom Promotion Programs." *American Journal of Public Health* 79(4):499–501.

Valdiserri, R.O., Lyter, D.W., Leviton, L.C., Callahan, C., Kingsley, L.A., and Rinaldo, C.R. 1989b. "AIDS Prevention in Homosexual and Bisexual Men: Results of a Randomized Trial Evaluating Two Risk Reduction Interventions." *AIDS* 3(1):21–26.

Valle, S.L. 1988. "Sexually Transmitted Diseases and the Use of Condoms in a Cohort of Homosexual Men Followed Since 1983 in Finland." *Scandinavian Journal of Infectious Diseases* 20(2):153–161.

Watkins, J.D., Conway-Welch, C., Creedon, J.J., Crenshaw, T.L., DeVos, R.M., Gebbie, K.M., Lee, B.J., Lilly, F., O'Connor, J.C., Primm, B.J., Pullen, P., SerVass, C., and Walsh, W.B. 1988. "Report of the Presidential Commission on the Human Immunodeficiency Virus Epidemic, June 24, 1988." Washington, D.C.: U.S. Government Printing Office.

Weinberg, D.S., and Murray, H.W. 1987. "Coping with AIDS: The Special Problems of New York City." *New England Journal of Medicine* 317(23):1469–1473.

Wiebel, W., and Altman, N. 1988. "AIDS Prevention Outreach to IVDUs in Four U.S. Cities." Abstract 8535, proceedings from the *IV International Conference on AIDS*, Book 2, page 392.

Wilkerson, I. 1987. "Town That Couldn't Evade Reality." *New York Times* October 16, 8.

Winerip, M. 1988. "AIDS Van's Day: Detox Coupons at the Projects." *New York Times* April 1, B1.

Winkelstein, W., Samuel, M., Padian, N.S., Wiley, J., Lang, W., Anderson, R., and Levy, J.A. 1987. "The San Francisco Men's Health Study: III. Reduction in Human Immunodeficiency Virus Transmission Among

Homosexual/Bisexual Men, 1982–86." *American Journal of Public Health* 77:685–689.

Wodak, A., Dolan, K., Imrie, A.A., Gold, J., Wolk, J., Whyte, B.M., and Cooper, D.A. 1987. "Antibodies to the Human Immunodeficiency Virus in Needles and Syringes Used by Intravenous Drug Abusers." *Medical Journal of Australia* 147(6):275–276.

Yarber, W.L., and Williams, C.E. 1975. "Venereal Disease Prevention and a Selected Group of College Students." *Journal of the American Venereal Disease Association* 2:17–24.

Yarber, W.L. 1977. "Teenage Girls and Venereal Disease Prophylaxis." *British Journal of Venereal Diseases* 53:135–139.

Chapter 6

The Role of HIV Testing in AIDS-Prevention Programs

DAVID W. LYTER

Soon after the discovery and description of the human immunodeficiency virus in 1983-1984 (Barre- Sinoussi et al. 1983; Gallo et al. 1984), tests for antibodies to the virus were developed as a research tool (Sarngadharan et al. 1984; Brun-Vezinet et al. 1984; Weiss et al. 1985). By the spring of 1984, licenses had been awarded to five American companies to develop commercial test kits for the detection of antibodies to HIV (Culliton 1984). In early March 1985, the first generation test kits were manufactured and made available to blood-banking organizations for the widespread screening of blood and blood products (Centers for Disease Control 1985b). Soon thereafter, testing was made available to individuals with a history of high risk behavior (Centers for Disease Control 1986c) as well as to selected segments of the general population, such as new military recruits (Centers for Disease Control 1986b). Initially, public health officials were reluctant to ascribe any significant role to testing in curbing HIV transmission among sexually active individuals (Centers for Disease Control 1985a). More recently, testing for HIV antibodies has come to be viewed by many as a cornerstone of national prevention efforts (Francis and Chin 1987; Goedert 1987).

In some respects, however, this growing emphasis on testing may be somewhat premature (Meyer and Pauker 1987). Limitations have shown up in the screening tests' technical validity for identifying

David W. Lyter, M.D., was Clinical Director of the Pittsburgh Multicenter AIDS Cohort Study, University of Pittsburgh.

true HIV infection, in their efficacy with respect to promoting behavioral change, and in the public health sector's ability to implement their widespread use. The subject of HIV testing has also instigated a complex debate that encompasses myriad political, legal, and psychosocial issues, including whether the public welfare may ever subsume individual rights. This chapter addresses the rationale behind the concept of screening, the technical aspects of HIV testing, guidelines for testing and results disclosure, various aspects of counseling and testing as they relate to different populations and to behavioral change, and the major areas of controversy over the role of HIV testing in AIDS-prevention efforts.

SCREENING AS A TOOL FOR DISEASE PREVENTION

Screening is defined as the "presumptive identification of unrecognized disease or defect by the use of tests, examinations, or other procedures which can be rapidly applied" (Wilson and Jungner 1968: 7). Screening has been used successfully to identify a variety of chronic and infectious diseases. Although it is not equivalent to diagnosis, screening is the first step in identifying individuals who have the greatest likelihood of being at risk for a particular disease. The goal of screening is to identify individuals with unrecognized or presymptomatic disease, whose morbidity and mortality may be reduced as a result of early detection. Through screening, carriers of an infectious agent may be identified; appropriate measures may then be taken to reduce the likelihood of transmission to others.

From a medical/public health perspective, the goal of screening for HIV infection is twofold. First is the objective of interrupting transmission by identifying infected individuals, body fluids and organs. The expectations are that virus carriers will stop or modify activities that might infect others and that biologic products identified as infectious will be discarded. Second is the goal of reducing the morbidity and mortality of asymptomatic victims of this infection. Individuals who are found to be HIV antibody positive (that is, to be infected) may seek medical care, which has the potential for altering the course of their disease. Periodic clinical evaluation, including physical examination, skin testing, chest X rays, and complete blood cell counts, can lead to earlier diagnosis and treatment of serious HIV-associated complications, such as mycobacterial infection (Centers for Disease Control 1986a), *Pneumocystic carinii* pneumonia, or thrombocytopenia (Morris et al. 1982). In the case of certain opportunistic infections, such as *Pneumocystis carinii* pneumonia, prophylaxis with antibiotics may be indicated (Hughes et al. 1987; Montgomery et al. 1987). Monitoring the absolute number of T helper (CD4) lymphocytes is especially helpful in identifying HIV-infected individuals who are at greatest risk of developing symptomatic disease in the near future (Polk et al. 1987). Abnormally low T cell levels can also be an indication for beginning the use of antiretroviral therapy such as zidovudine (Fischl et al. 1987; Physicians' Desk Reference 1988) or other experimental agents (Carter et al. 1987; Mitchell et al. 1987).

Experience working with a large cohort of HIV-infected men at the University of Pittsburgh Multicenter AIDS Cohort Study (Kaslow et al. 1987) has suggested that the medical and supportive care is of a higher quality and is better planned among individuals who have learned their HIV serostatus early in the course of their infection and have been followed by a physician who is familiar with their health history than it is for those who are unaware of their HIV serostatus until they are forced to enter the medical system, usually via an emergency room, in the midst of a health crisis. Finally, knowledge of HIV serostatus may reduce morbidity and mortality by encouraging infected individuals to modify behaviors that would reexpose them to HIV infection.

HIV TESTING AND ITS VALIDITY

In order to identify individuals who are infected with a microorganism, testing must be developed that detects the infecting agent directly or that identifies a marker of its presence. The most accurate tests identify the organism itself; examples are the throat culture for a streptococcal infection or the dark-field examination of fluid from a syphilitic chancre. However, in many instances, direct isolation of a virus is technically impossible or cost-prohibitive. In these cases, serological tests that assay the presence of viral particles or antigens are often used—as in the case of testing for hepatitis B surface antigen. In other cases, one can test for the presence of antibodies, which are surrogate markers of the virus. Antibodies are produced by an individual's immune system in response to the presence of a microorganism in the blood, and the antibody for each antigen, including viruses, is unique. In many cases, multiple antibodies are produced against different components of the same virus; for example, antibodies to the core, surface, and e antigens of the hepatitis

B virus. For antibodies to serve as an adequate marker for the presence of a virus, it is essential that the immune system produce an antibody response soon after exposure to the viral agent and that antibody production be maintained as long as the virus is present.

The validity of a screening test—its ability to separate those who have the disease or condition from those who do not (Wilson and Jungner 1968)—can be characterized on the basis of two parameters: sensitivity and specificity. *Sensitivity* is defined as the test's ability to give a positive finding when the person being tested is truly infected. *Specificity* is the test's ability to give a negative finding when the person being tested is truly free of infection (Vecchio 1966).

A test result that indicates antibodies are present is termed "reactive" or "positive," while the terms "negative" or "nonreactive" are used to signify that no antibodies were found. Ideally, a screening test would detect (that is, determine to be reactive or positive) all infected individuals or blood products (100 percent sensitivity) and would yield negative or nonreactive results for all uninfected samples (100 percent specificity). However, few if any screening tests are perfectly accurate, and the possibility of "false negative" (negative results in individuals who are infected) and "false positive" (positive results in persons who are not infected) results must be recognized as a limitation of screening. In addition to being accurate, a screening test needs to be inexpensive and easily performed.

Since direct detection of the human immunodeficiency virus is expensive and technically difficult, the most common screening test is an ELISA (enzyme-linked immunosorbent assay) procedure, which is used to detect HIV antibodies (Barrett 1978). ELISA techniques were performed by most clinical laboratories prior to the AIDS epidemic, and they had proven to be economically and technically suited to testing large volumes of samples for a variety of constituents.

Briefly, the ELISA technique involves placing a sample of diluted serum into a small well in a plastic microtiter plate, the base of which has been coated with purified, inactivated HIV antigens. If antibodies are present in the serum being tested, they are absorbed onto the floor of the well. The serum is removed, but if antibodies are present, they will remain bound to the antigen in the well. Next, a solution is added that contains antibodies against human antibodies. These antihuman antibodies, which are tagged with a peroxidase enzyme, attach to any HIV antibodies that may be present in the well. A second reagent is added that reacts with the peroxidase to produce a colored solution. Finally, the presence and intensity of color in the solution is measured by a spectrophotometer. The deeper the color (that is, the more intense the reaction), the more likely it is that the sample contains antibodies. A numerical reading of the solution's optical density (O.D.) is obtained. The sample's O.D. is compared with the O.D.s of a negative and positive control, which are run simultaneously. The negative control, which contains no HIV antibodies, will yield a colorless solution, with an O.D. close to zero. The positive control will produce a solution with an intense color and a high O.D. A cutoff value, calculated from the O.D.s of the controls, is used to determine the demarcation between a positive and negative test. Any sample O.D. that is greater than the cutoff is considered positive; if less, then negative. The higher the numerical value of a positive O.D., the greater the certainty that HIV antibodies are present.

Soon after their development, it became apparent that most test kits had sensitivities and specificities less than 100 percent (Mortimer et al. 1985; Reesink et al. 1986; Abb 1986; Courouce 1986) and were therefore prone to both false positive and false negative results. Since 1985, several articles have been published that suggest possible explanations for falsely positive results, including suboptimal laboratory techniques (Grunnet et al. 1985; Morgan et al. 1986), and possible cross-reactivity to other retroviral, treponemal (Fleming et al. 1987), malarial (Volsky et al. 1986), or HLA antibodies (Hunter and Menitove 1985; Kuhnl et al. 1985).

Predictive value is a concept closely related to the parameters of sensitivity and specificity. In fact, its derivation includes these two terms. The predictive value of a test result describes how likely it is that a particular individual's result is correct (Sivak and Wormser 1986). Mathematically, the predictive values of a positive result equals:

$$\frac{(\text{prevalence})\,(\text{sensitivity})}{(\text{prevalence})\,(\text{sensitivity}) + (1\text{-prevalence})\,(1\text{-specificity})}$$

Similarly, the predictive value of a negative test equals:

$$\frac{(1\text{-prevalence})\,(\text{specificity})}{(1\text{-prevalence})\,(\text{specificity}) + (\text{prevalence})\,(1\text{-sensitivity})}$$

Predictive value, therefore, depends on the sensitivity and specificity of a particular test, as well as on the prevalence of the infection in a given population. Predictive value is the parameter most important to individuals being tested, since the validity of their own results is of utmost concern.

Since the predictive value of a positive test depends on the prevalence of illness in a defined population, the lower the prevalence of an infection in a given population, or "risk group," the less likely that a particular positive result is valid. For example, for a gay man reporting a history of unprotected receptive anal intercourse in a city where the prevalence of HIV infection among homosexuals is 20 percent, the positive predictive value of an HIV ELISA test with a sensitivity of 99.0 percent and a specificity of 99.0 percent would be 96.1 percent. In contrast, however, the predictive value of a positive result from the same test kit would be only 2.0 percent for an individual, such as a blood donor, who was not known to have any risk factors for HIV infection, and who lived in a community where the prevalence of HIV infection in blood donors was only .02 percent. Therefore, in certain circumstances it may be difficult to provide individuals with an absolutely unequivocal diagnosis of infection or noninfection on the basis of a single test result. They may not realize that the validity of any individual test result depends significantly on the rate of infection in their population. And, for the person being tested, the level of confidence in the actual finding may be an important factor in motivating and sustaining behavioral change.

Given the presence of falsely positive results, especially among groups with a low HIV seroprevalence, it is necessary to perform another, confirmatory, test on all ELISA positive specimens. For the purpose of confirming the ELISA result, the immunoblot or Western blot is most often used (Martin et al. 1985). Immunoblots are designed to detect the presence of six or more unique antibodies against specific core, polymerase, or envelope components of the virus.

Briefly, an immunoblot is prepared by layering the various HIV antigens in distinct regions along a nitrocellulose strip. The strip is then incubated in a solution containing the diluted serum to be tested. If antibodies against the various HIV antigens are present in the serum, they will adhere to the layered antigens in their unique regions. As with the ELISA, ennzyme-linked antihuman antibodies are then added to the strip. A second reagent solution is added that contains a substrate that produces a colored reaction in the presence of the enzyme. Dark bands develop in regions of the blot strip where HIV antibodies have been bound. The number, intensity, and location of these bands are then recorded.

While significantly more expensive and technically more diffi-cult in comparison to the ELISA, the blot is a much more specific test (less prone to falsely positive results). The combined use of the ELISA as a screening test and the Western blot as a confirmatory test pro-vides the optimal balance between sensitivity and specificity. Since the main purpose of the ELISA is to serve as a screening test, it was designed to "err" on the side of optimal sensitivity (that is, identify as many antibody positive samples as possible), with the use of the Western blot as a confirmatory backup. It is much more cost effec-tive to identify any sample that has even a minimal chance of con-taining antibodies to HIV and in turn to test those samples with a highly specific confirmatory test, than it would be to test every sample by Western blot.

Unfortunately, the specificity, sensitivity, and predictive value of the "gold standard" Western blot are now known to be less than perfect (Taylor and Przybyszewski 1988). Key to this issue is the definition of a "positive" blot. Definitions for "positive" have varied from lab to lab (Centers for Disease Control 1988c). In some cases a blot with any single band present has been considered positive, while a more recent consensus is that one or more bands from two or more HIV antigenic regions (core envelope or polymerase) must be present for the blot to be called positive (Lundberg 1988).

While there is little doubt concerning the interpretation of a blot with strongly reactive bands against most or all of the HIV antigens, there is often uncertainty about the meaning of an immunoblot that displays only single bands or atypical band patterns. An atypical pat-tern may indicate very recent infection, or it may represent an idio-syncratic cross-reaction in an uninfected individual. Medical and public health professionals have expressed frustration concerning what recommendations to make to the small but significant num-bers of individuals whose results are indeterminant. Persons with indeterminant confirmatory tests should be advised that this pat-tern might indicate early HIV infection, and they should be retested within six months. In the interim, they should be urged to adopt risk-reduction behaviors. In some cases, these indeterminant tests become positive within six months, while in others they persist without change (Kleinman et al. 1988).

Other methods of detecting antibodies to HIV include immuno-fluorescence assays (Blumberg et al. 1986), red cell agglutination assays (Kemp et al. 1988), radio immunoprecipitation assays (Barre-Sinoussi et al. 1983), rapid latex agglutination assays (Quinn et al. 1988), and techniques designed to detect HIV IgM (Aiuti et al. 1985).

However, they are all somewhat limited in that they are designed to detect a marker of infection, namely antibodies, rather than the virus itself. It is now clear that there is not a 100 percent correlation between the presence or absence of antibody and the presence or absence of virus.

Discrepancies between infection status and antibody status are especially apparent in early infection. Although most individuals seroconvert from a negative to positive antibody status (that is, their tests become positive) within six to eight weeks after infection (Cooper et al. 1987), some individuals may remain "antibody negative" by conventional screening methods for several months following infection (Ranki et al. 1987). In fact, a small percentage of infected individuals may never elicit an antibody response (Groopman et al. 1985; Ward et al. 1988). Others who were known to be HIV antibody positive can lose their antibodies over time (Farzadegan et al. 1988).

It appears that "second generation" ELISA tests developed since 1987 may be better at detecting early infection than their predecessors (Lelie et al. 1987), and antibody testing protocols are being standardized to optimize their performance (Schwartz et al. 1988). But many newer testing methods focus on the detection of the virus itself, or one of its antigens, rather than on the antibody. The test for p24 antigen is an example. This assay was developed using a routine ELISA technique and has been instituted as a secondary screening tool in some blood banks (Stute 1987). Other techniques for antigen detection have been developed as well. Based on experience with these tests, it appears that the natural history of HIV antigen in the blood is diphasic. The antigen concentration peaks briefly in serum shortly after infection (and several weeks prior to antibody development), then no antigen can be detected for many months to years. Finally, antigen may return in the later stages of infection, in association with progressive immune deterioration (Gaines et al. 1987; Goudsmit et al. 1986). Since HIV antibody is also present during the second phase (when HIV antigen is not detectable), the only period during which antigen screening might detect infection more accurately than antibody testing is immediately prior to seroconversion, that is, shortly following infection. Because this period of time is relatively brief in most individuals, the cost-benefit ratio of antigen testing as a screening tool has been called into question (Backer et al. 1987; Peitrequin et al. 1987).

Culturing HIV has been an important research tool since the virus was first isolated (Gallo et al. 1984). Techniques have improved over time, especially with respect to this test's sensitivity. However, the cost and technical difficulty of culturing have, to date, prohibited it from becoming a practical diagnostic tool outside of large AIDS research centers. It is also less than ideal as a screening test in that the results of HIV cultures are not usually available for several weeks. Because it has a sensitivity of less than 100 percent, culturing may not always be able to clarify the true infection status of someone who has a negative or indeterminant immunoblot.

Other laboratory techniques, such as genetic probes (Shaw et al. 1984) and polymerase chain reaction (PCR) (Kwork et al. 1987) have been developed to detect the presence of HIV. However, they are currently too expensive and technically too complex for use in most routine situations. Although it is likely that additional testing modalities will become available to assist health care providers in making more accurate diagnoses of HIV infection (especially in persons who do not have any apparent symptoms of infection), uncertainty about a client's true infection status will remain in some situations.

GUIDELINES FOR HIV TESTING AND RESULT DISCLOSURE

While screening is usually applied to populations, the efficacy of any screening program is actually determined by the summation of its effects on each individual participant. Soon after HIV testing was made available, it became clear that the context within which testing was conducted was a very important factor in determining its impact on the individual being tested (Bayer et al. 1986).

In order to maximize the benefits and reduce the risks of undergoing testing for HIV, guidelines for conducting HIV counseling and testing have been developed. One of the earliest and most extensive sets of guidelines was published by the Centers for Disease Control (CDC) (1987b). Counseling and testing recommendations have also been published by other organizations, including the American Medical Association (1987) and the Presidential Commission on the HIV Epidemic (1988). Most subsequent guidelines offer slight variations or expansions of the original CDC recommendations.

Essential elements described in these guidelines include pretest counseling, informed consent, specimen handling precautions, testing procedures, confirmatory assays, client notification, posttest counseling, confidentiality, partner notification, and repeat testing.

These guidelines serve as standards to which all agencies and individuals performing the test should adhere. The following discussion summarizes the general content of the CDC guidelines and contains specific suggestions based on an HIV counseling and testing program conducted at the University of Pittsburgh as part of an HIV epidemiology study.

These guidelines emphasize the importance of linking the test with education about HIV and AIDS. Pretest counseling provides an opportunity for the health care provider or counselor to promote risk reduction at a time when individuals being tested may be more receptive emotionally to assimilating new information than they are after having been informed of a positive or negative result. Also, individuals who receive pretest counseling are better informed about the risks and benefits of the test prior to giving consent. In certain settings, such as blood-donation sites, a person may first consent to testing as part of the agreement to donate blood, and the test may be performed before counseling can take place. However, in most other settings, such as a physician's office or a sexually transmitted disease clinic, counseling should always occur prior to testing.

For the education and testing program to be well received, it is important that the testing site be arranged in such a way that persons who are seeking HIV counseling and testing can request it in a manner that is not obvious to other clients. The health care provider or counselor must be well informed about the various means of HIV transmission and should be sensitive to the circumstances of individuals who may practice riskful behaviors. The health care provider should elicit, in a nonjudgmental manner, the individual's motives for undergoing HIV testing, and should then obtain a history of the client's practice of behaviors known to transmit HIV. This is necessary in order to provide individualized pre- and posttest counseling. Additional factors should be assessed, including any symptoms the client has that might be related to HIV infection. After this assessment has been completed, the individual and the health care provider may mutually decide that HIV testing is not, in fact, indicated. However, providers should be aware that individuals who are involved in high-risk activities may not always be willing to admit to those behaviors (Potterat 1987). Therefore, testing may still be prudent despite a history that is ostensibly negative for risky behavior.

For the client, pretest counseling should clarify the meaning of various AIDS-related terms, including HIV, AIDS, ARC, incubation period, immunosuppression, chronic infection, and carrier state. Routes of HIV transmission, especially those germane to the individual's social circumstances and risk history, and the ways in which viral transmission can be prevented should be carefully discussed in language that the client understands. It is also essential to describe the actual testing process, including definitions of the following terms: *antibody* (as opposed to *virus*), *screening test* (ELISA), *confirmatory test* (Western blot or immunoblot), *reactive* or *positive* test result, *nonreactive* or *negative* test result, and *equivocal* or *borderline* test result. The limitations of the test should be reviewed, especially the concepts of false negative and false positive results, the inability of testing to detect recent exposure, and the inability of antibody testing alone to determine current health status or clinical outcome. Finally, it is important that the individual be aware that the test can have negative psychosocial consequences, including the possibility of significant adverse emotional reactions and discrimination by individuals or institutions, should the results of the test not be held in strictest confidence.

Sufficient opportunity should be allowed for questions and discussion. Adequate counseling and a question-and-answer period usually require a minimum of fifteen to twenty minutes. As with all other aspects of the testing process, pretest assessment and counseling should occur in a setting where privacy is assured.

In most situations, HIV-related testing should be performed only after pretest assessment and counseling have taken place and after the written, informed consent of the client has been received. At a minimum, the consent form should include an explanation of the test (including its purpose, potential uses, limitations, the meaning of its results, and the possibility of psychological and social consequences) and an explanation of the procedures to be followed throughout the testing and disclosure process. (A sample consent form can be found in Appendix 4).

Persons seeking HIV testing who wish to remain anonymous should be informed of the opportunity to do so if it exists in the community. A recent study by Fehrs and colleagues (1988) suggested that providing anonymous testing could increase the acceptance rate of testing by nearly 50 percent over confidential testing. In the case of anonymous testing, written, informed consent can be provided by using a coded system that does not link individual identity to the test request or results.

The necessity of an informed consent for HIV testing may not apply in the situation of a medical emergency when the subject of the test is unable to grant or withhold consent and when the test results are needed for medical diagnostic purposes. Another situation in which an informed consent may not be required is the case of HIV-related testing for research purposes, where testing is performed in a way that conceals the identity of the test subject so that it may not be retrieved by the researcher. An example of this scenario is the current CDC sentinel hospital program, in which the prevalence of HIV infection in America is being estimated by blinded HIV testing of all patients admitted to selected hospitals (Centers for Disease Control 1987a).

Institutions performing HIV testing may need to revise the way they label laboratory specimens in order to protect the confidentiality of clients. Optimally, personal identifying information should not appear on either the serum sample or the requisition sent to the laboratory for HIV antibody testing. Rather, a unique specimen code should be used. Only the health care provider should have access to information linking the identifying information with the specimen code, unless anonymous testing has been requested by the patient or client. Unfortunately this level of protection is difficult, if not impossible, to implement in most hospital and out-patient laboratory settings. However, ongoing staff education that emphasizes the importance of maintaining patient confidentiality, and limited access to clinical laboratory data and medical records should be considered as alternatives to special labeling procedures.

Universal precautions are now recommended for the protection of personnel who handle the specimens (Centers for Disease Control 1987c; Centers for Disease Control 1988d). These precautions stress that all body fluids should be considered potentially infectious and handled as such. These guidelines have replaced ones that advocated special labels only for specimens thought to contain an infectious agent.

A widely accepted algorithm also exists for the manner in which samples should be tested and results confirmed (Soloway 1986). While there are a number of different assays for detecting HIV antibodies, this protocol will refer to the most commonly used screening assay, the ELISA. Samples should be tested once with the most sensitive and specific ELISA testing system currently available. If the sample is found to be nonreactive, as defined by the testing kit manufacturer, it is recommended that the result be reported in writing to the health care provider as nonreactive.

If, on initial ELISA testing, the sample is found to be equivocal or reactive, as defined by the test kit manufacturer, the specimen should be retested in duplicate using the same technique. This strat-

egy provides a fast, reliable, and inexpensive way to recheck a potentially positive sample. If both repeat tests are nonreactive, the result
should be reported as nonreactive. If either or both repeat tests are
equivocal or reactive, an immunoblot should be performed. If antibody bands specific to antigens of HIV are detected on the immunoblot in sufficient number and of required type, as specified by the
immunoblot manufacturer, the sample should be reported as "ELISA
and immunoblot reactive." If a single antibody band or bands not of
sufficient type or number to meet the manufacturer's specifications
for a "positive" are detected on immunoblot, the sample should be
reported as "ELISA reactive, but immunoblot equivocal" and a repeat
blood draw and retesting within the next six months should be recommended. If the immunoblot shows no antibody bands, the result
should be reported as "ELISA reactive, but immunoblot nonreactive," and a repeat blood draw and retesting within six months
should be recommended. This is especially important if the person
gives a history of recent high-risk behavior, which might mean that
the possibility of early infection exists.

Once the result has been determined, the health care provider
must notify the client—a step that requires sensitivity to the issues
of confidentiality and an awareness of possible psychological reactions. Before the test is performed, the health care provider and the
client should mutually decide on the method of conveying the results and include their decision in the consent agreement. Results,
whether reactive or nonreactive, should not be reported by mail,
both to protect patient confidentiality and also to minimize the potential for psychological harm.

Optimally, all results should be disclosed in person. This is especially important if the individual has a history of high-risk behavior.
A face-to-face exchange will permit more effective posttest counseling and crisis intervention, including the opportunity to give medical or mental health referrals, for clients whose HIV antibody tests
are reactive (positive). For persons whose tests are nonreactive (negative), the health care provider needs to reinforce risk-reduction
recommendations and provide adequate posttest counseling concerning the meaning and limitations of a nonreactive test result.
Conducting these discussions in person acknowledges the individuality of clients and avoids creating the feeling that they are just "statistics" in a mass screening program. It is also important that the
testing site ensure prompt testing and client notification following
the client's visit. Long delays between the client's visit and notification can undercut the impact of the counseling.

In some cases, clients who have been tested for HIV cannot be reached or refuse to arrange an appointment to learn their results. In the course of providing counseling and testing to a cohort of more than 2,000 gay and bisexual men involved in a federally funded AIDS research project, instances of volunteers with positive HIV antibody results failing to arrange such an appointment happened rarely (Lyter et al. 1987). When they did, the clinic took the following steps. If a client could not be located, diligent attempts were made to notify the client by telephone or certified mail that the results were completed and available. All mailings were in opaque envelopes with only a post office box number for the return address. If the attempts by telephone were unsuccessful and certified mail was returned, efforts were discontinued—although these attempts were documented on the client's record. The results were not sent by mail, in order to protect the client's confidentiality should someone else open the letter. However, if the certified mail was accepted but the client failed to respond, the situation was handled according to the following guidelines.

If contact was made with the client but he refused to arrange an appointment to learn his results, the findings were offered by telephone. If this arrangement was accepted, referrals for follow-up care and posttest counseling were offered and the discussion documented in the client's medical record. If the client refused the results even by telephone, he was informed by telephone or certified mail that, unless he provided a written refusal of results, within two weeks of our request his results would be sent to him by mail. Along with this request, we enclosed literature reinforcing risk-reduction guidelines. If the client sent a letter of refusal, it was kept on file for documentation and no further action was taken. If we did not receive a letter of refusal, we sent a letter, by certified mail, which gave the results, urged risk-reduction practices, and offered posttest counseling and referral.

When clients return to learn the results of their tests, the health care provider or counselor should begin by reviewing the meaning of the test (but not their specific results) and the definitions of the terms *reactive* or *positive, nonreactive* or *negative,* and *equivocal* or *borderline.* This meeting should take place in private, so that the discussion cannot be overheard by other clients or staff members, and adequate time should be allowed for the client to ask questions before the results are disclosed.

If the results of the HIV test are negative (nonreactive), the counselor should present and interpret them clearly, making sure that the client understands the term *negative.* Next, the limitations of a negative result should be discussed, including its unreliability if a recent risky exposure has occurred. If such an exposure has occurred within the past five to six months, a repeat assessment should be planned within six month's time. The counselor should also stress that the client will remain uninfected only if he or she consistently follows risk-reduction guidelines, such as using safer sexual practices and, in the case of IV drug users, avoiding needle sharing. Clients must understand that the primary responsibility for preventing HIV infection is theirs, and not that of their partners. The counselor should give the client detailed risk-reduction information and be sure to elicit and respond to questions, as well as attempt to correct any client misconceptions about HIV infection and its prevention. It is especially important that seronegative clients not believe that they are "immune" to HIV because of a negative test result.

If the results of the test are positive (reactive), the counselor should present and interpret them in a clear and direct manner. If only the results of HIV testing are available to the health care provider (for example, if T helper cell counts have not been performed), the limitations of interpreting a positive test with respect to determining a patient's current clinical status or prognosis should be reviewed. It is essential that the client understand the need for further clinical evaluation, including T helper cell counts. If this testing is not available on site, appropriate referrals should be made. If more extensive clinical or laboratory information is available, the HIV test results should be discussed in light of these other findings. The counselor should also attempt to assess the client's level of understanding about the test results.

When disclosing a positive HIV test result, it is imperative that the counselor pay close attention to the client's affect, to determine and respond to his or her emotional state. Possible affective states in newly informed seropositive clients are shock, denial, fear, sadness, rage, self-pity, self-loathing, depression, and despair (Nichols 1985). Counselors should be prepared to spend time addressing these feelings and helping the client to accept the results of the test. Crisis intervention skills may be required: an increased rate of suicide has been documented in persons who are HIV seropositive (Marzuk et al. 1988). Since it is very likely that the seropositive individual will require ongoing emotional support, follow-up contact or supportive counseling should be recommended and arranged, if indicated. A referral list of qualified mental health practitioners or agencies should be made available to the client.

Next, the counselor should make health maintenance recommendations, stressing especially the importance of avoiding repeat exposure to HIV or to other infectious agents that could be detrimental to an infected individual (Johns et al. 1987). This is also an appropriate time to discuss the concept of cofactors and the interaction of nutrition, stress, and other aspects of life-style with the immune system. If the individual has a history of substance abuse, referral to a drug treatment program should be arranged.

It is essential to reinforce the importance of eliminating practices that could transmit the infection to others. The sexually active client should be urged to avoid unprotected intercourse and should be given clear instructions on condom and spermicide use. Client information on condoms should include the following specifics: wear condoms at all times during insertion; do not store them for prolonged periods of time in places where temperatures are elevated (for example, a wallet or glove compartment); use adequate water-based lubricants (never oil- or petroleum-based lubricants); use spermicidal compounds, such as nonoxynol-9 in conjunction with condoms; hold the base of the condom when withdrawing the penis to prevent slippage; and only ejaculate outside of the partner even if condoms are worn (since condoms can rupture or tear during intercourse).

If the client uses intravenous drugs, he or she should be counseled to enter treatment as soon as possible. In the interim, clients should be urged to stop sharing needles, but as an added precaution, clients should be given instructions on the importance of cleaning "works" before each use by flushing them twice with household bleach followed by flushes with clean water. Women of reproductive age should be reminded of the potential for perinatal transmission.

Seropositive clients must be urged to notify anyone with whom they have had recent riskful sexual contact or shared a needle that HIV testing is indicated. In fact, partner notification by the client is considered by many to be an important public health tool in reducing the spread of HIV infection (Centers for Disease Control 1988a). While there are limited data as yet on the efficacy of voluntary partner notification, the process of identifying infected people earlier (through partner notification), does have potential benefits: infected partners may in turn seek out medical evaluation sooner, change their own behaviors, and reduce the probability of their passing the virus to others. One must be careful, however, not to assume that a seropositive client's sexual or needle-sharing partner(s) will necessarily be infected with HIV themselves. When clients do refer partners for testing, it is preferable that they meet with the same person who counseled the index client.

Counselors and health care providers may be called upon to assist clients in informing a sexual or needle-sharing partner about their serostatus. Since many clients may feel threatened by the task of informing their partners, the health care provider or counselor should offer to assist in this process. Assistance may involve arranging an appointment with the client and his or her partner for the purpose of discussing HIV testing. This task should be handled in the manner described above. Testing should be made available to the referred partner, with the understanding that if the result is negative, repeat testing may be necessary in the future. Recommendations for risk reduction should again be reviewed.

A more aggressive form of partner notification, called contact tracing, has been a mainstay in controlling other sexually transmitted diseases in this country over the past several decades (Cutler and Arnold 1988). Contact tracing is usually carried out by trained health professionals who contact the identified partners of an infected client without naming the client. They inform these individuals of the possibility of a riskful exposure and urge follow-up counseling and testing.

Contact tracing can, potentially, identify infected individuals. Each new contact can lead investigators to additional persons at risk for HIV infection. One recent contact tracing identified eighty-three partners of HIV seropositive men by beginning with one infected client (Wykoff et al. 1988). Only four of these contacts had been tested previously; almost all agreed to be tested by the investigator.

Increasing numbers of health organizations are advocating notification of sexual partners of HIV-infected clients, either by the clients themselves or, if necessary, by contact tracing (Watkins et al. 1988; Wilkerson 1988). Some states are considering legislation, similar to that enacted for reporting suspected cases of child abuse, that would protect physicians who, contrary to the desire of their seropositive patients, deem it necessary to inform the patients' sexual partner (Barron 1988). While voluntary partner notification and contact tracing are becoming increasingly popular among health officials, they are not without their limitations (Rutherford and Woo 1988). The real impact of these efforts ultimately depends on the quality of the counseling and testing program. If these programs fail in the first place to promote behavioral change, contact tracing and partner notification are of little use.

There are many unanswered questions about the impact of contact tracing and partner notification on preventing the spread of HIV. Investigations can be very costly and time consuming. Wykoff and colleagues (1988) reported that contact tracing cost more than eight hundred dollars for each new infected individual identified. A study of heterosexual partners of people with AIDS from San Francisco (Woo et al. 1988:3565) reported that while only 7 percent of named contacts refused an interview, 44 percent of the individuals they attempted to contact were either deceased, had moved out of town, or simply could not be located.

There are other concerns about the impact of contact tracing on the named partners. Since there is currently no treatment to offer asymptomatic seropositive individuals, the public health benefits of contact tracing are largely dependent upon individuals' willingness to modify their behavior. This is distinctly different from contact tracing for syphilis, for example, where positive partners can be treated for their infection and rendered noninfectious. Contact tracing may also force the client's partners to learn about a "health problem" they may not have anticipated and that they may not be prepared to handle emotionally. Some people contacted this way may suffer severe psychological reactions that require additional support services. Finally, breaches of personal confidentiality could occur if the client discloses names of partners to providers who are not sensitive to privacy issues and protocols.

Health care providers and counselors need to talk with seropositive clients about the potential implications of disclosing results to others, including family, friends, employer, and insurers. It is helpful to review with the client the limitations of medical records confidentiality, including the fact that records can be subpoenaed by a court of law in most states. Clients should be informed that signing a blanket release of medical information, for example, in an application for life insurance, will give the recipient of that release access to all medical records—including HIV results, if they have been included in a medical record. However, in some circumstances local or state legislation may protect such information.

The commitment to confidentiality on the part of a counseling and testing program may be essential to its success. Many times, word-of-mouth is the most important advertisement for such programs. Clients who are satisfied that their test results are being handled confidentially are more likely to recommend the service to others. The commitment to confidentiality is especially important in smaller communities, where there may be close networking among members of the target groups. A negative experience for even one client might dissuade others from taking a similar risk. Individuals need to be assured that the benefits of coming forth for counseling and testing clearly outweigh the risks.

Finally, if the test results are equivocal (that is, if the ELISA and blot results cannot be interpreted as either negative or positive), the health care provider or counselor should present the findings and discuss the possible causes of an equivocal test, including recent in-fection or an idiosyncratic cross-reaction with an antigen other than HIV. If there is evidence in the client's history that the equivocal result may indicate recent HIV infection, it is necessary to allow sufficient time (about six months) for the full development of an an-tibody response before repeat testing is performed. However, the cli-ent should be informed that even after repeat testing, results may remain equivocal—especially if they are the result of a cross-reac-tion to a non-HIV antigen. Individuals with equivocal test results should be counseled according to the guidelines already presented for HIV seropositive persons until repeat testing or additional medi-cal and laboratory information clarifies their true serostatus.

The CDC guidelines for HIV testing were released in 1987. How-ever, it is unclear how widely implemented these standards are. A 1987 survey of 200 U.S. teaching hospitals and 171 general hospitals in Minnesota performing HIV testing found that less than half the hospitals in each group had established policies and working pro-tocols for informed consent, test ordering, confidentiality protec-tion, patient notification, or risk-reduction counseling (Henry et al. 1988). To optimize the potential for HIV counseling and testing to have a positive impact on AIDS prevention, it is essential that these guidelines be widely implemented.

HIV TESTING OF THE GENERAL POPULATION

In such settings as blood banks, military recruitment sites, and hos-pitals, the primary purpose of HIV testing does not usually include the enhancement of behavioral change among those being tested. For example, HIV screening programs have recently been instituted in numerous American hospitals for the purpose of surveying HIV seroprevalence among hospitalized patients (Baker et al. 1987; Dondero et al. 1988; Kerndt et al. 1988). In many of these settings, patient indentification information is not collected so that results cannot be linked to specific individuals. This blinded testing obvi-ates the need for informed consent of the patient, because findings remain anonymous and no potential exists for breaches of confiden-tiality or other adverse consequences. This allows researchers to gather more complete epidemiologic information by testing all patients being admitted to a particular institution, rather than only those who would be willing to be tested.

The first and most extensive use of HIV testing in the general population was implemented by the blood-banking system as a means of safeguarding the nation's blood supply. Within the first four months of using the ELISA test in 1985, over 1.1 million units of blood were screened (Centers for Disease Control 1985d). Of these, 2,831 units (.25 percent) proved to be repeatedly reactive by ELISA, one-third of which (.08 percent) were confirmed positive by Western blot or HIV culture. It was estimated that nearly 1,000 units of HIV-infected blood were detected and removed from the U.S. blood supply during that period of time. By the middle of 1987, the American Red Cross reported an HIV seroprevalence of approximately .012 percent in all of its donors (Centers for Disease Control 1987a). With an estimated 10 million blood donors in 1987, this screening would have identified about 1,200 infected donors by year's end.

The testing of donor blood to detect HIV infection has been hailed as a major step in the battle against AIDS, and justifiably so. Transfusion-related AIDS cases currently comprise only 2 percent of the cases reported in this country and will continue to decrease over time.

Although the major objective of screening donated blood is to prevent the occurrence of transfusion-associated HIV infection, blood banks are faced with the additional responsibility of notifying seropositive donors of their findings, and this provides them with an opportunity for preventing the further (behavioral) spread of HIV.

HIV seropositive donors are notified of their test results and prohibited from further donation. In most cases, interviews with these individuals yield histories of risk behaviors for HIV infection and failure of the self-deferral protocol (discussed in the next paragraph). As recommended by the CDC guidelines, these donors are to be counseled on the meaning of the test and given specific recommendations for medical follow-up and risk-reduction practices to prevent the future transmission of HIV to sexual and needle-sharing partners. However, there is limited published data as to whether the resources for counseling and referral at a blood bank are equivalent to those of an alternative testing site. To ensure the highest level of donor counseling, blood banks should establish referral networks with alternative testing sites, health care providers, and community resources so that seropositive donors can be referred for appropriate medical evaluation and ongoing counseling, as needed.

In addition to testing all units of donated blood prior to transfusion, blood banks also rely on voluntary donor deferral as a means of reducing the likelihood of transfusion-associated HIV infection. Voluntary deferral attempts to discourage all individuals at risk for HIV infection from donating blood. This can be accomplished by a variety of means. Public health officials, through widely distributed risk-reduction guidelines, have warned potentially infected persons not to donate blood. In the blood-donation setting, prospective donors are asked to read a pamphlet that requests them to refrain from donating if they belong to one of the high-risk groups. In some settings, donors are asked directly about their history of riskful behavior. Finally, many centers inform donors that they may call the blood bank after donation to request that their blood sample be discarded. This latter option can be helpful for individuals who feel pressured by family members or employers (who are not aware of their riskful behaviors) to donate blood.

It is possible that voluntary self-deferral (which was first instituted in March 1983, two years before HIV testing became available) (Centers for Disease Control 1983), may have encouraged less riskful behavior by calling attention to an individual's undesirability as a blood donor. It may also have prompted rejected donors to seek out evaluation at a more appropriate location once HIV testing was available. Unfortunately, it is impossible to determine how effective voluntary deferral has been or still is in promoting less riskful behavior. What is known, however, is that continued maintanence of this policy, supplemented by HIV testing, will succeed in reducing transfusion-related HIV infections to extremely low levels. The importance of stressing voluntary deferral is further supported by evidence that the majority of donors found to be HIV antibody positive have histories of riskful behavior (Centers for Disease Control 1985d).

Voluntary deferral's additional benefit over HIV testing of donated blood has been demonstrated by reports of transfusion-associated HIV infection resulting from the transfusion of HIV seronegative blood, donated by individuals who belonged to high-risk groups (Ward et al. 1988). More aggressive and consistent application of voluntary deferral might have prevented these infections, which were not detected by routine methods of antibody testing. In fact, the self-deferral criteria were changed in 1985 to include all males who reported same-sex sexual intercourse since 1977 (in place of males with multiple male sexual partners) as a result of confusion over the original criteria (Centers for Disease Control 1985e). Personnel at blood donation sites should provide explicit information about the criteria for and importance of self-deferral. They should offer referrals to alternative testing sites for donors whose main motivation for giving blood is the HIV test (Snyder and Vergeront 1988). Furthermore, it is absolutely essential that blood donation sites have routine procedures for deferring blood (even after it is donated) that do not embarrass a volunteer or make public the fact that his or her blood was rejected. This is necessary in light of the fact that individuals who are familiar with deferral criteria may still be pressured to donate blood because of personal, social, or job circumstances.

Another example of the use of HIV screening in the general population has been the testing of all potential recruits and active-duty personnel for the U.S. military. As part of their routine medical evaluation, each applicant is informed that HIV testing will be conducted. Seropositive applicants, who are denied entry into the service, are informed of their results and counseled by a physician or other staff member. Between the inception of the program in October, 1985, and the end of 1986, an HIV seroprevalence of .15 percent was found among the potential military recruits (Centers for Disease Control 1987d). A similar program for active-duty personnel found an HIV-infection rate of .13 percent out of 1.75 million individuals tested as of April 1988 (Centers for Disease Control 1988b).

Overtly, the Department of Defense's rationale for this screening is to eliminate the possibility of a person not known to be infected with HIV suffering serious health consequences as a result of receiving live-virus vaccines (Herbold 1986). These vaccines, which are routinely given to military personnel, can produce serious complications if they are inadvertently administered to immunocompromised individuals (Redfield et al. 1987). Another goal of this program is to ensure that all military recruits could serve as blood donors should emergency transfusions be needed in a crisis situation. Certainly some critics have accused the military of simply using HIV screening to identify homosexuals and IV drug users among its ranks and applicants, groups which have traditionally and legally been excluded from military service. Whatever the motivation, the primary purpose of the military's program is to identify individuals who are considered "undesirable" as a consequence of being HIV seropositive. As with the screening of donated blood, health promotion and enhancement of behavior change is not a primary objective of the military's screening program. There is no literature as yet on the impact of result notification by the military, especially on those who are found to be infected with HIV.

HIV TESTING TARGETED TO INDIVIDUALS WITH
HIGH-RISK BEHAVIORS

While the initial function of HIV testing was to screen the nation's blood supply and prevent transfusion-associated AIDS, by the spring of 1985 HIV testing was made available in settings other than blood banks (Centers for Disease Control 1986c). Public health officials conjectured that making testing available outside of the blood-banking system would further protect the blood supply by providing individuals who wished to learn their HIV serostatus an option other than blood donation. It was also believed that providing HIV testing at "alternate test sites" would help to promote behavioral change, especially among persons who were found to be seropositive.

Initially, the utility of alternate test sites was the subject of controversy and differing views. Some people believed testing would be a major tool in curbing the epidemic, in the same way that serologic testing had contributed to the control of syphilis. Others argued that the lack of antiretroviral therapy would dissuade persons who were likely to be infected from being tested. The inability to link test results with a clinical prognosis and the relative inexperience of most physicians in performing in-depth immunological evaluations of HIV seropositive persons also acted as impediments to widespread acceptance. Many people argued that behavioral modifications to reduce the risk of AIDS could take place in the absence of HIV testing, while others believed that testing and subsequent knowledge of HIV serostatus would be most significant in motivating permanent behavioral change. Factions of the gay community were squarely opposed to HIV testing because of potential breaches of confidentiality regarding both positive serostatus and sexual orientation. These fears were exacerbated by most alternate test sites being run by governmental agencies. This immediately raised anxiety about entrusting personal information to officials who might, at some future time, be empowered to use this information for mandatory reporting, contact tracing, or quarantine. In fact, one study on the effects of mandatory reporting of individuals found to be HIV positive revealed that attendance by gay men at an alternate test site in South Carolina dropped by 51 percent when mandatory reporting was instituted in 1986 (Johnson et al. 1988). Many people expressed concern about the emotional impact of a positive result disclosure. While the CDC had urged that all testing sites implement appropriate pre- and postdisclosure counseling, it was feared that these largely educational endeavors would not be adequate to deal with the long-term psychological needs of persons found to be seropositive.

The initial experience of the alternate test sites in 1985 was that requests for testing were less than expected (Centers for Disease Control 1986c). The reasons for this lower-than-expected demand are probably explained by many of the issues raised earlier. To date, most published information concerning the acceptance of testing is from research studies of homosexual or bisexual men. Since it is impossible to determine the size of these populations, it is equally impossible to know what portions of these groups have sought testing either through participation in research studies or alternate test sites.

Experience at the University of Pittsburgh in providing counseling and testing to a large cohort of gay and bisexual men enrolled in a prospective natural history study of HIV infection revealed that 54 percent of the men who joined the study between 1984 and 1986 had chosen to learn their HIV results (Lyter et al. 1987). More recently, the trend has been toward greater acceptance of HIV testing: nearly 90 percent of the participants who joined the Pittsburgh study in 1987-1988 wanted to learn their HIV serostatus. A national survey of 1,200 gay men in France in 1986 revealed that more than 30 percent of the respondents had been tested for HIV (Pollak et al. 1987). McCusker and her colleagues (1988) reported that 79 percent of their research subjects opted to learn test results, Farthing and colleagues (1987) reported 88 percent, Wiktor and colleagues (1988) reported 84 percent, and Van Griensven and colleagues (1987) reported 87 percent in similar cohorts of homosexual men. However, it is unlikely that the level of acceptance by well-educated volunteers in research studies (which have extensive confidentiality protection) is representative of how other gay men might react to the opportunity of being tested for HIV. If anything, it is probably an overestimate.

One study has examined factors related to learning HIV test results in clients of alternate testing sites in California (Rugg et al. 1988). Between March and May 1987, 2,196 consecutive clients were surveyed during their first appointment for HIV testing. However, 329 (11.3 percent) failed to keep a return appointment for result disclosure. Survey information found to be associated with the failure to learn results included a low level of social support for testing, an initial intention not to return for results, and dissatisfaction with the setting and services provided by the test site.

With time, many of the objections initially raised against HIV testing at alternate sites have noticeably lessened, and the availability of HIV counseling and testing is becoming more widespread. Many testing centers have gained reputations for handling results responsibly and have won the confidence of the gay community. Many states have passed legislation to provide higher levels of confidentiality or to make testing available on an anonymous basis. Mental health centers have gained expertise in providing emotional support, in individual or group settings, to seropositive individuals. Clinicians have become more adept at evaluating and treating HIV-infected individuals. Licensed and experimental anti-HIV therapies are becoming more widely available. It would appear that it is now much easier to endorse a position that recommends voluntary HIV testing, accompanied by appropriate pre- and posttest counseling, in a setting where confidentiality is assured, as generally beneficial.

What is still lacking, however, is clear evidence that HIV testing plays a substantial role in motivating behavioral change. Although there are many descriptive studies indicating that gay men are changing riskful behaviors to a significant degree (McKusick et al. 1985, Centers for Disease Control 1985c), research on the relative contribution of knowledge of HIV serostatus on sexual behaviors is sparse, and existing findings are often inconclusive or contradictory. Fox et al. (1987) found that men who learned that they were seropositive reduced their total number of sexual partners by a degree equal to men who failed to learn their results. In this same study, the men who learned that they were seronegative reduced their total number of partners to a significantly lesser degree. Seropositive men in this cohort did reduce their practice of insertive anal intercourse to a greater degree than the other two groups, while seronegative men decreased both receptive and insertive anal intercourse less than the other groups.

In contrast, Doll and colleagues (1988) found no difference in numbers of partners and no difference in the frequency of unprotected receptive or insertive anal intercourse with steady partners, comparing groups of homosexual men who knew their results to those who did not. She did find that seropositive men who did not know their results were more likely to engage in unprotected insertive anal sex with nonsteady partners. Ostrow and colleagues (1988) found no impact of results disclosure on subsequent sexual behavior, but did note a significant increase in anxiety and depression among those who learned they were infected with HIV. Wiktor and colleagues (1988) also found no effect of knowledge of HIV test results on sexual behavior, but did discover that if men learned that potential partners had a serostatus opposite to theirs, they were less likely to have sex with them. McCusker (1988) and her colleagues found that knowledge of HIV serostatus had no differential effect with respect to receptive anal intercourse in seronegative versus seropositive gay men. She did, however, confirm the finding that knowledge of a seropositive status was more often associated with the elimination of unprotected insertive anal intercourse.

Van Griensven and colleagues (1987) reported a decrease in numbers of sexual partners among gay men from the Netherlands who learned that they were seropositive, but no differences across groups with respect to self-reported change in specific sexual practices. Willoughby and colleagues (1987) found a greater reduction in sexual partners for seropositive than for seronegative gay men. Alarmingly, he also discovered a significantly greater percentage of seronegative men who reported never using condoms during receptive anal intercourse as compared with those who knew they were seropositive.

In summary, most of these studies report temporal reductions in the number of sexual partners regardless of HIV serostatus, with the greatest change occurring in seropositive men. However, when the frequencies of specific sexual practices are examined, there appears to be no consistent effect of knowledge of HIV serostatus on subsequent sexual behavior.

Again, the limitations of these studies must be kept in mind. Most are conducted within highly motivated and educated volunteer cohorts. The data collected are self-reported and therefore prone to recall bias and inaccuracy. Because many of these studies are not controlled (for both practical and ethical reasons), it is impossible to accept or reject the hypothesis that the same factors that motivate a person to learn his serostatus may also influence his subsequent sexual behavior. These studies are also limited in that sexual behavior is very complex and difficult to measure. Participants' decision to practice specific behaviors may be greatly influenced by the characteristics and serostatus of their sexual partners, on whom information is rarely available to the study investigators. The greater change noted in seropositive individuals may be related to their initially greater level of riskful behavior, which may permit "more room" to alter behavior. Change as a result of learning about a positive serostatus may also be secondary to decreased libido and depression, rather than a willful intention to pratice safer sex. Finally, because testing is usually conducted in a setting involving pre- and postdisclosure counseling, the independent effects of the actual result are very difficult to extricate from the entire process.

Studies addressing the acceptance of HIV testing and its impact on behavior change among intravenous drug users (ivdus) are scant in the scientific literature. A small study of ivdus in Minnesota revealed that 85 percent of clients enrolled in a methadone treatment program were willing to learn their hiv serostatus (Carlson and McClellan 1987). Another study of 962 ivdus who received pretest counseling at drug treatment clinics in Connecticut in 1987 (Cartter et al. 1988), found that 75 percent of the participants agreed to testing, but only 62 percent of those tested eventually requested their results. Marlink and colleagues (1987) reported that among ivdus in a methadone maintenance program who learned that they were hiv seropositive, nearly two-thirds returned to iv drug use as compared to a recidivism rate of 24 percent among seronegatives and a rate of less than 10 percent among untested individuals.

In contrast, a study of fifteen hiv seropositive and thirty-five hiv seronegative participants in a methadone program in New York in 1986 (Casadonte et al. 1988) found that both groups reported decreased iv drug use after learning their hiv serostatus. In fact, the hiv seropositive group reported a greater consistency of condom use in the follow-up period than did the seronegative individuals. This New York study also found that learning about a positive serostatus did not cause significant long-term emotional sequelae in subjects.

Van den Hoek and colleagues (1988) found, in their study of behavioral changes in 144 ivdus in Amsterdam from 1985 to 1987, that a greater proportion of the 77 hiv seronegative individuals stopped iv drug use in the six months after testing compared to the 42 hiv seropositives and the 25 untested individuals. They also found that both the seropositive and seronegative ivdus reduced their frequency of lending used needles to others, but that seronegatives failed to show any decrease in borrowing used needles, in contrast to the other two groups. Finally, the Amsterdam study failed to demonstrate an impact of testing on any of the three groups with respect to frequency of injections among those individuals who continued to use drugs. It is hoped that further research will clarify the relationship between hiv testing, needle-use behaviors, and sexual practices within this group.

Information on the acceptance and effects of hiv testing in sexually active heterosexuals is even more sparse. One study (Hull et al. 1988) examined the demographics of homosexual and heterosexual clients of a sexually transmitted disease clinic in New Mexico who chose to be tested for hiv antibody versus those who declined. Eighty-two percent of 1,401 patients at the clinic accepted hiv testing. Those who declined were more likely to be black, have a reactive syphilis serology, and be infected with hiv (determined by a blinded survey of refusers using blood collected for syphilis serology). There were no differences in age and sexual preference between those accepting and refusing testing.

It should be clear at this point that relying solely on HIV testing as a motivator for behavioral change is probably unrealistic. In fact, participation in pre- and posttest counseling may be just as important as the actual testing itself in terms of motivating behavioral change. Some AIDS-prevention programs, like those for intravenous drug users on methadone maintenance, may even opt to promote behavioral change without HIV testing. But, even if counseling and testing do not result in universal or complete behavioral change, they do serve to identify individuals who are at increased risk for HIV infection who might benefit from more intensive, perhaps individualized, risk-reduction interventions. Identifying this population will become increasingly important as biomedical treatment modalities move in the direction of treating HIV-infected individuals prior to the onset of symptoms.

Burgeoning research on the effects of HIV testing on subsequent behavior must be watched closely; data are still very scant. In the meantime, it might be a more effective strategy for the public health sector to emphasize the potential benefits of HIV testing for the individual, rather than the benefits to society at large. Seropositive individuals may benefit from earlier medical intervention as newer therapies become available. Seronegative individuals may benefit by a reduction in anxiety levels (Moulton et al. 1988). However, the limited data that exist suggest that seronegative individuals who are at potential risk for HIV infection are the very persons who have been least motivated to change. Perhaps, in the established tradition of STD control, too much attention has been focused on identifying and encouraging change in the seropositive carriers and not enough in the at-risk, uninfected population. Intervention techniques aimed at self-preservation of individuals not yet exposed may be more effective than techniques based solely on altruism or responsibility to society. Finally, it is clear that for any counseling and testing program to be accepted, there must be adequate legislation protecting confidentiality and prohibiting discrimination against those who are willing to participate.

REFERENCES

Abb, J. 1986. "Determination of Antibodies Against LAV/HTLV III: Comparative Evaluation of Four Different Commercial Test Kits." *AIDS Research* 2:93–97.

Aiuti, F., Rossi, P., Sirianni, M.C., Carbonari, M., Popovic, M., Sarngad-haran, M.G., Contu, L., Moroni, M., Romagnani, S., and Gallo, R.C. 1985. "IgM and IgG Antibodies to Human T-Cell Lymphotropic Ret-rovirus (HTLV III) in Lymphadenopathy Syndrome and Subjects at Risk for AIDS in Italy." *British Medical Journal* 291:165.

American Medical Association. 1987. "Prevention and Control of Acquired Immunodeficiency Syndrome: An Interim Report of the Board of Trustees." *Journal of the American Medical Association* 258:2097–2111.

Backer, U., Weinauer, F., and Gathof, G. 1987. "HIV Antigen Screening in Blood Donors." *Lancet* ii:1213–1214.

Baker, J.L., Kelen, G.D., Silverson, K.T., and Quinn, T.C. 1987. "Unsus-pected Human Immunodeficiency Virus in Critically Ill Emergency Pa-tients." *Journal of the American Medical Association* 257:2609–2611.

Barre-Sinoussi, F., Chermann, J.C., Rey, F., Nugeyre, M.T., Chamaret, S., Gruest, J., Dauget, C., Axler-Blin, C., Brun-Vezinet, F., Rouzioux, C., Rozenbaum, W., and Montagnier, L. 1983. "Isolation of a T-Lympho-tropic Virus from a Patient at Risk for Acquired Immunodeficiency Syndrome (AIDS)." *Science* 220:868–871.

Barrett, J.T. 1978. *Textbook of Immunology*. Saint Louis: C.V. Mosby.

Barron, J. 1988. "Bill to Provide Telling Mates about AIDS." *New York Times* March 10, B1.

Bayer, R., Levine, C., and Wolf, S.M. 1986. "HIV Antibody Screening: An Ethical Framework for Evaluating Proposed Programs." *Journal of the American Medical Association* 256:1768–1774.

Blumberg, R.S., Sandstrom, E.G., Paradis, T.J., Nuemeyer, D.N., Sarngad-haran, M.G., Hartshorn, K.L., Byington, R.E., Hirsch, M.S., and Schooley, R.T. 1986. "Detection of Human T-Cell Lymphotropic Vi-rus Type III-Related Antigens and Anti-Human T-Cell Lymphotropic Virus Type III Antibodies by Anticomplementary Immunofluores-cence." *Journal of Clinical Microbiology* 23:1072–1077.

Brun-Vezinet, F., Barre-Sinoussi, F., Saimot, A.G., Christol, D., Montagnier, L., Rouzioux, C., Klatzmann, D., Rozenbaum, W., Gluckmann, J.C., and Chermann, J.C. 1984. "Detection of IgG Antibodies to Lymphade-nopathy Associated Virus in Patients with AIDS or Lymphadenop-athy Syndrome." *Lancet* i:1253–1256.

Carlson, G.A., and McClellan, T.A. 1987. "The Voluntary Acceptance of HIV-Antibody Screening by Intravenous Drug Users." *Public Health Reports* 102:391–394.

Carter, W.A., Brodsky, I., Pellegrino, M.G., Henriques, H.F., Parenti, D.M., Schulof, R.S., Robinson, W.E., Volsky, D.J., Paxton, H., Kariko, K., Suhadolnik, R.J., Strayer, D.R., Lewin, M., Einck, L., Simon, G.L., Scheib, R.G., Montefiori, D.C., Mitchell, W.M., Paul, D., Meyer, W.A. III, Reichenbach, N., and Gillespie, D.H. 1987. "Clinical, Immunolog-ical, and Virological Effects of Ampligen, A Mismatched Double-Stranded RNA, in Patients with AIDS or AIDS-Related Complex." *Lancet* i:1286–1292.

Cartter, M., Petersen, L., Hadler, J., and Savage, R. 1988. "A New Approach: Providing HIV Counseling and Testing Services in Intravenous Drug Programs." Abstract 8537, proceedings from the *IV International Conference on AIDS*, Book 2, page 393.

Casadonte, P.P., Des Jarlais, D.C., Friedman, S.R., and Rotrosen, J. 1988. "Psychological and Behavioral Impact of Learning HIV Test Results in IV Drug Users." Abstract 8542, proceedings from the *IV International Conference on AIDS*, Book 2, page 394.

Centers for Disease Control. 1983. "Prevention of Acquired Immune Deficiency Syndrome (AIDS): Report of Interagency Recommendations." *Morbidity and Mortality Weekly Report* 32:101–103.

Centers for Disease Control. 1985a. "1985 STD Treatment Guidelines." *Morbidity and Mortality Weekly Report* 34:75s–108s.

Centers for Disease Control. 1985b. "Results of Human T-Lymphotropic Virus Type III Test Kits Reported from Blood Collection Centers—United States, April 22–May 19, 1985." *Morbidity and Mortality Weekly Report* 34:375–376.

Centers for Disease Control. 1985c. "Self-Reported Behavioral Change Among Gay and Bisexual Men—San Francisco." *Morbidity and Mortality Weekly Report* 34:613–615.

Centers for Disease Control. 1985d. "Update: Public Health Service Workshop on Human T-Lymphotropic Virus Type III Antibody Testing—United States." *Morbidity and Mortality Weekly Report* 34:477–478.

Centers for Disease Control. 1985e. "Update: Revised Public Health Service Definition of Persons Who Should Refrain from Donating Blood and Plasma." *Morbidity and Mortality Weekly Report* 34:547–548.

Centers for Disease Control. 1986a. "Diagnosis and Managment of Mycobacterial Infection and Disease in Persons with Human T-Lymphotropic Virus Type III/Lymphadenopathy-Associated Virus Infection." *Morbidity and Mortality Weekly Report* 35:448–452.

Centers for Disease Control. 1986b. "Human T-Lymphotropic Virus Type III/Lymphadenopathy-Associated Virus Antibody Prevalence in U.S. Military Recruit Applicants." *Morbidity and Mortality Weekly Report* 35:421–428.

Centers for Disease Control. 1986c. "Human T-Lymphotropic Virus Type III/Lymphadenopathy-Associated Virus Antibody Testing at Alternate Sites." *Morbidity and Mortality Weekly Report* 35:284–287.

Centers for Disease Control. 1987a. "Human Immunodeficiency Virus Infection in the United States: A Review of Current Knowledge." *Morbidity and Mortality Weekly Report* 36(S-6):1–48.

Centers for Disease Control. 1987b. "Public Health Service Guidelines for Counseling and Antibody Testing to Prevent HIV Infection and AIDS." *Morbidity and Mortality Weekly Report* 36:509–515.

Centers for Disease Control. 1987c. "Recommendations for Prevention of HIV Transmission in Health Care Settings." *Morbidity and Mortality Weekly Report* 36(S-2):3S–18S.

Centers for Disease Control. 1987d. "Trends in Human Immunodeficiency Virus Infection Among Civilian Applicants for Military Service—United States, October 1985–December 1986." *Morbidity and Mortality Weekly Report* 36:273–276.

Centers for Disease Control. 1988a. "Partner Notification for Preventing Human Immunodeficiency Virus (HIV) Infection—Colorado, Idaho, South Carolina, Virginia." *Morbidity and Mortality Weekly Report* 37:393–402.

Centers for Disease Control. 1988b. "Prevalence of Human Immunodeficiency Virus Antibody in U.S. Active-Duty Military Personnel, April 1988." *Morbidity and Mortality Weekly Report* 37:461–463.

Centers for Disease Control. 1988c. "Update: Serologic Testing for Antibody to Human Immunodeficiency Virus." *Morbidity and Mortality Weekly Report* 36:833– 840.

Centers for Disease Control. 1988d. "Update: Universal Precautions for Prevention of Transmission of Human Immunodeficiency Virus, Hepatitis B Virus, and Other Bloodborne Pathogens in Health Care Settings." *Morbidity and Mortality Weekly Report* 37:377–388.

Cooper, D.A., Imrie, A.A., and Penny, R. 1987. "Antibody Response to Human Immunodeficiency Virus After Primary Infection." *Journal of Infectious Diseases* 155:1113–1118.

Courouce, A. 1986. "Evaluation of Eight ELISA Kits for the Detection of Anti-LAV/HTLV III Antibodies." *Lancet* i:1152–1153.

Culliton, B.J. 1984. "Crash Development of AIDS Test Nears Goal." *Science* 225:1128–1131.

Cutler, J.C., and Arnold, R.C. 1988. "Venereal Disease Control by Health Department in the Past: Lessons for the Present." *American Journal of Public Health* 78:372–376.

Doll, L.S., O'Malley, P., Pershing, A., Hessol, N., Darrow, W., Lifson, A., and Cannon, L. 1988. "High-Risk Behavior and Knowledge of HIV-Antibody Status in the San Francisco City Clinic Cohort." Abstract 8102, proceedings from the *IV International Conference on AIDS*, Book 1, page 474.

Dondero, T.J., Rauch, K., Storch, G.A., Crane, L., Proffitt, M., Collinge, M.L., and White, C. 1988. "U.S. Sentinel Hospital Surveillance Network: Results of the First 20 Months." Abstract 6015, proceedings from the *IV International Conference on AIDS*, Book 1, page 357.

Farthing, C.F., Jesson, W., Taylor, H.L., Lawrence, A.G., and Gazzard, B.G. 1987. "The HIV Antibody Test: Influence on Sexual Behavior of Homosexual Men." Presented at the Third International Conference on AIDS in Washington, D.C., June 1–5, 1987.

Farzadegan, H., Polis, M.A., Wolinsky, S.M., Rinaldo, C.R., Sninsky, J.J., Kwok, S., Griffith, R.L., Kaslow, R.A., Phair, J.P., Polk, F.B., and Saah, A.J. 1988. "Loss of Human Immunodeficiency Virus Type 1 (HIV-1) Antibodies with Evidence of Viral Infection in Asymptomatic Homosexual Men." *Annals of Internal Medicine* 108:785– 790.

Fehrs, L.J., Foster, L.R., Fox, V., Fleming, D., McAlister, R.O., Modesitt, S., and Conrad, R. 1988. "Trial of Anonymous Versus Confidential Human Immunodeficiency Virus Testing." Lancet ii:379–381.

Fischl, M.A., Richman, D.D., Grieco, M.H., Gottlieb, M.S., Volberding, P.A., Laskin, O.L., Leedom, J.M., Groopman, J.E., Mildvan, D., Schooley, R.T., Jackson, G.G., Durack, D.T., and King, D. 1987. "The Efficacy of Azidothymidine (AZT) in the Treatment of Patients with AIDS and AIDS-Related Complex: A Double-Blind, Placebo-Controlled Trial." New England Journal of Medicine 317:185–191.

Fleming, D.W., Cochi, S.L., Steece, R.S., and Hull, H.F. 1987. "Acquired Immunodeficiency Syndrome in Low-Incidence Areas: How Safe Is Unsafe Sex?" Journal of the American Medical Association 285: 785–787.

Fox R., Odaka, N.J., Brookmeyer, R., and Polk, B.F. 1987. "Effect of HIV Antibody Disclosure on Subsequent Sexual Activity in Homosexual Men." AIDS 1:241–246.

Francis, D.P., and Chin, J. 1987. "The Prevention of Acquired Immunodeficiency Syndrome in the United States." Journal of the American Medical Association 257:1357–1366.

Gaines, H., Albert, J., von Sydow, M., Sonnerborg, A., Chiodi, F., Ehrnst, A., Strannegard, O., and Asjo, B. 1987. "HIV Anitgenemia and Virus Isolation from Plasma During Primary HIV Infection." Lancet i:1317–1318.

Gallo, R.C., Salahuddin, S.Z., Popovic, M., Shearer, G.M., Kaplan, J., Haynes, B.F., Palker, T.J., Redfield, R., Oleske, J., Safai, B., White, G., Foster, P., and Markham, P.D. 1984. "Frequent Detection and Isolation of Cytopathic Retroviruses (HTLV-III) from Patients with AIDS or at Risk for AIDS." Science 224:500–503.

Goedert, J.J. 1987. "Suggested Standards Linked to Testing for Human Immunodeficiency Virus." New England Journal of Medicine 316: 1339–1342.

Goudsmit, J., Paul, D.A., Lange, J.M.A., Speelman, H., van der Noordaa, J., van der Helm, H.J., de Wolf, F., Epstein, L.G., Krone, W.J.A., Wolters, E.C., Oleske, J.M., and Coutinho, R.A. 1986. "Expression of Human Immunodeficiency Virus Antigen (HIV-Ag) in Serum and Cerebrospinal Fluid During Acute and Chronic Infection." Lancet ii:177–180.

Groopman, J.E., Hartzband, P.I., Shulman, L., Salahuddin, S.Z., Sarngadharan, M.G., McLane, M.F., Essex, M., and Gallo, R.C. 1985. "Antibody Seronegative Human T-Lymphotropic Virus Type III (HTLV-III)-Infected Patients with Acquired Immunodeficiency Syndrome or Related Disorders." Blood 66:742–744.

Grunnet, N., Jersild, C., and Georgsen, J. 1985. "Photometric Reading of Anti-HTLV-III ELISA Kits." Lancet ii:1302.

Henry, K., Willenbring, K., and Crossley, K. 1988. "Human Immunodeficiency Virus Antibody Testing: A Description of Practices and Policies at U.S. Infectious Disease Teaching Hospitals and Minnesota Hospitals." *Journal of the American Medical Association* 259:1819–1822.

Herbold, J.R. 1986. "AIDS Policy Development Within the Defense Department." *Military Medicine* 151:623–627.

Hughes, W.T., Rivera, G.K., Schell, M.J., Thornton, D., and Lott, L. 1987. "Successful Intermittent Chemoprophylaxis for Pneumocystis Carinii Pneumonitis." *New England Journal of Medicine* 316:1627–1632.

Hull, H.F., Bettinger, C.J., Gallaher, M.M., Keller, N.M., Wilson, J., and Mertz, G.J. 1988. "Comparison of HIV-Antibody Prevalence in Patients Consenting to and Declining HIV-Antibody Testing in an STD Clinic." *Journal of the American Medical Association* 260:935–938.

Hunter, J.B., and Menitove, J.E. 1985. "HLA Antibodies Detected by ELISA HTLV-III Antibody Kits." *Lancet* ii:397.

Johns, D.R., Tierney, M., and Felsenstein, D., 1987. "Alteration in the Natural History of Neurosyphilis by Concurrent Infection with the Human Immunodeficiency Virus." *New England Journal of Medicine* 316:1569–1572.

Johnson, W., Sy, F.S., and Jackson, K.L. 1988. "The Impact of Mandatory Reporting of HIV Seropositive Persons in South Carolina." Abstract 6020, proceedings from the *IV International Conference on AIDS,* Book 1, page 358.

Kaslow, R.A., Ostrow, D.G., Detels, R., Phair, J.P., Polk, B.F., and Rinaldo, C.R. 1987. "The Multicenter AIDS Cohort Study: Rationale, Organization, and Selected Characteristics of the Participants." *American Journal of Epidemiology* 126:310–318.

Kemp, B.E., Rylatt, D.B., Bundensen, P.G., Doherty, R.R., McPhee, D.A., Stapleton, D., Cottis, L.E., Wilson, K., John M.A., Khan, J.M., Dinh, D.P., Miles, S., and Hillyard, C.J. 1988. "Autologous Red Cell Agglutination Assay for HIV-1 Antibodies: Simplified Test with Whole Blood." *Science* 241:1352–1358.

Kerndt, P., Sorvillo, F., Tormey, M., Run, G., Iwakoshi, K., Giles, M., and Waterman, S. 1988. "Human Immunodeficiency Virus (HIV) Seroprevalence in an Adult Medical and Pediatric Outpatient Population in Los Angeles County." Abstract 4197, proceedings from the *IV International Conference on AIDS,* Book 1, page 309.

Kleinman, S., Fitzpatrick, L., Secord, K., and Wilke, D. 1988. "Follow-up Testing and Notification of Anti-HIV Western Blot Atypical (Indeterminant) Donors." *Transfusion* 28:280–282.

Kuhnl, P., Seidl, S., and Holzberger, G. 1985. "HLA DR4 Antibodies Cause Positive HTLV-III Antibody ELISA Results." *Lancet* i:1222–1223.

Kwok, S., Mack, D.H., Mullis, K.B., Poiesz, B., Ehrlich, G., Blair, D., Friedman-Kien, A., and Sninsky, J.J. 1987. "Identification of Human Immonodeficiency Virus Sequences by Using In Vitro Enzymatic Amplification and Oligomer Cleavage Detection." *Journal of Virology* 61:1690–1694.

Lelie, P.N., Reesink, H.W., and Huisman, J.G. 1987. "Earlier Detection of HIV and Second-Generation Antibody Assays." *Lancet* ii:343–344.

Lundberg, G.D. 1988. "Serological Diagnosis of Human Immunodeficiency Virus Infection by Western Blot Testing." *Journal of the American Medical Association* 260:674–679.

Lyter, D.W., Valdiserri, R.O., Kingsley, L.A., Amoroso, W.P., and Rinaldo, C.R. 1987. "The HIV Antibody Test: Why Gay and Bisexual Men Want or Do Not Want to Know Their Results." *Public Health Reports* 102(5):468–474.

McCusker, J., Stoddard, A.M., Mayer, K.H., Zapka, J., Morrison, C., and Saltzman, S.P. 1988. "Effects of HIV Antibody Test Knowledge on Subsequent Sexual Behaviors in a Cohort of Homosexually Active Men." *American Journal of Public Health* 78:462–467.

McKusick, L., Wiley, J.A., Coates, T.J., Stall, R., Saika, B., Morin, S., Charles, K., Hostman, W., and Conant, M.A. 1985. "Reported Changes in the Sexual Behavior of Men at Risk for AIDS, San Francisco, 1982–84." *Public Health Reports* 100:622–629.

Marlink, R.G., Foss, B., Swift, R., Davis, W., Essex, M., and Groopman, J. 1987. "High Rate of HTLV-III/HIV Exposure in IVDA's from a Small-Sized City and the Failure of Specialized Methadone Maintenance to Prevent Further Drug Use." Presented at the Third International Conference on AIDS in Washington, D.C., June 1–5, 1987.

Martin, P.W., Burger, D.R., Caouette, S., and Goldstein, A.S. 1985. "Importance of Confirmatory Tests After Strongly Positive HTLV-III Screening Tests." *New England Journal of Medicine* 314:1577.

Marzuk, P.M., Tierney, H., Tardiff, K., Gross, E.M., Morgan, E.B., Hsu, M., and Mann, J.J. 1988. "Increased Risk of Suicide in Persons with AIDS." *Journal of the American Medical Association* 259:1333–1337.

Meyer, K.B., and Pauker, S.G. 1987. "Screening for HIV: Can We Afford the False Positive Rate?" *New England Journal of Medicine* 317:238–241.

Mitchell, W.M., Montefiori, D.C., Robinson, W.E., Jr., Strayer, D.R., and Carter, W.A. 1987. "Mismatched Double- Stranded RNA (Ampligen) Reduces Concentration of Zidovudine (Azidothymidine) Required for In Vitro Inhibition of Human Immunodeficiency Virus." *Lancet* i: 890–892.

Montgomery, A.B., Luce, J.M., Turner, J., Lin, E.T., Debs, R.J., Corkery, K.J., Brunette, E.N., and Hopewell, P.C. 1987. "Aerosolized Pentamidine as Sole Therapy for Pneumocystis Carinii Pneumonia in Patients with Acquired Immunodeficiency Syndrome." *Lancet* ii:480–483.

Morgan, J., Tate, R., Farr, A.D., and Urbaniak, S.J., 1986. "Potential Source of Error in HTLV-III Antibody Testing." *Lancet* i:739–740.

Morris, L., Distenfeld, A., Amorosi, E., and Karpatkin, S. 1982. "Autoimmune Thrombocytopenic Purpura in Homosexual Men." *Annals of Internal Medicine* 96:714–717.

Mortimer, P.P., Parry, J.V., and Mortimer, J.Y. 1985. "Which Anti-HTLV III/LAV Assays for Screening and Confirmatory Testing?" *Lancet* ii: 873–877.

Moulton, J., Stempel, R., Bacchetti, P., Temoshok, L., and Moss, A. 1988. "Results of a Longitudinal Psychosocial Study of the Impact of Antibody Test Notification." Abstract 6074, proceedings from the *IV International Conference on AIDS*, Book 1, page 372.

Nichols, S.E. 1985. "Psychosocial Reactions of Persons with the Acquired Immunodeficiency Syndrome." *Annals of Internal Medicine* 103: 765–767.

Ostrow, D.G., Joseph, J., Soucey, J., Eller, M., Kessler, R., Phair, J., Chmiel, J. 1988. "Mental Health and Behavioral Correlates of HIV Antibody Testing in a Cohort of Gay Men." Abstract 4082, proceedings from the *IV International Conference on AIDS*, Book 1, page 280.

Peitrequin, R., Graf, I., Lantin, J., Frei, P. 1987. "Routine Tests for HIV Antigen." *Lancet* ii:916–917.

Physicians' Desk Reference. 1988. Oradell, N.J.: Medical Economics Company.

Polk, B.F., Fox, R., Brookmeyer, R., Kanchanaraksa, S., Kaslow, R.A., Visscher, B., Rinaldo, C.R., and Phair, J. 1987. "Predictors of the Acquired Immunodeficiency Syndrome Developing in a Cohort of Seropositive Homosexual Men." *New England Journal of Medicine* 316:61– 66.

Pollack, M., Schiltz, M.A., Lejeune, B. 1987. "Safer Sex and Acceptance of Testing: Results of the Nationwide Annual Survey Among French Gay Men." Presented at the Third International Conference on AIDS in Washington, D.C., June 1–5, 1987.

Potterat, J.J. 1987. "Lying to Military Physicians About Risk Factors for HIV Infections." *Journal of the American Medical Association* 257:1727.

Quinn, T.C., Riggin, C.H., Kline, R.L., Francis, H., Mulanga, K., Sension, M.G., and Fauci, A.S. 1988. "Rapid Latex Agglutination Assay Using Recombinant Envelope Polypeptide for the Detection of Antibody to the HIV." *Journal of the American Medical Association* 260:510– 513.

Ranki, A., Krohn, M., Allain, J.P., Franchini, G., Valle, S.L., Antonen, J., Leuther, M., and Krohn, K. 1987. "Long Latency Precedes Overt Seroconversion in Sexually Transmitted Human Immunodeficiency Virus Infection." *Lancet* ii(8559):589– 593.

Redfield, R.R., Wright, D.C., James, W.D., Jones, T.S., Brown, C., and Burke, D.S. 1987. "Disseminated Vaccinia in a Military Recruit with Human Immunodeficiency Virus (HIV) Disease." *New England Journal of Medicine* 316:673–676.

Reesink, H.W., Huisman, J.G., Gonsalves, M., Winkel, I.N., Hekker, A.C., Lelie, P.N., Schaasberg, W., Aaij, C., van der Does, J.A., and Desmyter, J. 1986. "Evaluation of Six Enzyme Immunoassays for Antibody Against Human Immunodeficiency Virus." *Lancet* ii:483–486.

Rugg, D., Sweet, D., Hovell, M., and Fagan, R. 1988. "Factors Affecting the Decision to Learn HIV Test Results." Abstract 6075, proceedings from the *IV International Conference on AIDS*, Book 1, page 372.

Rutherford, G.W., and Woo, J.M. 1988. "Contact Tracing and the Control of Human Immunodeficiency Virus Infection." *Journal of the American Medical Association* 259:3609–3610.

Sarngadharan, M.G., Popovic, M., Bruch, L., Schubach, J., and Gallo, R.C. 1984. "Antibodies Reactive with Human T-Lymphotropic Retroviruses (HTLV-III) in the Serum of Patients with AIDS." *Science* 224:506–508.

Schwartz, J.S., Dans, P.E., and Kinosian, B.P. 1988. "Human Immunodeficiency Virus Test Evaluation, Performance and Use." *Journal of the American Medical Association* 259:2574– 2579.

Shaw, G., Hahn, M.B.H., Arya, S.K., Groopman, J.E., Gallo, R.C., and Wong-Stall, F. 1984. "Molecular Characterization of Human T-Cell Leukemia (Lymphotropic) Virus Type III in the Acquired Immune Deficiency Syndrome." *Science* 226:1165–1171.

Sivak, S.L., and Wormser, G.P. 1986. "Predictive Value of a Screening Test for Antibodies to HTLV- III." *American Journal of Clinical Pathology* 85(6):700– 703.

Snyder, A.J., and Vergeront, J.M. 1988. "Safeguarding the Blood Supply by Providing Opportunities for Anonymous HIV Testing." *New England Journal of Medicine* 319:374–375.

Soloway, H.B. 1986. "Matrix Analysis for Interpretation of Human Immunodeficiency Virus Panels." *Laboratory Medicine* 17:694–695.

Stute, R. 1987. "HIV Antigen Detection in Routine Blood Donor Screening." *Lancet* i:566.

Taylor, R.N., and Przybyszewski, V.A. 1988. "Summary of the Centers for Disease Control Human Immunodeficiency Virus (HIV) Performance Evaluation Surveys for 1985 and 1986." *American Journal of Clinical Pathology* 89:1–13.

Van den Hoek, J., Van Haastrecht, H., Goudsmit, J., and Coutinho, R.A. 1988. "Influence of HIV-Ab Testing on the Risk Behavior of IV Drug Users in Amsterdam." Abstract 4541, proceedings from the *IV International Conference on AIDS*, Book 2, page 197.

Van Griensven, G., Tielman, R., Goudsmit, F., Van der Noordaa, J., De Wolf, F., and Coutinho, R.A. 1987. "Effect of HIV-AB Serodiagnosis on Sexual Behavior in Homosexual Men in the Netherlands." Presented at the Third International Conference on AIDS in Washington, D.C., June 1–5, 1987.

Vecchio, T.J. 1966. "Predictive Value of a Single Diagnostic Test in Unselected Populations." *New England Journal of Medicine* 274:1171–1173.

Volsky, D.J., Wu, Y.T., Stevenson, M., Dewhurst, S., Sinangil, F., Merino, F., Rodriguez, L., and Godoy, G. 1986. "Antibodies to HTLV-III/LAV in

Venezuelan Patients with Acute Malarial Infections." *New England Journal of Medicine* 314:647–648.

Watkins, J.D., Conway-Welch, C., Creedon, J.J., Crenshaw, T.L., DeVos, R.M., Gebbie, K.M., Lee, B.J., Lilly, F., O'Connor, J.C., Primm, B.J., Pullen, P., SerVass, C., and Walsh, W.B. 1988. "Report of the Presidential Commission on the Human Immunodeficiency Virus Epidemic, June 24, 1988." Washington, D.C.: U.S. Government Printing Office.

Ward, J.W., Holmberg, S.D., Allen, J.R., Cohn, D.L., Critchley, S.E., Kleinman, S.H., Lenes, B.A., Ravenholt, O., Davis, J.R., Quinn, M.G., and Jaffe, H.W. 1988. "Transmission of Human Immunodeficiency Virus (HIV) by Blood Transfusions Screened as Negative for HIV Antibody." *New England Journal of Medicine* 318:473– 478.

Weiss, S.H., Goedert, J.J., Sarngadharan, M.G., Bodner, A.J., Gallo, R.C., and Blattner, W.A. 1985. "Screening Test for HTLV-III (AIDS Agent) Antibodies—Specificity, Sensitivity and Applications." *Journal of the American Medical Association* 253(2):221–225.

Wiktor, S., Biggar, R., Melbye, M., Ebbesen, P., and Goedert, J. 1988. "Effect of Knowledge of HIV Status Upon Sexual Activity Among Homosexual Men." Abstract 4073, proceedings from the *IV International Conference on AIDS*, Book 1, page 278.

Wilkerson, I. 1988. "A.M.A. Urges Breech of Privacy to Warn Potential AIDS Victims." *New York Times* July 1, A1.

Willoughby, B., Schechter, M.T., Boyko, W.J., Craib, K., Weaver, M.S., and Douglas, B. 1987. "Sexual Practices and Condom Use in a Cohort of Homosexual Men: Evidence of Differential Modification Between Seropositive and Seronegative Men." Presented at the Third International Conference on AIDS in Washington, D.C., June 1–5, 1987.

Wilson, J.M.G., and Jungner, S. 1986. "Principles and Practice of Screening for Disease." *World Health Organization Public Health Papers* 34: 7–163.

Woo, J.M., Neal, D.P., Geoghegan, C.M., Rauch, K.J., Barnhart, J.L., Lemp, G.F., and Rutherford, G.W. 1988. "Evaluation of Heterosexual Contact Tracing of Partners of AIDS Patients." Abstract 6002, proceedings from the *IV International Conference on AIDS*, Book 1, page 354.

Wykoff, R.F., Health, C.W., Jr., Hollis, S.L., Leonard, S.T., Quiller, C.B., Jones, J.L., Artzrouni, M., and Parker, R.L. 1988. "Contact Tracing to Identify Human Immunodeficiency Virus Infection in a Rural Community." *Journal of the American Medical Association* 259: 3563–3566.

Chapter 7

Evaluating AIDS-Prevention Programs

In its most elemental sense, *evaluation* describes the process by which activities, objects, or actions are judged with respect to other known reference points. Very few human activities occur in the absence of some form of evaluation, either formal or informal, planned or spontaneous, objective or subjective. As sapient beings we are predisposed to make judgments about most of our experiences, whether personal, professional, political, or commercial, by comparing them to other similar experiences or to predetermined expectations. For example, when shopping for a new home, prospective buyers judge their potential choices against a series of objective and subjective criteria that are predetermined to be of importance to them. Some buyers may place more importance on objective criteria (for example, whether the home is in a particular school district or neighborhood) while other buyers may place more importance on subjective criteria (whether it reminds them of the home in which they were raised or "feels" comfortable). Certainly, potential buyers who have been through the process before incorporate their past experience into the evaluation process.

When we move from the realm of personal experience into the realm of organized, premeditated activity involving large numbers of people, evaluation takes on a more complex and objective character. This evolution relates to resource expenditures and the subsequent need for accountability being of a much higher magnitude in these situations than they are in most personal situations—where the results of decision making are likely to have only a limited sphere of influence. When we evaluate organized efforts, such as AIDS-prevention programs, for example, we are interested in answering a number of questions, not the least of which is "did the program accomplish what it set out to accomplish?" If it did not, we

246

are interested in learning why. We are also interested in assessing the relative costs and benefits of the program, for although it may have accomplished its stated goals, the costs required to meet those goals may have been prohibitive. Finally, we are interested in looking at the results of our program evaluation for indicators of how existing service systems might be modified to incorporate our findings, and to determine whether the evaluation results suggest additional areas of inquiry. Evaluation therefore represents an essential step in the following sequence of program development: planning, implementation, evaluation, and modification. This sequence is circular, not linear, in that information provided by the evaluation process should be incorporated into new planning efforts, which begin the cycle anew.

SETTING PROGRAM GOALS

The process of program evaluation begins at the outset of the program, when goals are set. Certainly, the ultimate goal of any AIDS-prevention program is to prevent infection with or transmission of HIV. But, given the wide variety of forms that prevention activities can take, and the multiplicity of specific target audiences in need of AIDS-prevention services, this goal, as stated, is too general to be of much practical value. An analogous goal in business would be "to make a profit." While this might be the ultimate intent of most business ventures, it does not provide adequate detail in terms of how the profit will be made, over what period of time the profit will be realized, what resources will be necessary to achieve this profit, and what existing evidence supports the likelihood that the enterprise can make a profit. In order to translate abstract, general goals into reality, all organizations, whether private, nonprofit, or public, rely on objectives to describe the specific operational activities they must undertake to accomplish their desired purpose.

In AIDS-prevention programs, the development of specific objectives serves a variety of functions. First and foremost, these objectives represent the tangible product of collaboration between program planners, technical experts, and target group members in determining, by consensus, what the output of the program should be. The consensual process by which these objectives are elaborated is extremely important, as it enables all of the parties who have a significant stake in AIDS prevention to participate in shaping and directing prevention efforts. The importance of joint participation has been a recurrent theme throughout this book and, according to the American Public Health Association, it is an absolutely essential criterion of health promotion and education programs (1987). Second, these mutually agreed upon objectives act as a nidus for planning efforts and enable the project team to develop a meaningful estimate of the level of resources necessary to achieve programmatic goals. Finally, these objectives function as standards to gauge the success or failure of the program, and in this capacity, represent the initial step in the process of evaluation.

When service-oriented programs set objectives, they usually consider three distinct levels: process (formative), impact, and outcome. Outcome objectives are best thought of as long-range goals. In their book on evaluation of health-promotion programs, Green and Lewis define outcome objectives as the "ultimate goal or product of a program," indicating that they are "generally measured in the health field in terms of morbidity or mortality statistics in a population" (1986:364). Impact objectives are short-range or intermediate goals that describe the "immediate, observable effects of a program" (Green and Lewis 1986:363). Process or formative objectives relate to activities that must be completed prior to and during the early phase of program implementation. In order for these three levels of objectives to achieve the functions described above, it is important that they be "specific, realistic, time-phased, and measurable" (Centers for Disease Control 1987:6).

In its 1987 publication, "Guidelines for AIDS Prevention Program Operations," the Centers for Disease Control listed a series of examples for each of the three levels of objectives we have described. For AIDS-prevention programs targeting school-aged youth, appropriate process objectives might include the following: determining how many schools in the region already have an acceptable AIDS curriculum; developing an AIDS-prevention curriculum for those schools without such a program; obtaining consensus on this curriculum from teachers, students, parents, and school administrators; training teachers to deliver this curriculum; and measuring baseline levels of drug use and unsafe sexual activity (sexual intercourse without the use of condoms) among the target audience, prior to implementing the curriculum. Specific impact and outcome objectives would be set after the process objectives have been agreed upon and after "process objectives are achieved to gather and analyze baseline data which will define the problem" (Centers for Disease Control 1987:6).

Continuing with our example of a school-based AIDS-prevention program, a typical impact objective might be stated as follows: "By the end of the current budget period, increase from [baseline percent] to [projected percent due to program impact] the high schools in the three largest cities that provide a quality unit of education on AIDS, sexually transmitted disease, and drug abuse, emphasizing positive health behaviors rather than biomedical details" (adapted from Centers for Disease Control 1987:8).

The outcome objectives identified in these guidelines address long-term goals, and generally gauge effect by looking for decreases in the level of HIV seroprevalence in regions where programs have been implemented or among groups who have attended prevention programs: "By April 30, 1991, no more than [percent projected from baseline seroprevalence] of new patients attending STD clinics in the three largest cities will be positive for HIV antibody" (Centers for Disease Control 1987:8).

Identifying the three levels of objectives marks the beginning of the evaluation process by creating the standards against which program results will be measured. Seemingly, evaluation now becomes a relatively straightforward process of comparing observed to expected outcomes. This description, while accurate in the most general sense, does not address the specific difficulties that program managers face in actually conducting an evaluation. Our discussion will now turn to addressing the two major difficulties inherent in program evaluation. The first considers the limitations of measurement itself, while the second relates to the innate complexity of the objects we are evaluating and the multiple functions that evaluation can fulfill.

LIMITATIONS OF MEASUREMENT

The limitations we face in evaluating the effects of AIDS-prevention programs are not dissimilar from obstacles we face in evaluating the effects of other complex phenomena, whether naturally occurring or humanly mediated. Most often, these limitations result from the restrictions placed upon us by the quality of the measurements available to us, rather than from an ignorance of the issues involved or an inability to appreciate the complexity of the phenomena. According to Green and Lewis, measurement is "the assignment of numbers to objects, events, or people, according to specified rules" (1986:58). Measurement may also be considered a universal activity of intelligent life. In fact, refinements in the process of measurement permitting a higher degree of accuracy and precision within existing forms of measurement, and extending the act of measurement to different and more complex phenomena, can be viewed as a primary marker of cultural and scientific evolutionary development. This observation is suggested by Rossi and Freeman's description of evaluation as "a response to efforts to move toward a more perfect world" (Rossi and Freeman 1985:105).

Limitations notwithstanding, the need to measure is a sine qua non in the process of evaluation, since, generally speaking, changes in inaccurate information, "obstructive" attitudes, and unsafe behaviors are the desired outcomes of AIDS-prevention activities (except, of course, for programs in which maintenance of healthy behaviors is the desired outcome, and in those instances we would measure the absence of change). Public education campaigns attempt to change persistent incorrect beliefs that human immunodeficiency virus is highly contagious. Poster campaigns targeted at sexually active gay men attempt to change negative attitudes about condoms, especially by encouraging change in group norms relating to condom use. Outreach workers visiting "shooting galleries" encourage IV drug users to change drug-using behaviors, either through entry into treatment programs or by the routine practice of cleaning needles and syringes with bleach. Health educators in publicly funded clinics for the treatment of sexually transmitted diseases educate clients about the manner in which HIV is transmitted and attempt to change the attitudes of those heterosexual clients who believe that AIDS is a disease limited to gay men.

To determine the success of these activities, we must be able to measure specified parameters of interest before and after our intervention. These parameters might include attitudinal and factual information about the transmission and prevention of HIV collected by telephone survey; self-reports of condom-use practices collected by written survey from the patrons of a gay bar; quarterly reports on the number of referrals made to drug treatment facilities by outreach workers visiting "shooting galleries"; or staff assessments of the degree of self-perceived risk of HIV infection based on personal interviews with STD clinic clients.

To better appreciate the limitations of measurement, let us examine this task using a relatively simple construct of what we measure, how we measure it, when we measure it, and on whom we conduct our measurements.

In considering what to measure in evaluating an AIDS-prevention program, it would seem eminently logical to measure behavior, since the extinction of behaviors that are "unsafe" and the maintenance of "safe" behaviors are key objectives of AIDS-prevention activities. However, the simplicity of this approach belies the complexity of health behavior and its change. In recognition of this complexity, programmatic attempts to influence health-related behavior are generally multifactorial and include strategies to increase knowledge, change attitudes, enhance skills, influence health-related group norms, and provide services that will support or enable the desired behavior (Centers for Disease Control 1987:6). Therefore, measuring behavior change alone may not take adequate note of the important elements that contribute to it.

For example, when evaluating an AIDS-prevention program targeted to intravenous drug users who are receiving methadone maintenance, we may have an impact objective that states that "within six months after the program's implementation, condom use among men enrolled in the program should increase by 25 percent from baseline levels." Let us assume further that information about condom-use behavior, which is being collected routinely at each client visit, is accurate, and that these data unequivocally demonstrate that this impact objective has not been met. In order to understand the reason(s) for failure to meet this impact objective, we would clearly need additional information. Does the health educator present information about the importance of condom use in an effective way? Do these men have attitudes of fatalism or denial that interfere with their use of condoms? Are they resistant to using condoms because they feel that sexual pleasure would be impaired? Or do their partners object to their use of condoms? Is the problem that the men do not know how to discuss the subject of condoms with sexual partners, and are concerned that doing so would make a partner think that they are infected? Or is it that they have intentions to use condoms, but do not have access to a readily available supply?

Questions such as these indicate that the parameters we choose to measure in evaluating prevention programs must coincide with the theoretical and programmatic approaches undertaken to promote behavioral change and the impact objectives that reflect this theoretical underpinning.

Earlier we identified the misperception that AIDS is a disease limited to gays as a barrier to prevention campaigns within racial and ethnic minority communities. Therefore, an AIDS-prevention program targeted to African-American adolescents may strive to personalize the risk of HIV infection as a means of enabling black youth to internalize and act upon AIDS-prevention information, as described in the following impact objective: "By the end of the current

budget period, reduce by 75 percent from baseline percent the number of African-American adolescents who believe that AIDS is something 'that only happens to gays.' " Evaluation in this context would
include not only measurements of behavior, but also the measurement of variables that gauge the perception of risk of HIV infection—
as this has been identified as an important theoretical component
and as a potential barrier to change that the program has targeted as
an impact objective. Although the specific variables to be measured
will vary on the basis of these two parameters (theory and objectives), many programmatic evaluations rely on the traditional approach of measuring knowledge, attitudes, and behavior to address
the major elements in the "mix" of health behavior change.

After the variables that reflect programmatic theory and objectives have been determined, the next issue is how to measure them.
In discussing the limitations of measurement, we must begin by accepting the premise that all measurement is approximation, and
some approximations are more accurate than others. We may be
fairly confident in estimating clients' knowledge of the cause of
AIDS, how the human immunodeficiency virus is transmitted, what
body fluids contain HIV, or how a condom should be lubricated, on
the basis of their answers to a series of true and false questions. But,
when we attempt to assess relevant attitudes, such as feelings about
the pleasurability of "unsafe" sexual practices, or personal concerns
about the confidentiality of HIV counseling and testing, or the importance of cleaning "works" before injecting drugs, we usually rely
on a participant's self-ranking of a statement on some form of continuum scale (for example, "strongly agree," "agree," "mixed feelings," "disagree," and "strongly disagree"). Though widely used,
these scales "manifest some degree of unreliability because of the
different meanings attributed to the same statements by different
subjects" (Rossi and Freeman 1985:198).

One way to improve the predictability of these attitudinal measures is to frame the statement containing the attitude of interest as
a hypothetical situation (Wicker 1972:269). For instance, to develop
a measure of an individual's intent to discuss condoms with a new
sexual partner, we might posit an imaginary encounter in which the
subject meets someone new and is sexually aroused by that person.
We would then ask the subject to rank or rate the likelihood of talking about condoms with the imaginary sexual partner.

Our inability routinely to employ observational approaches for
the measurement of sexual and drug-using behaviors forces us to
rely extensively on self-reported measurements, and this is yet an-

other source of potential error. Clients may not always accurately depict their sexual and drug-using behaviors, for reasons of privacy, fear of disclosure, fear of social or legal sanction, or fear of censure if they engage in "unsafe" behaviors. It is well known that "response effects in surveys increase as questions become more threatening," and may take two forms: "the overstatement of desirable behavior" and "the understatement of behavior perceived to be less socially acceptable" (Blair et al. 1977:316).

There are techniques to lessen the "response effects" to questions dealing with extremely personal subjects, such as sexual behavior and drug use. One such strategy is the randomized response method, which links the response to the item of interest to a chance occurrence, such as the toss of a coin (Kolata 1987). Although it has been proven to improve the "honesty" of responses to personal questions, it is time consuming and may thus be prohibitive for hard-pressed personnel in community-based organizations.

Serologic tests for HIV infection may also serve as markers to measure the behavioral effects of a program, but they, too, have limitations. In addition to the technical limitations discussed earlier, there are other reasons the HIV antibody test may not always be appropriate as a means of evaluating program effects. At a procedural level, if clients must be referred elsewhere for HIV counseling and testing, test results will not be available to program staff. Merely monitoring serologic status of individuals already infected with HIV will not tell us whether they have modified their behaviors to prevent transmission of the virus or reinfection with other viral strains. In certain populations, the incidence of new infection may be so low that it would be impossible to gather a sample large enough to assure statistical validity.

For example, if the prevalence of HIV infection among female contraceptors in a low-incidence AIDS area is in the range of 1 in 1,000 or less, using the absence of serologically documented HIV infection as a means of assessing the impact of a prevention program conducted among 500 sexually active women with multiple partners does not really indicate whether or not these women have modified their behaviors: probability would lead us to expect all of these women to be HIV seronegative regardless of their behaviors (because of the low HIV seroprevalence).

Finally, there may be individuals who are interested in participating in a prevention program but who are not willing to be tested, whether for personal reasons or fear of untoward consequences should they learn that they are infected.

From an epidemiologic perspective, measuring changes in HIV seroprevalence is an appropriate and meaningful way to evaluate long-term or outcome objectives of activities to prevent the spread of HIV (Allen and Curran 1988). However, practical considerations are likely to limit the application of measurement to research settings or ongoing surveillance activities funded by federal and state governments.

VALIDITY, RELIABILITY, AND INTERVALS OF MEASUREMENT

Given that we are often forced to depend upon nonobservational, self-reported forms of measurement, usually through the administration of a survey instrument, we must be able to recognize the degree of error inherent in these instruments. In describing the limitations of measurement, the parameters of validity and reliability are especially important. *Validity* refers to the degree of assuredness "that results obtained from measurement or evaluation are an accurate reflection of reality" (Green and Lewis 1986:367). *Reliability* refers to the dependability and consistency of measurement. Reliable instruments "can be relied on to rank order a person similarly on the characteristic of interest with repeated measures under like conditions" (Green and Lewis 1986:99). When these two parameters are fully realized, the instrument is able to make an extremely accurate measurement of a phenomenon or quantity with great precision.

There are techniques for evaluating the reliability and validity of survey instruments, and the reader is referred to an excellent discussion of this subject in Green and Lewis's book on evaluation of health promotion programs (1986:82–115). Detailed descriptions of techniques that can be used to determine internal consistency reliability, split half reliability, stability reliability, content validity, criterion validity, and construct validity are clearly beyond the focus of this chapter, yet their importance as technical issues germane to the subject of evaluation should not be minimized. In reality, many of the technical issues related to the process of evaluation, including program design, survey development and pretesting, and interpretive analysis of data, are best addressed through the input of expert consultants.

Whenever the issue of measurement is raised it is invariably followed by questions about interval. For example, how often and over what period of time do we measure in order to make inferences about the results of our program? Do positive effects have to last for a certain period of time in order to be considered significant, or do we consider any positive effects, regardless of their duration, to be desirable? Furthermore, the parameters we wish to measure are not static. Increasing media attention to AIDS, ongoing legislative and policy development at the state and federal level, and the changing circumstances of the epidemic itself are undoubtedly influencing levels of knowledge, attitudinal postures, and sexual and drug-using behaviors. As the number of persons who are diagnosed with AIDS or other HIV-related diseases increases, so too will the number of individuals who have some first-hand knowledge of the illness increase. The degree to which this first-hand experience influences knowledge, attitudes, and behaviors—and whether its effects can be separated from the results of programmatic efforts—are significant evaluation concerns.

Finally, we must consider the sources of measurements. Obviously, information is obtained from program participants, but who are these individuals? In programmatic situations where the target group is obliged to participate, such as prevention programs in prisons or school-based programs in states where legislation mandates AIDS-prevention curricula, we can be assured that our efforts are reaching a majority of the intended audience (although this, by itself, does not imply efficacy). However, when we evaluate programs in which participation is voluntary, we must consider the distinct possibility that persons who are participating are different from those who are not participating, and therefore, findings resulting from the evaluation may not be generalizable.

Let us consider a hypothetical AIDS-prevention workshop targeted to gay men, which employs group process and peer influence to endorse safer sexual behavior as a caring and responsible adaptation to the threat of AIDS. Let us assume that participants attending this workshop were recruited by flyers and posters distributed in gay bars, bookstores, and adult cinemas, and that demographic information collected on the participants upon enrollment reveals that most are white, college educated, and in a middle- or upper-middle-class income range. Suppose further that the men who attend this hypothetical workshop report a decrease in unprotected receptive anal intercourse six months after their participation. Although this observation is compatible with one of the explicitly stated impact objectives of the program, it does not necessarily follow that the program itself was responsible for this change because we do not have comparable information on the sexual practices of gay men who did not attend our program over the same period of time (that is, we do not have a control or comparison group). Nor does it mean that similar approaches would produce analogous results with other gay men, especially those belonging to ethnic/racial minorities, or those of a lower socioeconomic class, since we know that the men who attended our program were not demographically representative of these subcategories of gay men.

Fortunately, there are ways of minimizing most of the limitations of measurement as it pertains to program evaluation—and again, the reader is referred to texts devoted exclusively to the subject of program evaluation (Green and Lewis 1986; Rossi and Freeman 1985). However, the difficulties imposed by the measurement process are only part of the reason program evaluation can be so complicated. The other major reason has to do with the diversity and complexity of the object of our interest, namely, the AIDS-prevention program itself.

VARIETY OF AIDS-PREVENTION PROGRAMS

Although all AIDS-prevention initiatives may have the same "outcome" objective—preventing the spread of HIV—the target audience, theoretical basis, program design, program setting, impact objectives, available resources, and existing constraints vary greatly from one program to another. AIDS-prevention activities can be found in public, private, and nonprofit organizational settings. In our discussion of AIDS-prevention programs in Chapter Five, we documented a variety of programmatic approaches to the problem of AIDS prevention. Some prevention programs may be carried out within the context of state or federally funded health departments, with significant service components subcontracted to local community-based organizations. Other AIDS-prevention programs may be part of a larger organizational effort to address AIDS, and thus may fall under the direct purview of agencies providing medical, psychosocial, and practical support services to persons already infected with HIV. Still other programs may be grafted onto existing organizations that provide health-related, social, or educational services to persons who, on the basis of sociodemographic parameters, are at increased risk of becoming infected with HIV. This wide array of programmatic permutations makes it difficult to standardize the process of evaluating AIDS-prevention programs. And activities that are not easily standardized are not often routinely undertaken.

The variety of programmatic incarnations that the desire to prevent HIV infection can manifest is nearly unlimited. But, even if the programmatic approaches to preventing HIV infection were fewer in number, we would still have to reckon with the reality that program evaluation is not straightforward, for programs are not simple entities. A close examination of the structure of medical/public health programs, reveals that they consist of a number of different but related areas of expertise and foci melded together for the purpose of addressing particular needs through the provision of services. Certain elements of the blend are readily identified because of their visibility, while other components, which are equally important for success, may be less readily identified or quantified.

In a methadone maintenance treatment program, for example, the pharmacological component of the program (the provision of methadone) is the most highly visible, while the supportive components—job counseling, legal aid, or family group therapy—are often less visible. The training process and referral system that buttress the supportive components may be even less visible. However, for the program to function successfully, all of its elements are necessary. Each of the individual elements in our hypothetical methadone maintenance program lends support to the others and contributes to the outcome of the treatment in ways that are not purely additive.

In describing programs as complex integrative systems, which consist of components that influence and support one another toward a common goal, we are reminded of the oft-quoted maxim of Gestalt psychology: "the whole is greater than the sum of its parts." Gestalt psychology interprets phenomena as organized wholes rather than aggregates of distinct parts, and holds that each individual element of a group is altered in its individuality by its membership in that group. Although Gestalt theory applies primarily to the process of perception, an analogous construct could be applied to describe the relationship between the individual components that constitute a service-oriented program.

Choosing to describe service programs as wholes that are greater than the sums of their individual parts is more than an intellectual exercise in analogy. In considering AIDS-prevention program evaluation, this concept acts as a premise which (a) recognizes the complexity of programs; (b) reinforces the importance and interrelatedness of each of the programmatic components; (c) views program outcome as a synergistic effect; and (d) cautions that evaluating a complex, integrative structure, such as an AIDS-prevention program, is more than a reckoning of "inputs" versus "outcomes."

In addition to the variety of AIDS-prevention programs and the complexity of programmatic activity per se, we must also keep in mind that evaluation itself can have a variety of functions. As explained by Rossi and Freeman, evaluation can be undertaken for a number of reasons, including achievement of management and administrative purposes; assessment of the impact of program changes; identification of ways to improve service delivery; satisfaction of accountability requirements of funding sources; planning and policy purposes; testing of new approaches to health/social problems; or testing of a particular social science hypothesis (1985:38). Although some of these functions are likely to be considered important in almost all programmatic settings (for example, management and accountability), others will be considered essential only in specialized environments (for example, testing a social science hypothesis).

Programmatic context is therefore likely to influence the process of evaluation, both in terms of how evaluation is conducted and also in terms of what the results of the evaluation are expected to achieve. Because the ethos of community-based organizations is service provision, administrators are likely to view evaluation primarily as a reckoning of the units of service delivered and the number of individuals who were reached by the program. To a social scientist, evaluation is likely to be seen as a primary means of testing a hypothesis. Because the scientist is intent on being able to accept or reject a series of hypotheses dealing with program design, content, or impact, evaluation becomes much more than a reckoning of service delivered. It is instead a process expressly undertaken to answer predetermined questions of scientific interest.

To illustrate these two perspectives, let us return to the example of the safer sex workshop for gay men, which was described earlier. First and foremost, a social scientist would be intent on finding out how much of the behavioral change observed in participants was due to their attending the workshop. This would require designing the intervention so that the sample of men attending was representative of the entire gay male population. This would include attempts to ensure the participation of racial/ethnic minorities as well as persons of lower educational levels and socioeconomic status. It would also require the inclusion of a control or comparison group, so that the scientist could assess the degree of sexual behavior change in a similar group of gay men who had not attended the workshop. With a large enough sample, the scientist would be able to look for differential program effects on the basis of selected features, such as age, educational level, race, ethnic background, and years of homosexual experience. In order to test hypotheses about the effects of the workshop, the social scientist would design the workshop and its evaluation to incorporate the five essential elements of a true experiment: the sample would be representative of the target population; preintervention measures of the variable of interest would be available; an unexposed group of similar individuals would be used for comparison purposes; individuals would be randomly assigned to either the experimental (intervention) or control group; and one or more postintervention measures of the variable of interest would be available to the scientist (Green and Lewis 1986:198).

If this same workshop were conducted by a community-based organization, the director would probably be primarily concerned about the number of men participating and the quality of the actual workshop sessions as rated by the participants. For the director, the evaluation process would be mainly a means of assuring the quality of the actual intervention, by relaying feedback from the health educators and clients to the administrative component of the program. Issues relating to the scientific implications of the program, such as the representativeness of the sample, the ability to generalize results to different settings, or the generation of new theory, are likely to be considered of secondary importance. If behavioral data were collected before and after the workshop, it is likely that success would be defined simply as a descriptive decrease in unsafe behaviors, without concern about the degree of comparable change among men who had not attended a session.

These generalizations are not meant to denigrate the capabilities of service-oriented community-based AIDS-prevention programs or to suggest that all prevention programs must be designed to test scientific hypotheses about behavioral change. Nor should they be construed to imply that the directors of community-based programs are never concerned about issues of efficacy or theory. They merely address the reality that the evaluation process is likely to be substantially influenced by the programmatic context in which it is embedded.

DETERMINING THE NEED FOR EVALUATION

For readers using this book as a means of learning more about AIDS prevention or improving the quality of their own programmatic endeavors, such philosophizing is unlikely to be of much comfort.

What unifying theme or message is contained within this litany of the limitations of measurement and the difficulties of evaluating AIDS-prevention programs?

To address practical concerns relating to the need for concrete recommendations about the role of evaluation in AIDS-prevention programs, let us begin by reiterating the recommendation of the American Public Health Association (APHA) that "not every health promotion program needs to be evaluated." Instead, the APHA explains, if a health promotion program is designed "so that it can be evaluated" it is "more likely to be an effective program" (American Public Health Association 1987:91). This recommendation is by no means a minimization of the importance of program evaluation. To justify their recommendation, the American Public Health Association explains that "the process of making certain that a program is implemented in a manner conducive to evaluation assures that its structure and operation are more orderly and predictable," and that "when a program is set up in such a way that achievement of its expected and intended effects can be determined, the program is more likely to operate in an efficient manner" (1987:91).

These statements from the APHA recall a theme alluded to throughout this chapter; namely, that program evaluation is synonymous with competent program management. Gathering information about the intended recipients of a service and specifying objectives for the delivery of that service are examples of the kind of rational planning that should guide any form of organized, premeditated activity, whether it is health related, as in the case of AIDS-prevention programs, or commercially motivated—as in the case of marketing management. When we describe the use of client- and staff-generated feedback to provide us with information about the quality of the services we are delivering, we are really describing a form of quality assurance, an activity ubiquitous in any competently managed endeavor, regardless of its focus. Keeping track of the personnel, time, and supplies expended in providing a service is likewise a universally accepted standard of good management practice and is in no way unique to program evaluation. Certainly, the whole idea of conducting an objective assessment of an activity in order to compare its expected performance to its actual performance, to uncover its weaknesses and strengths, and to suggest modifications that capitalize on these findings, is nothing more than a generic description of strategic planning.

The fifth criterion for the development of health promotion and education programs—that programs be organized from the outset so that their operations and effects can be evaluated—recognizes this association between competent program management and program evaluation. Another way to interpret this criterion is to say that programs that are competently administered, in the most comprehensive sense of that phrase, are less likely to be in need of evaluation as a separate and distinct activity because many of the functions of the evaluation process have already been incorporated into the routine workings of the program.

Therefore, this criterion does not suggest the minimization of evaluation (in its recommendation that not all programs need be evaluated) as much as it suggests that competent, ongoing program management can assume many of the functions of program evaluation. This, then, becomes a concrete recommendation: To improve the overall quality of health-promotion programs and to ensure that they are meeting the needs of the persons for whom they are targeted, improve the quality of program management.

Another approach to program evaluation that may be particularly helpful to community-based organizations is, whenever possible, to endow evaluation activities with therapeutic or, in the case of AIDS-prevention efforts, with health-promotional qualities. From the previous discussion of behavioral theories (see Chapter Three), it is apparent that the process of health behavior change is more often gradual than precipitous and that persons attempting such change may require ongoing support. By fusing the procedure of providing ongoing support and the activity of gathering information for the purpose of program evaluation, we not only improve the level of follow-up information available for future decision making, we also extend the level of prevention service delivery beyond a single encounter.

Let us consider the example of an AIDS-prevention program in a family planning setting to illustrate this recommendation. Suppose that such a program targets heterosexually active women who are considered to be at increased risk for HIV infection on the basis of a confidential, self-ranked risk assessment instrument. Women who are so identified are provided with information about HIV transmission, educated about the proper use of condoms as prophylactics, informed about the local availability of HIV counseling and testing services, and encouraged to discuss these subjects with their sexual partners. Information is supplied by the medical staff of the clinic, usually a nurse practitioner, in a-one-on-one encounter. The impact objectives of this intervention include increasing the frequency of condom use for the prevention of HIV infection and promoting the discussion of AIDS prevention among couples.

There are several ways in which an evaluation of the impact objectives of this program could be undertaken. Most simply, the organization might opt to measure the number of condoms dispensed to its clients before and after the period of the program. Alternatively, women could be asked to fill out a questionnaire before and after the intervention in order to document any change in the frequency of condom use. This same questionnaire could also be used to document whether women had discussed AIDS-prevention issues with their sexual partners.

Returning to our recommendation, however, we suggest that the collection of follow-up information on women who attended this program be conducted as a "therapeutic" counseling session with a trained counselor, during which each woman could share her experiences regarding the use of condoms and relate any difficulties she has had in discussing the subject of AIDS prevention with her sexual partner. This format would allow the staff person not only to make an assessment of programmatic impact on the client but also to provide the client with ongoing support, reinforcement, and, when necessary, specific recommendations regarding barriers she might be encountering in the adoption of safer sexual practices.

Follow-up information would be fed into the developmental arm of the program for the purpose of modifying the intervention to meet client needs. For example, after counseling fifty women who attended this program over several months, a health-care worker may become aware that many women require specific training in how to bring up the subject of condoms with a sexual partner. Based on this information, the program manager may decide to incorporate a role-playing session into the intervention. This would afford women the opportunity of rehearsing the discussion of condom use before undertaking such a discussion with a partner who is resistant to the idea.

In summary, evaluation should not be considered an ancillary component of AIDS-prevention programs. When it is integrated into existing programmatic structure, it can fulfill a variety of functions. But, before we conclude our discussion of evaluating AIDS-prevention programs leaving the reader with the impression that evaluation can always be addressed in therapeutic encounters or through consistent management practices, we must emphasize that there are also circumstances requiring that programs be designed and evaluations conducted along recognized scientific lines. The decision to undertake such a task should, as in all instances of evaluation, be based on an awareness of need.

The need to employ scientifically designed evaluations is apparent when dealing with hard-to-reach populations, where specialized sampling procedures may be necessary (Sudman et al. 1988), or when testing the use of controversial prevention modalities (for example sterile needle distribution, erotic safer sex films and videos for gay men, or school-based distribution of condoms). In such cases, only a clearcut demonstration of improved efficacy in outcome can enable policy makers and legislators to support the promotion of such approaches.

Evaluation is not a static technique or quantity. Like good management in general, evaluation should be dynamic and responsive to the circumstances surrounding it. To be most fully effective, evaluation activities should be integrated into the fabric of prevention programs. They should not be superimposed after the last client has participated in an intervention and the last questionnaire has been completed. Like the other components of AIDS-prevention programs reviewed in this book, evaluation is best considered in relationship to all of the variables that surround and influence the programmatic effort.

REFERENCES

Allen, J.R., and Curran, J.W. 1988. "Prevention of AIDS and HIV Infection: Needs and Priorities for Epidemiologic Research." *American Journal of Public Health* 78(4):381–386.

American Public Health Association. 1987. "Criteria for the Development of Health Promotion and Education Programs." *American Journal of Public Health* 77(1):89–92.

Blair, E., Sudman, S., Bradburn, N.M., and Stocking, C. 1977. "How to Ask Questions About Drinking and Sex: Response Effects in Measuring Consumer Behavior." *Journal of Marketing Research* 14:316–321.

Centers for Disease Control. 1987. *Guidelines for AIDS Prevention Program Operations.* Atlanta, Ga.: U.S. Department of Health and Human Services.

Green, L.W., and Lewis, F.M. 1986. *Measurement and Evaluation in Health Education and Health Promotion.* Palo Alto, Calif.: Mayfield.

Kolata, G. 1987. "How to Ask About Sex and Get Honest Answers." *Science* 236:382.

Rossi, P.H., and Freeman, H.E. 1985. *Evaluation: A Systematic Approach.* Beverly Hills, Calif.: Sage.

Sudman, S., Sirken, M.G., and Cowan, C.D. 1988. "Sampling Rare and Elu-
   sive Populations." *Science* 240:991–996.
Wicker, A.W. 1972. "Processes Which Mediate Behavior-Environment Con-
   gruence." *Behavioral Science* 17:265–276.

Chapter 8

Barriers to AIDS-Prevention Programs

Barriers, by definition, impede advancement or prevent access. Circumstances as well as objects can function as barriers, and throughout this book *barriers* has been used to refer to the many obstacles, whether cultural, financial, political, or legal, that are capable of interfering with programmatic attempts to prevent the transmission of HIV infection. Although there are many different kinds of barriers to AIDS-prevention programs, a significant proportion appear to be related to social issues that develop as a consequence of people living together in groups. This final chapter will explore socially related circumstances that can interfere with or prevent the planning, implementation, or operation of AIDS-prevention programs.

Considering social circumstances alone as barriers to AIDS-prevention programs is somewhat restrictive, since there are undeniably nonsocial circumstances that can obstruct programmatic response and effectiveness. Uncertainty about the extent of the epidemic—owing to the difficulty of obtaining reasonably complete information about the number of individuals infected—has hampered planning efforts (Lambert 1988b). Although the paucity of such information is not a social circumstance per se, some of the reasons individuals are not willing to be tested for HIV infection are related to social issues, especially fear of discrimination (Dickens 1988).

As in any programmatic effort, incompetence is a not uncommon cause of inefficient program functioning (Lambert 1988a). Incompetence is not discussed here as a socially related barrier because it tends to be an individual rather than a group problem—and because it is potentially remediable by replacing the inept person or persons. Such is not the case with societal barriers.

The current lack of an effective vaccine with which to immunize against HIV infection is another uncontested barrier to prevention, yet it too is excluded from this discussion. This is not because the process of vaccine development is devoid of societal influence. On the contrary, the vigorous funding of biomedical research aimed at developing a vaccine is proof positive of society's support for such an endeavor. However, the current lack of an effective vaccine is primarily a consequence of the complexity of the virus under study rather than the consequence of a societal circumstance acting as a barrier.

Many of the societal barriers to AIDS-prevention programs can be grouped together in a category that includes those obstacles resulting from deficits or inadequacies in societal structures. The term *structures* as used here refers to a society's physical and organizational products. The lack or underdevelopment of structures through which AIDS-prevention services could be delivered is a major societal barrier to preventing HIV infection. In the United States, the most frequently cited structural barrier to AIDS-prevention activities is the lack of an adequate system to treat intravenous drug users (Boffey 1988b; Hubbard et al. 1988). In the absence of such a system, it is extremely difficult and costly to reach active users with information about AIDS prevention. And without adequate treatment opportunities for intravenous drug users, there is little hope of extinguishing needle-using behaviors and no guarantee that even those drug users who have been educated about AIDS prevention will not resort to needle sharing because of the demands of their addiction.

However, it is not just in the direct provision of AIDS-related services that structures can exert an influence on AIDS-prevention activities. Even structures whose primary function does not include the provision of AIDS-related services can influence AIDS-prevention programs. For example, a major goal of the World Health Organization's plan of action for AIDS control in Africa is to strengthen the health infrastructure of African nations in order to support AIDS-related activities, including prevention efforts (World Health Organization 1986).

Acknowledgment of the influence that a society's structures can exert on AIDS-prevention programs is actually recognition of the interrelatedness of every component of a social system. The structural elements of a society, like the systems of the human organism, influence one another, sometimes in a positive manner and sometimes in a negative manner. This interactiveness is not unique to AIDS-prevention programs, and its consequences have been observed in other health- and service-oriented programs. For example, a nationwide immunization campaign in Nigeria conducted in the mid-1970s failed because of the lack of motor vehicles with which to distribute vaccines and the lack of electricity in remote villages with which to keep the vaccine refrigerated (Brooke 1988). Biomedical solutions were not lacking in this situation, but the structures necessary to deliver the vaccine and maintain its integrity prior to immunization were not in place.

ATTITUDES, VALUES, AND RESOURCE ALLOCATION

Another major category of societal barriers to AIDS-prevention programs are those barriers that develop as a result of value conflicts. Even in a homogeneous society, it is unlikely that values are shared universally, and in a pluralistic society, people can attach very different values to the same issue. If a significant proportion of society shares a common value relating to a problem, their state of consensus facilitates decision making about the problem and allocation of societal resources to solve it. However, when a society is divided in its values about a particular problem, the expenditure of resources may be delayed while factions debate approaches to solving the problem.

The development of consensus on any issue is influenced by such variables as the type of society in which the process is occurring, the legal ramifications of the issue under consideration, the number of persons having direct personal experience with the issue, and other cultural circumstances that might influence people's perceptions of the issue. For example, Americans hold differing views on the subject of homosexuality. Some people accept it as a valid form of sexual expression, while others view it as a perversion. An individual's attitudes about homosexuality are influenced by the person's ethnic, social, and religious background and whether he or she personally knows someone who is homosexual. Laws about homosexuality, especially those that consider it a crime, both reflect and influence individual values. This continuum of reactions, from acceptance of homosexuality to its unequivocal rejection, indicates that different people attach opposing values to the same activity — there is a lack of consensus as to the "worth" of homosexuality. This lack of consensus can act as a barrier to programmatic efforts targeted to gay men if prevention activities are perceived as endorsements of homosexuality by those holding negative values about the behavior (Booth 1987).

These two categories of societal barriers are not mutually exclusive. The values of a society influence its structural achievements, usually through the process of resource allocation. If there is a consensus that removing a structural barrier to a health problem will help to solve that problem, resources are likely to be so applied. The recommendation of the President's Commission on the Human Immunodeficiency Virus Epidemic to expand the nation's drug treatment programs, along with support from both the medical community and government health officials, strongly suggest that future budget appropriations will reflect this consensus (Boffey 1988b; "Increased Treatment . . ." 1988; Watkins et al. 1988).

However, not all structural barriers can be remedied by the application of additional resources, especially if value conflict barriers are responsible for underdevelopment of the structure. Creating a system of school-based health clinics in every junior and senior high school in this country would greatly facilitate attempts to control the spread of HIV among sexually active adolescents by providing them with AIDS-prevention information along with counseling and reproductive health services (Hirsch et al. 1987). However, attempts to develop such a structure are likely to encounter organized opposition because of our society's lack of consensus relating to teenage sexuality and contraception (Brozan 1986). Some parents, administrators, students, and teachers are bound to oppose such a system because of their convictions that providing services of this nature would induce students who were not sexually active to become so (Harris et al. 1983) and that promoting condom use as a means of preventing HIV transmission would "undermine moral resistance to premarital sex and contraception" (Barron 1987:18).

The recognition of barriers to the work of AIDS prevention is not new. The fact that the epidemic was first recognized in gay men virtually guaranteed that the issues surrounding prevention activities would become entangled in the subject of homosexuality, often with negative consequences (Shilts 1987). AIDS-prevention programs for intravenous drug users have also been affected by the larger debate on drug use prevention and treatment. Although sociologists and policy analysts may be fascinated with such phenomena, program staff may come to view the societal variables influencing AIDS-prevention programs as secondary to their major role of "providing a service." Nothing could be further from the truth. Programs, in addition to their functional capacity to provide services, are also products of the society that creates them. Because they are microcosms of the universe in which they exist, they are prey to the same controversies, barriers, and restraints that occur in the larger world around them. Wearying though it may be to hear about the conflicts that often accompany AIDS-prevention activities, it is important to remain receptive to the lessons they can teach.

The term *barrier* itself is not value neutral. Given our pluralistic society and the laws of probability, it is unlikely that readers of this book will view the circumstances described here as barriers in a consistent way. This is not unexpected, since part of what contributes to these circumstances acting as barriers to AIDS-prevention programs is the lack of an unequivocal consensus as to their worth. Regardless of where the reader's values may fall on the continuum of responses to such issues as homosexuality, teenage sexuality, or drug use, it is still possible to recognize that the lack of value consensus on these issues has had an impact on programmatic efforts to prevent HIV infection, and will probably do so for some time in the future.

BARRIERS TO AIDS PREVENTION IN DEVELOPING COUNTRIES

Structural barriers to AIDS-prevention programs do not occur only in societies of the industrialized world. Countries whose economic, political, and social development is still evolving are especially vulnerable to epidemic HIV infection, precisely because the societal structures that are called upon to lend support in combatting the epidemic are not as highly developed in these countries as they are in industrialized nations. While it may be a challenge for industrialized nations to integrate AIDS-prevention activities into existing societal structures for health care, education, and social service, it is an even greater challenge for developing nations to elaborate these structures in order to provide adequate support for AIDS-prevention programs. The kinds of structural barriers to AIDS-prevention programs that can be found in the societies of the developing world are exemplified in Africa.

Much has been written about AIDS in the African nations, sometimes to the consternation of Africans who believe that reports in the world press suggesting their continent as the "birthplace" of the human immunodeficiency virus have fueled prejudices and perpetuated stereotypes about Africans (Sabatier 1987). Such sensitivities are not uncommon nor are they ungrounded. In fact, enumerating the limitations of organizational structures in African societies that interfere with efforts to prevent HIV infection might also be misconstrued to imply negligence or blame. Such is not the intent of this discussion. Nor is it the intent to imply that these societies are somehow less credible or valuable than those of the Western world because their social and economic resources are less fully developed. Yet, they are different, and this discussion will focus on how some differences are manifested in the epidemiology of HIV infection and in the resources available to combat the epidemic in Africa.

As discussed earlier, the vast majority of Africans who have developed AIDS have become infected as a result of heterosexual intercourse (Piot et al. 1988). Prostitutes play an important role in spreading the infection (Carael et al. 1988; Kreiss et al. 1986; Vittecoq et al. 1987). In addition to heterosexual intercourse and the attendant probability of vertical transmission from mother to child, HIV infection through untested blood or blood products remains a significant mode of transmission in Africa (Piot et al. 1988). The use of nonsterile needles and syringes for medical purposes undoubtedly accounts for some cases of infection, but the exact proportion is undetermined at present (Von Reyn and Mann 1987). Male homosexuality is reportedly quite rare in Africa, and most studies echo the belief that this behavior is an unlikely mode of HIV transmission in Africa (Hrdy 1987; Piot et al. 1988).

This epidemiologic description gives an adequate account of how the virus is transmitted in Africa, but does not begin to suggest the difficulties inherent in mounting national campaigns to prevent its spread. In describing the structural barriers faced by many of the African nations, experts point to the "recent rapid increase in urbanization" in many parts of Africa, which has had both economic and sociological consequences for individuals' health status and has "severely affected the health infrastructure" (Quinn et al. 1986:982). In short, many countries in which malaria, diarrheal diseases, and malnutrition may be "more important" than AIDS "in terms of morbidity and mortality" are now not only forced to confront HIV-infected individuals who are symptomatic but must also take on the added responsibility of preventing new infections (Piot et al. 1988:577). These burdens are extreme, given that existing systems of care delivery are frequently poorly or inconsistently developed.

Expanding services to diagnose, treat, and prevent sexually transmitted diseases would be a logical step to take in combatting the spread of HIV infection in Africa. We know that the human immunodeficiency virus itself is sexually transmissible, and convincing evidence suggests that concurrent venereal disease plays a role in HIV infection—especially genital ulcer disease (Cameron et al. 1988a; Greenblatt et al. 1988), which is common in the tropics (Fast et al. 1984). The rate of genital ulcer disease for African prostitutes whose clients use condoms is much lower than for women whose clients seldom or never use condoms (Cameron et al. 1988b). Cameron and his colleagues concluded that condom use is "not only important to prevent transmission of HIV, but may be synergistic in reducing the heterosexual transmission of HIV by reducing the prevalence of genital ulcer disease in prostitutes" (1988b:276).

That the "annual health budget of many African governments is less than $5 per capita" and a year's supply of condoms "costs $5 wholesale" presents the dilemma in terms that anyone can understand (Tinker 1988:44). Furthermore, condom education and distribution programs are just one component of AIDS-prevention activities. Although such activities are critical to the successful interruption of HIV transmission, they do not address the underlying problem of prostitution, which contributes significantly to the sexual transmission of HIV infection in Africa.

The circumstances surrounding prostitution in Africa underscore the close association between socioeconomic factors and health status. The relationship between prostitution and the spread of sexually transmitted diseases in Africa has long been recognized (D'Costa 1985; Meheus et al. 1974). In an analysis of sexually transmitted diseases in Ethiopia in 1981, Plorde identified a number of socioeconomic circumstances responsible for an increase in prostitution, including migration and urbanization, leading to weakening of family and community organizations; nationalization of all farm lands, which forced many farmers to abandon their farms and families; and issues relating to the status of women, including the paucity of ways for a woman to support herself in traditional Ethiopian society (p. 361). Plorde viewed the increase in prostitution as a primary manifestation of women's needs to support themselves and urged the development of programs to educate women and to provide them with alternative job opportunities in order to break the cycle of prostitution and the transmission of sexually transmitted diseases. Hrdy reiterated these circumstances in his analysis of cultural practices contributing to the transmission of HIV in Africa when he identified the "destitution of poor migrant women" and the "rootlessness of young male migrants and soldiers" as primary contributors to the apparent increase in promiscuity "as people leave rural villages and migrate to urban areas" (1987:1112).

Therefore, a major structural barrier to preventing the sexual transmission of HIV among African prostitutes is the paucity of viable economic options for women to support themselves, especially after they leave a rural village and settle in an urban area. While it is important to educate prostitutes about the dangers of HIV infection, and to encourage the use of condoms, these findings suggest that a more permanent solution to AIDS prevention in this group would result from programs that provide these women with alternative ways to support themselves.

Breast-feeding provides another example of how difficult it is to extricate AIDS-prevention activities from other socially relevant health issues in the developing world. The ability of a woman to transmit HIV infection postnatally to her child through breast milk has been demonstrated (Bucens et al. 1988). Although breast-feeding is considered a potential mode of HIV transmission (Colebunders et al. 1988), studies in Haiti suggest that the risk of HIV transmission through breast-feeding is low (Stanback et al. 1988). It may be that the greatest risk of HIV infection for the breast-fed infant occurs if the mother or wet nurse experiences a primary HIV infection in the postnatal period (Ziegler et al. 1988). The World Health Organization suggests that if a mother is "considered to be HIV infected," the "known and potential benefits of breast-feeding should be compared to the theoretical, but apparently small, incremental risk to the infant of becoming infected through breast-feeding" (1987). Because of the "anti-infective" properties of breast milk and its ability to indirectly shield the infant from exposure to "contaminated food and water sources," breast-feeding "offers strong protection against death from diarrhea and respiratory infections" in the developing world (Victoria et al. 1987:320–321).

Studies of the risk of HIV infection through breast-feeding are ongoing, but it is apparent that the elimination of this small, but potential, risk of infection would depend on making clean water supplies and breast milk substitutes available. Both are likely to be in short supply in areas of extreme poverty. These structural deficits (lack of adequate water supply and resources to provide breast milk substitutes) are significant barriers that impinge upon efforts to prevent the transmission of HIV through breast-feeding in the developing world.

It is clear that the overall objective of preventing the transmission of HIV can be severely hampered by societal circumstances. Population movements of migrant workers, armies, and refugees weaken family ties, undercut many of the normal sanctions on sexual activity, negate access to consistent health care services, disrupt local economies, and contribute to the number of women who become prostitutes for "purely monetary reasons" (Hrdy 1987:1112). Furthermore, HIV infection is only one of many potential untoward health consequences of these societal circumstances. Tinker explains how these factors have contributed to the creation of a "global underclass" living in "urban shantytowns," with "little or no access to health clinics," and unreached "by family planning advice" (1988:46). The nations of the developing world exemplify, incontrovertibly, that attempts to limit the spread of HIV infection are often indistinguishable from efforts to improve the overall health status of a society. In the broadest sense, the difficulties in doing so can be considered as structural barriers to AIDS-prevention activities.

Many of the specific program needs in terms of AIDS-prevention activities in Africa can be traced to a lack of resources. Adequate resources, appropriately managed, could result in an expansion of treatment facilities for sexually transmitted diseases, widespread condom distribution programs, increased laboratory services for screening blood and blood products and testing individuals for the presence of HIV, contraceptive services for HIV-infected women of child-bearing age, the implementation of ongoing surveillance activities to gauge the spread of the epidemic and the effect of AIDS-prevention campaigns, training opportunities for medical and nursing personnel, and facilities to sterilize medical equipment. But, in addition to providing the specific programmatic services described here, resources must also be applied to correct the underlying socioeconomic circumstances that contribute to the spread of the virus, especially in terms of rectifying the structural barriers which reflect these circumstances.

The technical and financial support of the World Health Organization's Special Programme on AIDS has assisted many of the world's nations in developing national AIDS programs (Mann 1987). In fact, the World Health Organization has entered into an alliance with the United Nations Development Program in an effort to "persuade third world countries to build AIDS-prevention measures into their development strategies" (Lewis 1988:A-12). This alliance addresses the importance of cultivating societal structures to provide tangible support to AIDS-prevention program activities. By mobilizing the "resources of education ministries, planning ministries and health ministries as well as the authorities in charge of family planning, child care and urban development" it is hoped that the spread of AIDS in developing countries will be substantially retarded (Lewis 1988:A-12).

Although structural barriers to AIDS-prevention activities in the developing world are significant, it would be a mistake to infer that they have precluded prevention initiatives. Many countries in Africa are active in addressing the problem of AIDS prevention (Okware 1987), and according to some analysts, "did so before some Western states" (Nunn 1987:54). Africans have conducted much of the pioneering work on risk-reduction education among prostitutes and have made substantial scientific contributions to our understanding of the heterosexual and perinatal transmission of HIV (Piot et al. 1988:578).

VALUE CONFLICTS AND
PROGRAM DEVELOPMENT

Societies can be categorized not only by their level of organizational development but also by the values they endorse. Values that are not held in consensus and that invoke completely opposite viewpoints can act as barriers to AIDS-prevention programs. Such barriers can be just as durable as those resulting from inadequate societal structures.

In considering how conflicting values affect AIDS-prevention activities, there are many fertile fields for analysis. To understand effects at a programmatic level, consider the value conflicts that can accompany efforts to prevent HIV infection in adolescents.

No one disputes that adolescents are a crucial target for AIDS-prevention activities. Although the number of American teenagers who have been diagnosed with AIDS is currently minimal (Centers for Disease Control 1988:12), there is no doubt that a significant proportion of adolescents engage in activities that place them at risk for HIV infection. Studies show that about "28 percent of persons aged 12 to 17 are currently sexually active," and that "about 70 percent and 80 percent of teenage girls and boys, respectively, have had at least one coital experience" (Yarber 1987:1). Nearly 2.5 million American teenagers "are affected with a sexually transmitted disease each year," and 17 percent of boys aged 16 to 19 report at least one homosexual experience (Centers for Disease Control 1988:11). An estimated 5 million teenagers have "used a stimulant intravenously" (Yarber 1987:1). Furthermore, surveys among adolescents

have documented an incomplete understanding of both HIV transmission and the precautions necessary to prevent infection (DiClemente et al. 1986; DiClemente et al. 1988; Helgerson et al. 1988;
Strunin and Hingson 1987). It is even more ominous that because
adolescents and young adults may not perceive themselves to be
at risk for HIV infection they may continue to engage in high-risk
behaviors without adopting appropriate behavioral modifications
(Landefeld et al. 1988: Strunin and Hingson 1987).

Obtaining access to the "captive" population of American adolescent school students to educate them about AIDS prevention makes
good sense; it is an obvious example of how preexisting societal
structures can be integrated into the effort to promote AIDS-prevention activities. Because "more than 47 million students attend
90,000 elementary and secondary schools" in America on a daily basis (Yarber 1987:1), this system has tremendous potential for reaching a large number of young people prior to the onset of behaviors
that could place them at risk for HIV infection. In fact, a majority of
American adults are in favor of students learning about AIDS in
school, and a number of states have already passed legislation man-
dating school-based AIDS education (Centers for Disease Control
1988:12).

From the foregoing, it would seem that there is little, if any,
disagreement about developing AIDS-prevention programs in the
schools. This is true enough, of itself, for the conflict is not so much
whether or not AIDS education should take place in a school setting
as it is about what that education should entail. When conflicts
arise in the development and implementation of AIDS-related curricula, they usually center around the specific approaches advocated
for the prevention of HIV infection (Perlez 1988). Few people disagree
that students should learn that AIDS is the result of a virus that is
transmitted sexually and through needle sharing. But beyond that
fundamental information, opposing values about adolescent sexuality come into conflict. Those who believe that any sexual experimentation in adolescence should be discouraged and repressed are
directly opposed to others who take sexual experimentation as a
given and opt for educating adolescents about responsible decision
making regarding sex.

Exploring the ramifications of value conflicts surrounding AIDS-
prevention programs targeted to adolescents is difficult because it is
a complex topic fraught with ambiguities. The value-laden subjects
of human sexuality, reproduction, contraception, and drug use are

difficult enough for adults to discuss, without the added sensitivities that derive from including adolescents in the process. Based on their individual value systems, parents are likely to have strong feelings about how AIDS education should be undertaken, and some may be uncomfortable in delegating to a teacher what they perceive to be their sole responsibility—teaching their children about such personal topics as sex, drug use, contraception, and venereal disease prophylaxis.

The value conflict between those who believe that sexual expression should be limited to the confines of marriage and those who endorse the position of responsible premarital sexual behavior can be found at every level of decision making: the home; the school board; and local, state, and federal government. Initially, the federal government's response to AIDS education in the schools emphasized the importance of "teaching restraint as a virtue" and presenting sex education "within a moral context" (U.S. Department of Education 1987:9). More recent recommendations from the Centers for Disease Control, while still emphasizing the values of abstinence and a "mutually monogamous relationship within the context of marriage," recognize that "despite all efforts, some young people may remain unwilling to adopt behavior that would eliminate their risk of becoming infected" and suggest that programs include specific prevention information for students who are sexually active or who use illicit drugs (1988:4).

Because HIV infection is sexually transmissible, it is not surprising that the value conflicts that can arise during attempts to develop curricula for its prevention are similar to those that have accompanied the more general topic of sex education in the schools. Although a majority of American adults favors sex education in the schools, conflicts may still arise "over the inclusion of specific controversial topics such as contraception, abortion, or homosexuality" (Hayes 1987:143–144).

In America, it is currently estimated that fewer than "10 percent of all students take comprehensive sex education courses." The majority of school-based sex education programs are "10 hours or less" and "tend to focus on the basics of anatomy, human reproduction, and physical and psychological changes during puberty" (Hayes 1987:144). While sex education courses that are "mechanical" in orientation are better than none at all, they may not meet the practical needs of students. In a retrospective survey of students and alumni from two schools with sex education programs identified as "exemplary" by the Centers for Disease Control, half of the program alumni "believed they did not obtain a greater ability to make decisions or communicate their feelings verbally as a result of their school's sex education program." Both of these skills have been identified as important in coping with peer pressure to become sexually active (Klein et al. 1984:813).

Because adolescents need more than information about how sexual intercourse is accomplished and what the negative consequences of sexual activity are, increased attention is being focused on a cognitive-behavioral approach, which recognizes that adolescents need "cognitive skills to understand the consequences of their actions" and behavioral skills for communicating with other adolescents about issues pertaining to sexuality (Mitchell and Brindis 1987:423).

In the cognitive-behavioral model there are four essential steps: the need for accurate information on which to base decisions and behavior; the ability to "perceive, comprehend, and store information accurately"; the need to "personalize" information; and behavioral skills "to implement these decisions in social situations" (Mitchell and Brindis 1987:423). It is not difficult to understand how parents, teachers, and administrators who associate adolescent sexuality with negative values might perceive this model as one that teaches teenagers how to have sex.

Developing school-based AIDS-prevention programs in light of value conflicts about adolescent sexuality is not a simple matter of determining who is "right" and who is "wrong." Instead, it is a group process in which individuals with opposing views must work through their differences in perspective and settle upon a reasonable plan that is acceptable to the majority and that incorporates accepted standards of public health and education.

The Centers for Disease Control (CDC) recommend that this process begin by convening a broad-based group representing the salient factions of the community in which the program is to be implemented. This group should include "representatives of the school board, parents, school administrators and faculty, school health services, local medical societies, the local health department, students, minority groups, religious organizations, and other relevant organizations." The CDC further recommends that this group be given the responsibility for developing "school district policies on AIDS education" that are "consistent with parental and community values" (1988:2).

Group process is rarely an easy process. Commenting on developing curricula for teaching about AIDS, one analyst observed, "if community members are involved, the educator must be prepared to deal with difficulties in reaching consensus on curriculum content and methodology." Creating community committees to develop AIDS-related curricula can also give the impression that there are controversies and problems to resolve at the outset, even if this is not the case. No less thorny are questions about the responsibility of the school to provide AIDS education to students even if their parents have refused to give the teacher permission to talk about sensitive topics, such as condom use and needle sharing (Yarber 1987:3).

There are no easy solutions to any of these problems, and each circumstance must be judged and acted upon individually. As a general guideline, however, it is most prudent to incorporate some mechanism by which the community can help in shaping the policies and curricula for AIDS-prevention activities. However, because of our lack of societal consensus on the issue of adolescent sexuality, the process of curriculum development and program implementation may be interrupted by the need to resolve ongoing value conflicts. Values not held in consensus can slow the entire process of school-based AIDS-prevention programs, from goal setting and planning to implementation. Exceptions to this scenario may be found in communities where the school has previous experience working with community groups, especially in the development of sex education programs, or in communities having a large number of AIDS cases, where the level of concern and the perception of risk is great.

Another major source of ambiguity that can overlay the issue of school-based AIDS-prevention programs relates to the complexity of human behavioral change—especially change in sexual behavior. Experience in the area of teenage pregnancy prevention programs suggests that "diversified strategies" for pregnancy prevention are necessary to address the "tremendous diversity among adolescents" (Mitchell and Brindis 1987:424). Past pregnancy prevention strategies, which reasoned that given "enough information and services, adolescents would be sufficiently motivated to take positive action," have shown that "only a small portion of the teen population responded to this approach" (Mitchell and Brindis 1987:401).

A study of repeat pregnancy in 675 economically disadvantaged teenage mothers revealed that "half of the teenagers went on to become pregnant again" in the two-year study period, despite adequate information and access to contraceptives (Polit and Kahn 1986:170).

This does not mean that improved education and access to contraceptive counseling and services are inappropriate responses to teenage pregnancy prevention, only that they may not address the other issues involved in bearing a child. In explaining their findings, the authors suggested that the "opportunity costs" of bearing a second child out-of-wedlock "may be negligible," and that "having a baby is likely to confer upon the teenager a number of social and personal rewards" (Polit and Kahn 1986:171).

Policy analysts on the subject of teenage pregnancy prevention suggest that "multipronged" and "comprehensive" approaches must be instituted to prevent teenage pregnancy (Mitchell and Brindis 1987:433). These should be directed to teenage girls, teenage boys, and their families, and should be integrated with "all of the various aspects of an adolescent's life" (Mitchell and Brindis 1987: 434). These approaches might include programs that "assist adolescents in delaying the initiation of sexual activity"; programs that "facilitate the sexually active adolescent's access to contraceptive services"; and "programs that maximize adolescents' ability to be responsible decision makers about sexual activity in the context of their lives" (Mitchell and Brindis 1987:416).

Offering a variety of options in recognition of the different needs of adolescents is consistent with the acknowledgment of peoples' different motives for behavioral change and different needs in terms of initiating and maintaining that change (see Chapter Three). In concrete terms, it means that in the same classroom there may be sexually active students who require access to contraceptives and support in the consistent use of them, and sexually inactive students who need to develop skills that can help them resist pressure from peers and significant others to initiate sexual activity until they can engage in it responsibly. The same generalities can be made about AIDS-prevention programs. While every student needs to know about the manner in which HIV is transmitted, sexually active students may need more specific information about condom use and skills training in discussing the subject of condoms with sexual partners. Students who deny the risk of AIDS may need special assistance in understanding and personalizing their risk of HIV infection. Gay adolescents who "hide, deny, or dismiss their homosexual feelings" may also "avoid confronting the reality and risks of their sexual experimentation" (Remafedi 1988:140).

School-based health promotion programs, including those that attempt to prevent the transmission of HIV, are not without their limitations. Bartlett (1981) identified a number of constraints to school health education programs, including an emphasis on cognitive and educational psychology, with inadequate attention paid to social and behavioral psychology; undue emphasis on lecture-oriented learning, which deemphasizes skills training; lack of administrative support; inadequate coordination with community programs that address the same health concerns; lack of consensus as to the goals of the program; and competing influences on the students' behavior. And, of course, school-based health promotion programs do not address the needs of adolescents who are not part of that system. In some communities, adolescents who are at greatest risk of HIV infection may no longer attend school (Remafedi 1988:141).

Distinguishing industrialized from developing nations on the basis of societal barriers is an arbitrary exercise. Barriers relating to value conflict can be just as significant in the developing world as they are elsewhere. Traditional African values, which emphasize procreation (Okware 1987:727), sexual mores "rooted in tribal traditions" (Sabatier 1987:714), and the traditional view that a woman's worth may be "judged by the number of children she can bear" (Rule 1987:15), can impede AIDS-prevention efforts in Africa the same way that conflicting values about teenage sexuality can interfere with American prevention programs.

In the same vein, the United States is not without its own significant structural barriers, despite the collective mass of our resources. For example, the World Health Organization has recommended that HIV prevention and control programs "be integrated with primary health care" (Mann 1987:733). As a general goal in health care, integrating services is laudable, and it is important that all primary health care providers receive education about AIDS and the special social and behavioral circumstances of those who are at increased risk of infection. However, relying on the structure of primary health care delivery systems to prevent HIV infection may not be effective in inner-city neighborhoods where primary health care services are underdeveloped. Individuals who engage in high-risk behaviors may be inaccessible to the primary health care system or may present to that system only after symptomatic infection has become manifest.

Poverty has long been associated with illness, and evidence continues to accumulate reinforcing the link between economic disadvantage and poor health status. The American drug problem, in particular, seems to be taking a divergent path on the basis of socioeconomic status, with the educated and affluent tending to decrease their use of drugs, while the poor, especially those in the inner city, are increasing their use of drugs, especially "crack," the smokable form of cocaine (Kerr 1988a). The accelerating problem of drug use in poor inner-city American communities is made all the more difficult because of the lack of community-specific resources to confront it. Crack use and its subsequent "periods of heightened sexual activity with many partners" is believed to have been a significant contributor to the national increase in syphilis cases observed between 1985 and 1987; it has also been identified as a potential accelerator of the spread of HIV infection in these same communities (Kerr 1988b:B-1).

Looking at the societally mediated barriers to AIDS prevention, whether they are related to structural inadequacies or value conflicts, whether they are present in a developing nation or an industrialized one, is really just another way of emphasizing the close relationship between disease and society, a perspective that is often attenuated by a biomedical approach to illness.

Emphasizing the significance of societal barriers to AIDS-prevention programs is not an attempt to deride particular values, to lay blame, or to embrace pessimism. It is an attempt to reiterate that disease is more than the infection of an organism by a microbe or the biochemical effects of substance X on cell structure. Disease is also a reflection of how we live as a society, what values are important to us, how well we plan and allocate resources, and how sophisticated we are in our understanding of the interrelatedness of all of society's elements.

The awareness gained in the process of understanding the relationship between illness and society is not limited to prevention programs. Many of the issues of consequence for AIDS-prevention programs are no less important for programmatic initiatives aimed at individuals who are already infected with HIV. Understanding how people communicate with one another, how new information spreads within a particular group of people, the multiplicity of supports that people may need throughout the process of health behavioral change, the organizational structures available in a community to support service delivery, and the special concerns of minority group members, whether racial, ethnic, or sexual, are exceedingly important whether we are planning programs to prevent HIV infection, to administer an AIDS vaccine, or to treat asymptomatic HIV infection.

More than anything else, AIDS prevention requires an understanding of the consequences of people living together in groups. This book has attempted to develop the commonality of the issues involved in AIDS-prevention activities rather than focus exclusively on the needs of a particular group of individuals. When we understand that preventing HIV infection is synonymous with improving the health and quality of life of all of our citizens, then we will truly understand AIDS prevention.

REFERENCES

Barron, J. 1987. "Learning the Facts of Life." *New York Times* November 8, L16–19.

Bartlett, E.E. 1981. "The Contribution of School Health Education to Community Health Promotion: What Can We Reasonably Expect?" *American Journal of Public Health* 71:1384–1391.

Boffey, P.M. 1988a. "AIDS Panel Backs Wide Drive in U.S." *New York Times* March 3, B5.

Boffey, P.M. 1988b. "More Drug Treatment Centers Are Urged." *New York Times* June 5, Y15.

Booth, W. 1987. "Another Muzzle for AIDS Education?" *Science* 238:1036.

Brozan, N. 1986. "School Project Cuts Pregnancy Rates." *New York Times* July 10, C3.

Brooke, J. 1988. "Technology Aids Vaccination Effort." *New York Times* April 26, C3.

Bucens, M., Armstrong, J., and Stuckey, M. 1988. "Virological and Electron Microscopic Evidence for Postnatal HIV Transmission Via Breast Milk." Abstract 5099, proceedings from the *IV International Conference on AIDS*, Book 1, page 339.

Cameron, D.W., D'Costa, L.J., Ndinya-Achola, J., Piot, P., and Plummer, F.A. 1988a. "Incidence and Risk Factors for Female-to-Male Transmission of HIV." Abstract 4061, proceedings from the *IV International Conference on AIDS*, Book 1, page 275.

Cameron, D.W., Plummer, F.A., Ndinya-Achola, J., Ngugi, E., and Ronald, A.R. 1988b. "The Use of Condoms by the Clients of Prostitutes Reduces the Prevalence of Genital Ulcer Disease." Abstract 6517, proceedings from the *IV International Conference on AIDS*, Book 1, page 276.

Carael, M., Van De Perre, P.H., Lepage, P.H., Allen, S., Nsengumuremyi, F., Van Goethem, C., Ntahorutaba, M., Nzaramba, D., and Clumeck, N. 1988. "Human Immunodeficiency Virus Transmission Among Heterosexual Couples in Central Africa." *AIDS* 2:201–205.

Centers for Disease Control. 1988. "Guidelines for Effective School Health Education to Prevent the Spread of AIDS." *Morbidity and Mortality Weekly Report* 37(S-2):1–14.

Colebunders, R.L., Kapita, B., Nekwei, W., Bahwe, Y., Baende, F., and Ryder, R. 1988. "Breast Feeding and Transmission of HIV." Abstract 503, proceedings from the *IV International Conference on AIDS*, Book 1, page 340.

D'Costa, L.J., Plummer, F.A., Bowmer, I., Fransen, L., Piot, P., Ronald, A.R., and Nsanze, H. 1985. "Prostitutes Are a Major Reservoir of Sexually Transmitted Diseases in Nairobi, Kenya." *Sexually Transmitted Diseases* 12(2):64–67.

Dickens, B.M. 1988. "Legal Rights and Duties in the AIDS Epidemic." *Science* 239:580–586.

DiClemente, F.J., Zorn, J., and Temoshok, L. 1986. "Adolescents and AIDS: A Survey of Knowledge, Attitudes, and Beliefs About AIDS in San Francisco." *American Journal of Public Health* 76:1443–1445.

DiClemente, F.J., Boyer, C.B., and Morales, E.S. 1988. "Minorities and AIDS: Knowledge, Attitudes, and Misconceptions Among Black and Latino Adolescents." *American Journal of Public Health* 78:55–57.

Fast, M.V., D'Costa, L.J., Nsanze, H., Piot, P., Curran, J., Karasira, P., Mirza, N., Maclean, I.W., and Ronald, A.R. 1984. "The Clinical Diagnosis of Genital Ulcer Disease in Men in the Tropics." *Sexually Transmitted Diseases* 11(2):72–76.

Greenblatt, R.M., Lukehart, S.A., Plummer, F.A., Quinn, T.C., Critchlow, C.W., Ashley, R.L., D'Costa, L.J., Ndinya-Achola, J.O., Corey, L., Ronald, A.R., and Holmes, K.K. 1988. "Genital Ulceration as a Risk Factor for Human Immunodeficiency Virus Infection." *AIDS* 2(1):47–50.

Harris, D., Baird, G., Clyburn, S.A., and Mara, J.R. 1983. "Developing a Teenage Pregnancy Program the Community Will Accept." *Health Education* 14(3):17–20.

Hayes, C.D. 1987. *Risking the Future.* Washington, D.C.: National Academy Press.

Helgerson, S.D., Petersen, L.R., and the AIDS Education Study Group. 1988. "Acquired Immunodeficiency Syndrome and Secondary School Students: Their Knowledge Is Limited and They Want to Learn More." *Pediatrics* 81(3):350–355.

Herron, K. 1987. "The Teen Years: Time of Mixed Messages." *New York Times* November 8, L20–22.

Hirsch, M.B., Zabin, L.S., Street, R.F., and Hardy, J.B. 1987. "Users of Reproductive Health Clinic Services in a School Pregnancy Prevention Program." *Public Health Reports* 102(3):307–316.

Hrdy, D.B. 1987. "Cultural Practices Contributing to the Transmission of Human Immunodeficiency Virus in Africa." *Reviews of Infectious Diseases* 9(6):1109–1119.

Hubbard, R.L., Marsden, M.E., Cavanaugh, E., Rachal, J.V., and Ginzburg, H.M. 1988. "Role of Drug-Abuse Treatment in Limiting the Spread of AIDS." *Reviews of Infectious Diseases* 10(2):377–384.

"Increased Treatment for Addicts Is Urged." *New York Times* June 28, C11.

Kerr, P. 1988a. "The American Drug Problem Takes On Two Faces." *New York Times* July 10, E5.

Kerr, P. 1988b. "Syphilis Surge and Crack Use Raising Fears on Spread of AIDS." *New York Times* June 29, B1 and B5.

Klein, D., Belcastro, P., and Gold, R. 1984. "Achieving Sex Education Program Outcomes: Points of View from Students and Alumni." *Adolescence* 19(76):805–815.

Kreiss, J.K., Koech, D., Plummer, F.A., Holmes, K.K., Lightfoote, M., Piot, P., Ronald, A.R., Ndinya-Achola, M.B., D'Costa, L.J., Roberts, P., Ngugi, E., and Quinn, T.C. 1986. "AIDS Virus Infection in Nairobi

Lambert, B. 1988a. "New York Faulted on Tuberculosis." *New York Times* January 24, 1 and 20.

Lambert, B. 1988b. "Puzzling Questions Are Raised on Statistics on AIDS Epidemic." *New York Times* July 22, B4.

Landefeld, C.S., Chren, M.M., Shega, J., Speroff, T., and McGuire, E. 1988. "Students' Sexual Behavior, Knowledge, and Attitudes Relating to the Acquired Immunodeficiency Syndrome." *Journal of General Internal Medicine* 3 (March/April):161–165.

Lewis, P. 1988. "WHO Joins Campaign for Coordinated AIDS Programs in Third World." *New York Times* March 27, A12.

Mann, J.M. 1987. "The World Health Organization's Global Strategy for the Prevention and Control of AIDS." *Western Journal of Medicine* 147(6):732–734.

Meheus, A., DeClercq, A., and Prat, R. 1974. "Prevalence of Gonorrhoea in Prostitutes in a Central African Town." *British Journal of Venereal Disease* 50:50–52.

Mitchell, F., and Brindis, C. 1987. "Adolescent Pregnancy: The Responsibilities of Policymakers." *Health Services Research* 22(3):399–437.

Nunn, P. 1987. "AIDS, Africa and Education." *Health Education Journal* 46(2):53–55.

Okware, S.I. 1987. "Towards a National AIDS-Control Program in Uganda." *Western Journal of Medicine* 147(6):726–729.

Perlez, J. 1988. "School Board Rejects Book on AIDS." *New York Times* March 19, A29.

Piot, P., Plummer, F.A., Mhalu, F.S., Lamboray, J.L., Chin, J., Mann, J.M. 1988. "AIDS: An International Perspective." *Science* 239:573–579.

Plorde, D.S. 1981. "Sexually Transmitted Diseases in Ethiopia." *British Journal of Venereal Disease* 57:357–362.

Polit, D.F., and Kahn, J.R. 1986. "Early Subsequent Pregnancy Among Economically Disadvantaged Teenage Mothers." *American Journal of Public Health* 76:167–171.

Quinn, T.C., Mann, J.M., Curran, J.W., and Piot, P. 1986. "AIDS in Africa: An Epidemiologic Paradigm." *Science* 234:955–963.

Remafedi, G.J. 1988. "Preventing the Sexual Transmission of AIDS During Adolescence." *Journal of Adolescent Health Care* 9:139–143.

Rule, S. 1987. "To Cut Births, Kenya Turns to TV Show." *New York Times* June 14, 15.

Sabatier, R. 1987. "Social, Cultural and Demographic Aspects of AIDS." *Western Journal of Medicine* 147(6):713–715.

Shilts, R. 1987. *And the Band Played On: Politics, People and the AIDS Epidemic*. New York: St. Martin's Press.

Stanback, M., Pape, J.W., Verdier, R., Jean, S., and Johnson, W.D. 1988. "Breast Feeding and HIV Transmission in Haitian Children." Abstract 501, proceedings from the *IV International Conference on AIDS*, Book 1, page 340.

Strunin, L., and Hingson, R. 1987. "Acquired Immunodeficiency Syndrome and Adolescents: Knowledge, Beliefs, Attitudes and Behaviors." *Pediatrics* 79(5):825–828.

Tinker, J. 1988. "AIDS in the Developing Countries." *Issues of Science Technology* 4(2):43–48.

U.S. Department of Education. 1987. *AIDS and the Education of Our Children: A Guide for Parents and Teachers*. Washington, D.C.: U.S. Government Printing Office.

Victoria, C.G., Vaughan, J.P., Lombardi, D., Fuchs, S.M., Gigante, L.P., Smith, P.G., Nobre, L.C., Teixiera, A.M., Moreira, L.B., and Barros, F.C. 1987. "Evidence for Protection by Breast Feeding Against Infant Deaths from Infectious Diseases in Brazil." *Lancet* ii(8554):319–322.

Vittecoq, D., Roue, R.T., Mayaud, C., Borsa, R., Armengaud, M., Autran, B., May, T., Stern, M., Charanet, P., Jeantils, P., Modai, J., Rey, F., and Chermann, J.C. 1987. "Acquired Immune Deficiency Syndrome After Travelling in Africa: An Epidemiological Study in Seventeen Caucasian Patients." *Lancet* I(8533):612–615.

Von Reyn, C.F., and Mann, J.M. 1987. "Global Epidemiology." *Western Journal of Medicine* 147(6):694–701.

Watkins, J.D., Conway-Welch, C., Creedon, J.J., Crenshaw, T.L., DeVos, R.M., Gebbie, K.M., Lee, B.J., Lilly, F., O'Connor, J.C., Primm, B.J., Pullen, P., SerVass, C., and Walsh, W.B. 1988. "Report of the Presidential Commission on the Human Immunodeficiency Virus Epidemic, June 24, 1988." Washington, D.C.: U.S. Government Printing Office.

World Health Organization. 1987. "Statement from the Consultation on Breast-Feeding/Breast Milk and Human Immunodeficiency Virus (HIV)." *Special Programme on AIDS*, June 23–25, 1987.

World Health Organization. 1986. "Acquired Immunodeficiency Syndrome." *Weekly Epidemiologic Record* 61(13):93.

Yarber, W.L. 1987. "School AIDS Education: Politics, Issues, and Responses." *SIECUS Report* 15:1–5.

Ziegler, J.B., Stewart, G.J., Penny, R., Stuckey, M., and Good, S. 1988. "Breast-Feeding and Transmission of HIV from Mother to Infant." Abstract 5100, proceedings from the *IV International Conference on AIDS*, Book 1, page 339.

Appendix 1

Individuals Interviewed for This Book

Name	Organization	Date of Interview
Rashidah L. Hassan, Executive Director	Blacks Educating Blacks About Sexual Health Issues (BEBASHI)	February 16, 1988
Mr. Curtis Wadlington, Program Director	BEBASHI	February 16, 1988
Ms. Ann McFarren, Executive Director	AIDS Action Council	February 27, 1988
Ms. Pamela Nimorwicz, Social Worker	Hemophilia Center of Western Pennsylvania	March 3, 1988
Ms. Anne Wilson, Clinical Specialist	Development Associates, Inc.	March 8, 1988
Ms. Nina Peyser, Administrator	Beth Israel Methadone Maintenance Treatment Program	March 14, 1988
Mrs. Glorice Sanders, Comprehensive Care Manager	Beth Israel Methadone Maintenance Treatment Program	March 14, 1988
Ms. Yolanda Serrano, Executive Director	Association for Drug Abuse Prevention and Treatment (A.D.A.P.T.)	March 14, 1988
Ms. Casey Horan, Volunteer	A.D.A.P.T.	March 14, 1988
Mr. Richard Dunne, Executive Director	Gay Men's Health Crisis	March 15, 1988

287

Dr. Charles McKinney, Education Director	Gay Men's Health Crisis	March 15, 1988
Ms. Joyce Jackson, Clinical Operations Specialist	New Jersey State Health Department	March 22, 1988
Dr. Michele Rigaud, Project Coordinator	Health Education and Risk Reduction Program	April 4, 1988
Ms. Marilyn Volker, Director of Community Education	Health Crisis Network	April 4, 1988
Dr. Tim Wolfred, Executive Director	San Francisco AIDS Foundation	April 11, 1988
Mr. Charles Frutchey, Assistant Director of Education	San Francisco AIDS Foundation	April 11, 1988
Mr. Ernesto Hinojos, Assistant Director of Campaign Development	San Francisco AIDS Foundation	April 11, 1988
Ms. Carolyn Wean, General Manager	KPIX-TV 5	April 11, 1988
Dr. Phyllis Simpson, Director of AIDS Education	Dallas Independent School District	May 9, 1988
Dr. Charles Haley, Epidemiologist	Dallas County Health Department	May 10, 1988
Ms. Anne Freeman, Manager of AIDS Prevention Project	AIDS Prevention Project Dallas County Health Department	May 10, 1988
Ms. Jo Ann Valentine, AIDS Educator	AIDS Prevention Project Dallas County Health Department	May 10, 1988
Ms. Yolanda Rivera, AIDS Educator	AIDS Prevention Project Dallas County Health Department	May 10, 1988
Mr. Barry Skiba, AIDS Educator	AIDS Prevention Project Dallas County Health Department	May 10, 1988

Mr. Marc Lero, AIDS Educator	AIDS Prevention Project Dallas County Health Department	May 10, 1988
Mr. Craig Hess, Volunteer Director	AIDS Resource Center	May 10, 1988
Mr. William Seals, Fundraising Coordinator	AIDS Resource Center	May 10, 1988
Mr. Marc Chandler, AIDS Educator	AIDS Resource Center	May 10, 1988
Dr. Anthony Meyer, Chief, Health Promotion Unit	World Health Organization Global Programme on AIDS	June 15, 1988

Appendix 2

Names and Addresses of Organizations Referred to in Chapter Five

AIDS Resource Center
3920 Cedar Springs
Dallas, Texas 75219
(214) 521-5124

ADAPT (Association for Drug
    Abuse Prevention and
    Treatment)
85 Bergen Street
Brooklyn, New York 11201
(718) 834-9585

Blacks Educating Blacks About
    Sexual Health Issues
    (BEBASHI)
1319 Locust Street, 3rd Floor
Philadelphia, Pennsylvania 19107
(215) 546-4140

Beth Israel Medical Center
Methadone Maintenance Treat-
    ment Program
245 East 17 Street
New York, New York 10003
(212) 420-2073

Health Education and Risk Reduc-
    tion Program
Dade County Public Health Unit
1350 N.W. 14th Street
Miami, Florida 33125
(305) 324-2491

AIDS Prevention Project
Dallas County Health Department
1936 Amelia Court
Dallas, Texas 75235
(214) 920-7960

Dallas Independent School District
3700 Ross Street
Dallas, Texas 75204-5491
(214) 824-1620

Gay Men's Health Crisis
Box 274
132 West 24 Street
New York, New York 10011
(212) 807-7035

Health Crisis Network, Inc.
P.O. Box 42-1280
Miami, Florida 33242-1280
(305) 326-8833

Hemophilia Center of Western
    Pennsylvania
Central Blood Bank of Pittsburgh
812 Fifth Avenue
Pittsburgh, Pennsylvania 15219
(412) 622-7273

KPIX-TV 5
855 Battery Street

San Francisco, California
  94111-1597
(415) 765-8874

New Jersey State Department of
  Health
Division of Narcotics and Drug
  Abuse Control
20 Evergreen Place
East Orange, New Jersey 07018
(201) 266-1910

San Francisco AIDS Foundation
P.O. Box 6182
San Francisco, California
  94101-6182
(415) 864-5855

World Health Organization
Global Programme on AIDS
CH-1211
Geneva, 27 Switzerland

Appendix 3

Criteria for the Development of Health-Promotion and Education Programs: Prepared by an Ad Hoc Work Group of the American Public Health Association

Criterion 1: A health-promotion program should address one or more risk factors which are carefully defined, measurable, modifiable, and prevalent among the members of a chosen target group, factors which constitute a threat to the health status and the quality of life of target group members.

Criterion 2: A health-promotion program should reflect a consideration of the special characteristics, needs, and preferences of its target group(s).

Criterion 3: Health-promotion programs should include interventions which will clearly and effectively reduce a targeted risk factor and are appropriate for a particular setting.

Criterion 4: A health-promotion program should identify and implement interventions which make optimum use of available resources.

Criterion 5: From the outset, a health-promotion program should be organized, planned, and implemented in such a way that its operation and effects can be evaluated.

Appendix 4

Example of a Consent Form for Testing for Antibodies to Human Immunodeficiency Virus

Please read the following carefully.

Purpose and Benefits of the test:

This test is used to determine whether a person is infected with HIV, the human immunodeficiency virus, by testing blood for the presence of antibodies to HIV. An antibody is a protein that blood cells make in response to an infection. The purpose of this test is to help individuals and their doctors understand and more effectively treat symptoms that may be caused by HIV. This test can also identify persons who are infected with the virus and who can therefore spread the infection to others through sexual intercourse, needle sharing, donating body fluids such as blood and semen, or childbirth.

Interpretation of the test:

First your blood will be tested using a screening test. If necessary, a second, confirmatory, test will be performed. If your test result is a *confirmed* "positive" it means that you are infected with HIV and are capable of spreading the infection to others—through sexual intercourse and by sharing needles to inject drugs. If your test is "negative" it means that there is no laboratory evidence at this point in time that you are infected with HIV.

Limitations of the test:

As with many other blood tests, some individuals' test results will be what is called "false positive." This means that the screening test was "positive," but the confirmatory test was "negative." For some reason, the screening test indicates that HIV antibody is present when, in fact, it is not. There are also "false negative" results in which no antibodies are detected on the screening test even though the virus is present. This is especially likely to happen if a person has just been infected with the virus. Some persons may have test results that are "indeterminant" (that is, it is not certain whether they are infected or not), and they will be asked to return at a later time to be retested.

Another limitation of this test is that it does not predict whether a person will remain healthy, have mild symptoms, or develop AIDS. Further medical evaluation and testing can help to determine a person's risk of developing medical problems as a result of HIV infection.

Risks of the test:

Individuals who are told that they have antibodies to HIV (whose tests are "positive") can have strong emotional reactions to this information, including severe anxiety and depression. "Positive" results might also be used as a basis for discrimination by other individuals or institutions.

Consent:

I certify that I have read the preceding or it has been read to me and that I understand its contents, including the limitations, benefits, and risks of this test. I have received additional pretest counseling, including information on how to reduce the risk of infecting myself and others. I have also discussed with the testing facility the procedures that I will be required to follow in order to learn my results and I agree to this process. I understand that this testing is voluntary and that I may withdraw my consent at any time. I have been informed of the steps that will be taken to protect the confidentiality of my results. Any questions I have pertaining to this test have been and will be answered by _____.

Date   Client Signature

_____   _____

Health Care Provider Signature

_____

Witness

_____

Index

acquired immune deficiency syndrome (AIDS): in heterosexuals, 111, 115, 156; in homosexuals, 2, 3, 95; incidence of related to duration of seropositivity, 11; in intravenous drug users, 9–10, 111, 115; minorities and, 111, 113, 115; risk groups and, 1; women and, 5, 115, 156

adolescents: AIDS in, 274; AIDS prevention in, 111, 112–113, 140, 141, 142–143, 160, 161–162, 192, 251–252, 268, 274–276, 279; condom use and, 160–161, 162, 163, 166, 268; drug use and, 108, 109–110, 111–112, 274, 276; hemophilia and, 108–109, 146, 159; homeless, 110, 112, 143; homosexuality in, 97–99, 139, 145, 149, 274, 279; pregnancy and, 108, 115–116, 278–279; pregnancy prevention and, 278–279; risk taking and, 108–109, 161, 163, 274; sex education and, 276–277; sexual behavior and, 163, 274, 275–276, 277; sexually transmitted diseases and, 274

Africa: AIDS and, 2, 6, 269–270; AIDS prevention and, 266, 270–274, 280; condom promotion campaigns in, 271, 273; epidemiology of HIV infection in, 270; health problems in, 270, 273; prostitution and, 6, 270, 271–272, 273, 274; sexually transmitted disease in, 270–271

African-Americans: AIDS prevention and, 101, 113, 115, 116, 117, 140, 141, 142–143, 152, 158, 160, 188, 235, 251–252; adolescents, 109, 111–112, 142–143, 160, 251–252; drug use and, 109, 111, 112; economic disadvantage and, 112, 140; homosexuality in, 101, 113–114, 115; women, 115, 116, 168

AIDS. See acquired immune deficiency syndrome

AIDS Lifeline (KPIX-TV), 129, 189

AIDS prevention programs: barriers to, 38, 116, 117, 136, 265–281; community input into, 277–278; developing world and, 266, 269–274, 280; evaluation of, 193–196, 253, 259–263; goals of, 247; HIV testing and, 135–136, 162, 182, 233–236, 253; implementation of, 185–186, 194, 196, 247; importance of involving target groups in, 95, 117–118, 120, 137–146, 247; marketing campaigns and, 143, 144–146, 149–150; media and, 80, 91–94, 150–151, 183, 188–193; minorities and, 113–117, 140, 141, 142, 144; objectives of, 193, 247–249; outreach workers in, 64, 70, 75, 76, 80, 81; planning of, 117–